Health Empowerment of Women

Health Empowerment of Women

A Desirable Strategy in 21st Century Hospitals –

Volume - II

Gynecological Health

Editors

Dr. Amarjeet Singh
Dr. Vanita Suri
Dr. Sukhpal Kaur

KALPAZ

ISBN: 978-93-5324-051-6 (Vol. II)
978-93-5324-024-0 (Set)

First Published, 2020

Published by

Kalpaz Publications
C-30, Satyawati Nagar,
Delhi – 110052
Ph.: 011-47034999, 9811692060
www.kalpazpublications.com
E-mail: kalpaz@hotmail.com

Printed at: G. Print Process, Delhi

Contents

Volume - II

Gynecological Health

Chapter - 1

Self-Instruction Module for the adolescent girls for puberty related changes 7

—Risha Gupta, Seema Chopra, AK Sinha, Jugal Kishore, Amarjeet Singh

Chapter - 2

Dealing with Menstrual cramps/Painful menses 23

— A. Chaudhuri, LK Dhaliwal, AJ Singh

Chapter - 3

A Woman's Guide to Deal with Polycystic Ovary Syndrome (PCOS) . 39

— Ishwarpreet Kaur, Dr. Amarjeet Singh, Dr. Vanita Suri

Chapter - 4

Infertility Management in OPD Setting 89

—Davinder Kaur, Vanita Suri, Rupinder Kaur, AJ Singh, LK Dhaliwal

Chapter - 5

Training Package for Minor Disorders in Pregnancy 143

— Avinash Rana, Vanita Suri, LK Dhaliwal, Amarjeet Singh

Chapter - 6

Intervention package for the Health and Fitness of Ante - And Post-Natal Women 163

— Pradeep Sarkar, MS Dhillon, Paramveer Singh, Vanita Suri, Amarjeet Singh

Chapter - 7

Behavior Therapy for Urine Leakage (Urinary Incontinence) 175

— S Kumari, V Jain, AK Mandal, AJ Singh

Chapter - 8

Promoting Health of Women – Conservative Management of Pelvic Organ Prolapse 197

— R Kashyap, AJ Singh and V Jain

Chapter - 9

Empowering Women to Deal with Menopause Related Problems 211

— Dr. Purnima Kaushal, Dr. Ruchi Sharma, Dr. Neelam Aggarwal, Dr. Seema Chopra, Dr. Amarjeet Singh

Chapter - 10

Dealing with therapy related issues of cervical cancer- A guide for patients/family caregivers 245

— Dr. Amudeep Singh, Dr. Vanita Suri, Dr. Sushmita Ghoshal, Dr. Sukhpal Kaur, Dr. Amarjeet Singh

Chapter - 11

Dealing with diagnosis and therapy related issues of ovarian cancer - A guide for patients/family caregivers 325

— Dr. Janavi , Dr. Bhavana Rai, Dr. Vanita Suri and Dr. Amarjeet Singh

Chapter - 1

Self-Instruction Module for the adolescent girls for puberty related changes

—Risha Gupta, Seema Chopra, AK Sinha, Jugal Kishore, Amarjeet Singh

Puberty attainment is a very important phase of life for both the boys and the girls. This is the phase of their transition into adulthood. This phase is called **adolescence** i.e. the age of 11-18 years. Girls have more physiological and psychological changes during adolescence than boys. They suffer from fear, apprehension and confusion about these changes much more than boys. This is due to many reasons. Plenty of myths, taboos and superstitions are linked to bodily changes in girls at puberty. Ignorance about various puberty related issues and lack of intra-family communication further complicates the situation for girls. Because of this, many girls feel constrained in their career or study related pursuits. But now the time has changed. Girls have to compete with boys. So today there is a great need for girls to know the intricacies of puberty related changes.

Before starting any further discussion, let's introduce you with some terms:

Puberty occurs due to various hormonal changes. Hormones are chemicals which regulate and control many of our body processes. The sex hormones become activated and make a child's body to mature into an adult human body. Now a girl is capable of reproduction and fertilization. She is now becoming ready to give birth to another human being. Age of attain puberty in girls can vary from 8 - 13 years.

Vagina is the opening / entry point to the uterus that leads from external genitals (between your legs).The part between vagina and uterus is called **cervix** (the neck of uterus).

Uterus is commonly known as the womb. It is a hollow muscular organ of the female reproductive system. It is responsible for the development of the baby during pregnancy. The baby (fetus) grows in uterus. It stays there for 9 months of pregnancy.

There are many puberty related issues. Many girls do not discuss these issues even with their mothers. The reasons for this are

- Shyness: Even mothers may not share all the things with their daughters. One woman said, "we are not supposed to discuss this stuff with our daughters, What will they think of us".
- They want to give respect to their mothers.
- They think that this is the very much private thing of a person, not to be shared with anyone.
- This is the test of a girl's ability and she has to tolerate it alone.

Their most easy source of information is their friends and cousins. Many girls came to know about puberty and related issues from television, magazines and other social media also. But quite often the information they get is incomplete. Even they are given incorrect information by their peer group or relatives. The best source is mother or elder sister. In case of any further doubt, you should consult your doctor. Having done that you should guide your friends also.

Menstruation

The major worry for most of the girls of 11-18 years of age is the periodic monthly bleeding from their vagina. This is called menstruation, commonly known as monthly/ periods/cycles/date etc. This is accompanied with the feelings of fear, tension and apprehension in them. They need to get an advice on:

(1) Menarche

(2) Regularity/ irregularity of periods

(3) Absorbent material (pads) to be used

(4) Associated conditions/ disorders

(5) Myths/ misconceptions

Changes before the onset of menarche: Few weeks or months before starting of the first menstrual period, a girl might notice an increased amount of clear or whitish fluid from the vagina. This is commonly known as 'Vaginal Discharge'. This discharge is a part of normal changes of puberty. It shows that a girl may get menstrual periods in few weeks. It can be irritating or itching also, if hygiene is not maintained.

The most troublesome aspect of menarche is its unpredictability. When it will start? Where it will start (in school, in market, while playing etc.)? This bothers a girl/ her mother very much. Onset of vaginal discharge signals a girl that she should "be ready". She will get menses in the near future.

Management

- Regularly clean your genitalia. Frequent washing of genitalia, especially when you go to toilet, will be helpful. Do not try to clean it with any piece of cloth or your finger.
- Wear clean and cotton undergarments.
- Take bath regularly at least once every day.
- Start carrying sanitary pads with you. Keep these either in the bag or in the lockers.

(1) Menarche ***(first menstrual period):*** When a girl gets her first menstrual period, doctors call it 'menarche'. It is an important milestone in a girl's life. This prepares her to bear a baby in the future. It usually starts between 11 and 14 years. Most of the girls do not have any knowledge about menstruation prior to first menstrual bleeding. This leads them to a state of fear, apprehension, shame and disgust. Thus it is very important for a girl to know about it before the first menstrual bleeding begins.

At menarche, you will notice a spot of blood on your undergarment or you may notice drops of blood after/before urination. It's the time when you should start using an absorbent such as sanitary pads or cloth menstrual pads. You should soon consult a woman you trust the most (whether your mother, aunt, *bhabhi, massi* or elder sister). If you are in the school and notice red spots on your dress, ask immediately your female teacher for help. She will provide you all the stuff and guide you.

The initial flow consists of fresh and clotted blood. It is usually brighter in color than mature menstrual flow. It is often scanty in amount. Initially it may be very brief, even a single instance of spotting.It can confuse or scare a girl. They may develop a fear of getting some disease. They may feel that something abnormal is happening. But do not be afraid of this. It is a part of a natural maturation process. It happens to every girl. If menarche does not occur beyond the age of 16 years, ask your mother to consult a doctor.

Some girls may worry that they are losing too much blood. But it is unlikely. It is an undue fear. It is only seen in 1 in 1000 girls. This occurs only if there is any underlying disease. Though the blood loss may look like a lot, it is not so. The average amount of blood loss is usually about 2 tablespoons (30 ml) for an entire period. The first period is sometimes followed by no periods for few months. No need to worry. It may take your body a while to sort out all the changes going on. Within a year or so, your periods will become regular.You may feel tense or emotional during your menses. There may be cramps in lower abdomen, legs and back. You may also feel tenderness in your breasts. All these problems may last only a few hours or so.

(2) Regularity/irregularity of periods: After menarche, you get periodic monthly bleeding from your vagina. It lasts for 3 to 7 days every month. It occurs approximately after every 28 days (range anywhere from 21 to 45 days). That's why we call it as menstrual cycle or periods. Actually each menstrual cycle in females is an attempt of the body to bear a child. Every month an egg is released from ovaries of the girls. It occurs in the middle of the cycle. Side by side uterus thickens. It is prepared every month to receive a fertilized egg. Since pregnancy does not occur every month, the bleeding occurs due to the shedding of the lining of the uterus. This monthly bleeding lasts from menarche until menopause (the end of bleeding @ ~ 45-50 years).

Failure to bleed at expected dates usually means that a woman is pregnant. During 9 months of pregnancy, no menses come.

Irregularity of periods: After menarche i.e. after first menstrual period, sometimes your few months go without any menstrual bleeding. *For example, you may start to bleed in the month of November. After that, you may not bleed for 5 months. You get your next cycle in May, next year.* Please note, this is not a matter of worry. Your body is trying to adapt to the hormonal changes taking place. If this problem still continues, then you should consult a doctor.

Sometimes you may have very little bleeding (for instance, only a spot in the whole day) or too much bleeding (if you have to change the pad every 2-3 hrs). Don't worry. Initially you may face these problems. But later on, your cycle will surely normalize after few months. If the problem continues, then consult a doctor.

(3) Products to be used as absorbents:

"*You can't change periods, but you can change the way you feel about them.*"

At puberty when periods start, girls should learn to manage their menses. For this daily bleeding during periods, girls need to use something to absorb it. Otherwise blood will soil the legs and thighs or even the clothes. These

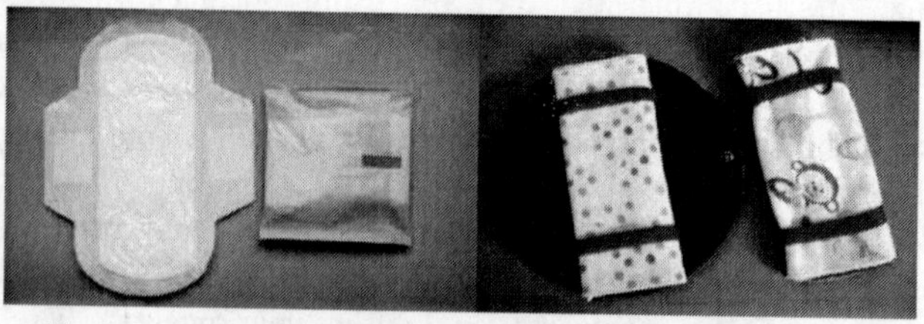

Pix 1: Sanitary napkin/ pad ***Pix 2: Cloth menstrual pad***

days **Sanitary napkins** are available in the market for this purpose. Other absorbent material commonly used by girls is **cloth menstrual pad**.

Sanitary napkins/ pads are the most commonly used absorbent. It is worn externally, between the genitalia and a woman's undergarment. These are disposable items. Thus these are single use items. These are designed to be disposed of by placing these in a paper bag/ wrap, then to be thrown into a bin. There are generally two types of pads- thicker one for heavy flow days and thin one for the days you are just spotting. Select a pad based on how your period is and what kind of clothes you will be wearing.

How to use a sanitary pad

Choose a pad of the appropriate shape, thickness, absorbency and size as per your flow. Stay away from scented pads, especially if your skin is sensitive. These can be irritating.

I. Remove any wrapper or boxes and take out the pad. You can discard them. But it is better to use them to dispose of the used pad you are replacing. Remember not to throw it in the toilet. It can flood the commode. Even the toilet can get blocked.

II. Stick the adhesive part of pad to your undergarments and keep the absorbing part facing upwards. Regularly check it. Change the pad after every 4 to 8 hours as per the need to avoid odors. If your pad is itching or irritating you at all, remove it. Use a different brand.

III. It is necessary to change the pad after every 4-8 hours. Menstrual blood gets contaminated with the body's own organisms. This rule applies for even those days when you don't have much bleeding. This is because your pad may be still damp. Even sweat from your genitals may contaminate it also. When these organisms remain in a warm and moist place for a long time they tend to multiply. It can lead to conditions like urinary tract infection, vaginal infections and skin rashes.

IV. Opt for more comfortable clothes. You will feel better wearing loose pants or skirts. It will give you a peace of mind.

V. Do not use pads as a routine (when not bleeding). Some girls think that it keeps them fresh. No, please don't do it. Your vagina needs to breathe. Use of pad all the time can lead to bacterial and fungal infections. This occurs because of lack of air circulation in the inner thigh area.

VI. Dispose of your pad by putting it in the wrapper of new one. If wrapper is unavailable, wrap it in a paper bag. Even toilet paper may be used. Don't flush it in the toilet. It can lead to blockage of sewer system.

VII. Always wash your hands two times after changing pads. Stay hygienic.

VIII. Keep a ready supply of pads. Reserve stock will help.

IX. Always carry extra pads with you during expected dates. Don't hesitate in asking another girl for it. If you do not have sanitary pad when needed, you can use toilet paper also. But has to be changed after every 1 to 2 hours.

X. Avoid embarrassment. Use red/ brown *salwars/ pajamis/* trousers during expected dates of period.

XI. If your school dress is light colored/ white during expected dates of period, confide in few of your classmate girls. They will check and warn you if there is any spot.

Those allergic to pads can use reusable pads (cotton wrapped in a piece of cloth).

Cloth menstrual pads Washable menstrual pads do not need to be disposed of after use. Therefore, these offer a more economical alternative for girls. This is the practice in most homes where ready cash is not a part of girl's life. They are allergen and perfume free. These can be more comfortable for women who suffer from irritations from using disposable pads. After each use, it should be soaked in cold and mildly salty water. If you use hot water, then it can cause the blood to set in and leave a permanent stain. After soaking, it should be properly washed and dried in the sun. Sun rays are natural sterilizers that kill germs and bacteria.

(4) Associated conditions/ disorders: Girls may also face following problems linked with menses. They need to know that these can be managed easily.

(a) Pre-menstrual syndrome *(pain/discomfort 1 or 2 days before periods)*: Pre' means 'before' and 'syndrome' means 'collection of signs and symptoms'. Thus, Pre-menstrual syndrome is a set of physical and emotional symptoms related to a girl's menstrual cycle. Thus, before the periods (bleeding) starts every month girls may experience various symptoms. These can be mild (or tolerable) or sufficiently severe (that can interfere with your work). Their severity and pattern varies from girl to girl.

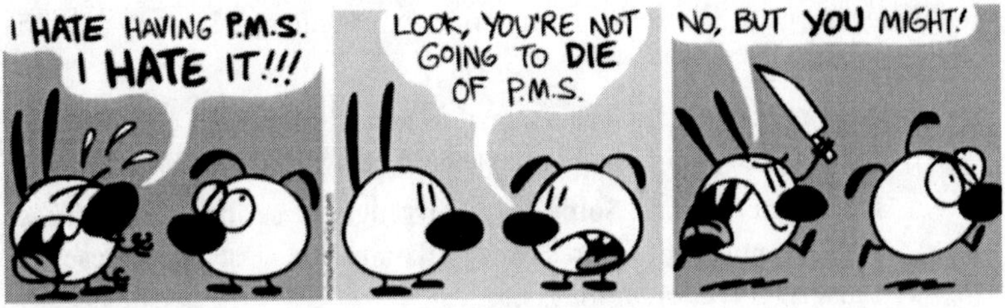
I HATE HAVING P.M.S.
I HATE IT!!!
LOOK, YOU'RE NOT GOING TO DIE OF P.M.S.
NO, BUT YOU MIGHT!

Emotional symptoms	Physical symptoms
- Irritability	- Bloating
- Tension	- Cramps
- Dysphoria (unhappiness)	- Constipation
- Stress	- Swelling/ tenderness in breasts
- Anxiety	- Joint/ Muscle pain
- Insomnia	- Weight gain
- Headache	
- Food cravings	
- Mood swings	

Most (85%) of the menstruating girls experience some of these symptoms. Only 2-10% experience severe symptoms. Following factors may cause or aggravate existing condition. lxxxii

- Cyclical changes in hormones
- Stress and depression
- Family history (if your mother/ sister also had these symptoms).
- Dietary factors (low levels of vitamins and minerals particularly Magnesium, vitamin B6, Manganese, Zinc, vitamin E & vitamin D)

Management: These symptoms can be managed by simple dietary and lifestyle changes (see related chapter)

(b) Acne (*blackheads, whiteheads or pimples*): '*Muhanse*' or acne also trouble girls a lot. These appear on face due to increased secretion of oil at puberty. It increases the susceptibility of the skin to acne. It varies greatly in severity in different people. Acne is characterized by areas of blackheads, whiteheads, pimples and greasy skin. Scarring may occur if it is scratched and healing does not occur properly. Face is the most common site involved by acne. Back, chest, neck and arms are the other areas commonly affected. It often causes impaired psychological development. Girls may experience reduced self-esteem. Many suffer emotional distress. This may be due to perceived disfigurement i.e. they may feel their facial beauty spoiled. The root cause of such feeling is the importance given in our society to sense of beauty and good looks.

Management: It is a self-limiting condition. Acne usually stop after the age of 25 years.

- Routine cosmetics (chemicals used in oil based cold creams, moisturizers and foundations) should be avoided.
- Do not use steroids. Some doctors wrongly prescribe steroids. These may temporarily suppress the inflammation. But later these can cause aggravation of the acne.
- Stress is to be avoided. Tension will only make the acne worse. Girls should take good diet. Try to get sufficient sleep (not less than 8 hours).
- Food with high fat content and high glycemic index i e.g. burgers, chocolates, ice creams etc. need to be avoided. Take lots of fluids. Fruits and vegetables also help. Keep more focus on natural food.
- It is better to avoid direct exposure to sunlight.
- Girls should ensure adequate cleaning of their face (and body). Face and hands should be washed 3-4 times a day. Before going to sleep make it a habit to wash your face. Always wash your face with a mild cleanser. Do not use soaps. These will excessively dry your face and make your acne worse.
- Local application of Retino A cream may help. Vitamin B complex tablets should also be taken for 10-15 days.

(b) PCOD (Polycystic Ovarian Disorder): Now I wish to introduce you to a problem many girls are facing today. In gynae clinics, many girls come with a problem of missed periods. Many develop hair on face (moustache). PCOD has emerged as an important cause for this. Because of PCOD women are not able to bear a child after marriage. But the good news is that it is easy to manage it. We can rectify it by using simple measures.

PCOD is the most common endocrine disorder seen in girls these days. It is the leading cause of oligomenorrhea (scanty menstrual periods). It is characterized by presence of two or three of the following criteria:

- An-ovulation/ oligomenorrhea: longer menstrual cycles (or <8 cycles per year).
- Clinical hyperandrogenism: presence of male like features like excess hair growth, alopecia (lack of hair), acne etc.
- Polycystic ovaries: cysts in the ovaries which can be detected by ultrasound examination.

Causes: Evidence suggests that it is likely to be caused by genetic factors and lifestyle factors. It will also have a negative impact on future pregnancy outcomes. There is also an increased risk of diabetes, hypertension and other chronic diseases. Thus its management is very crucial for us. We can modify our lifestyle and control the worst outcome.

Management: Certain lifestyle changes are the first-line treatment for you. Medications are reserved for the further complications. The lifestyle changes include change in diet, reduction in weight by exercise etc such as:

- Weight loss is an essential modality. Even a small amount of weight loss help balance your hormones. You may start up your menstrual cycle again. It is also seen that adequate weight loss may help childless women to bear a child.
- Eat a balanced diet that includes lots of fruits, vegetables, whole grains and low fat dairy products. Avoid fast food. Focus on natural food.
- Get regular exercise to help you lose weight and feel better.

Consult a doctor if no relief is there.

(c) Obesity (overweight/*motapa*): is a medical condition in which excess fat accumulated in the body. It has negative consequences on the health. It may lead to various health problems such as heart diseases, diabetes etc. Sometimes death also may result. The obesity in adolescent girls can be due to the early menarche (girls who menstruate earlier have short stature and are fatty). Increased fat intake and sedentary lifestyle also cause obesity. Hormonal changes associated with adolescence may also be involved. The most immediate consequence of obesity is the psychological impact. Fat girls often develop a feeling of rejection about themselves. They acquire a "fat phobia".

Some girls are ignorant and careless about their body fat. You should note that some amount of abdominal body fat gets distributed during your growth. But excess fat does not get distributed. This obesity may continue into adulthood. Obese girls may also face retarded growth in the future. You can also check whether you are obese or not by calculating your BMI (Body Mass Index) from the following formula:

BMI = weight (kg)/ height (m2)

Weight category classification	***BMI (kg/ m2)***
Underweight	<18.5
Normal weight	≥18.5-24.9
Overweight	≥25.0-29.9
Obesity	≥30.0
Obesity Class I	30.0-34.9
Obesity Class II/ morbid obesity	35.0-39.9
Obesity Class III/ grossly morbid obesity	≥40

For example, BMI of a girl of 50 kg weight and 5 feet height comes out to be 22.2 (kg/m2). She comes in the category of normal weight.

Keeping this in view obesity should be managed by dietary and exercise modifications.

- Strengthening exercises like dancing, cycling, walking, running, swimming etc. should be done to reduce the weight
- **Diet plan for an obese/ overweight girl:** you should not stop eating to reduce weight. But you should have a planned eating. Starving hinders your digestion process. It doesn't help you in losing weight.
    - Take a glass of water or green tea before and after every meal. It will fill you up. This way you will not feel the need to eat as much. This will also help digest the food faster.
    - Replace one of your meals with fruits and salads.
    - Include green vegetables in your diet most of the time.
    - Take proteins in the form of meat, fish, etc. (if you are a non-vegetarian) or dairy (milk, cheese, yoghurt, etc.) daily.
    - Eat carbohydrates sparingly. Eating carbohydrates and sugars will make weight loss harder.
    - Avoid rice, potatoes, fried and sweet things.
- **Diet plan for an underweight girl:** As soon as girls reach puberty, they acquire fat phobia. They start losing weight by restricted eating. Some girls are excessively thin. As a result their growth interrupts. Foods that they should include daily to gain weight are:
    - Full-cream milk at least 2 times a day.
    - Meat, fish, eggs etc. if you are a non- vegetarian.
    - Bread and cereals. Eat at least 2-3 chapattis every meal.
    - Fruits like 1 or 2 bananas every day.
    - Fats and oils: like butter, *ghee*, cream etc.
    - Healthy desserts: 1-2 servings (e.g. *Halwa, Kheer* etc.)
    - Avoid fast foods. These will only increase fat, not strength in your body.

(5) Myths/ misconceptions about menstruation:

1. Menstrual blood is impure.

   It is not so. Actually it is your own blood. How it can be impure?

2. Your first few periods come exactly after 28 days.

   It is not so always. Inter-menstrual period can vary from 21 to 45 days. Even at beginning, it is common for your periods to be irregular.

3. You cannot do your usual activities.

   You can do your day to day activities. The only restriction is that you should not carry heavy weights. You should also do not do strenuous exercises during menstrual days.

4. Menarche signals that a girl will not gain growth in height further.

   This is not so. The reality is that the average gain in height after menarche is about 7 cm (3 inches).

5. Do not visit holy places, relatives and friends.

   In reality do not restrict yourself from going anywhere. This is only a psychological restriction in our minds. So there's a great need to change our mindset.

6. Drinking more milk and eating healthy foods causes early puberty.

   Some people restrict them from eating nutritious food. They think that they will mature and attain puberty earlier. Do not do this. You are compromising your health only. Take a good diet.

CHANGING BODY SHAPE

A girl's body starts showing changes in shape as well as size as soon as you enter in this phase. Since these changes are many and occur within a short span of time, this can disturb you. But do not worry. This happens to every girl. The only difference is the extent and the time of onset of these changes. All these changes mould a girl's body to acquire a womanly shape. It is a part of being a woman. You should welcome these changes. It increases your attraction. The changes are as follows:

(1) **Hips broaden**: Girls experience more widening of the pelvic bones. There is changed distribution in weight and fat. Due to this, there is now fatter around buttocks, thighs and hips. This may cause considerable anxiety in girls. Often they may start a diet plan to lose weight. This may be a significant reason for weakness in girls seen these days. The deposition of fat is a part of the normal development. The body will soon redistribute the fat.

(2) **Breast development**: This is the very first sign of puberty. Breast appears as a firm, tender lump on both the sides of chest. Usually it starts at the age of 10-11 years. In some girls it may be much earlier and in others it may occur somewhat later.

It can make girls somewhat worried especially when they feel tenderness or soreness in their breasts. They may be unable to sleep on their stomach. This is normal. It is just a part of normal growing process.What you really need is to start wearing a soft, gentle and supportive undergarment (commonly known as bra). It should be made up of cotton. Initially, you should talk with your mother or elder sister. They can guide you well about the size and stuff of bra you should wear. Never feel shy in buying this from market even if you are alone. Be cautious about the size of the bra. Too loose and too tight bra will disturb the shape of your breasts.

In the early stages of puberty, one breast may be larger than the other. This usually resolves within a year or so. Breast size may become equal in due course of time.

(3) **Appearance of pubic hair:** This is the second physical change you may observe in your body. In some girls, these can appear before the breasts develop. These are few and soft in the beginning. Eventually these become thicker and curlier. First they will appear in the pubic area (from lower abdomen to the inner thighs). Then the hair will develop under the armpits also.

All these changes are natural and normal. You need to remember that for each girl, the change in shape of legs, thighs, breast, shoulder and abdomen is different. It is the inner beauty which is more important. You need not hate your body.

PERSONAL HYGIENE

Keeping a good personal hygiene helps to prevent the development and spread of infections. Diseases and odor are also controlled. It generates a feeling of self-esteem in girls. It gives them confidence. It is also pleasant for others around you. Maintenance of hygiene is even more important for girls. They have to give birth to a new life. Chances of getting infections to the mother and the baby are much more, if hygiene is poor.

1. **Sweat and body odor:** Sweat glands become more activated at the onset of puberty. Because of this, there is increased production of sweat. Also there is increased production of body oil (sebum) from the skin. It can lead to a different new kind of body odor. Use an appropriate deodorant/ anti-perspirant.
2. Take a bath or shower with a mild soap at least once a day.
3. Maintain your oral hygiene i.e. brush your teeth twice daily. Girls are susceptible to oral diseases when they attain puberty.

4. Cut your nails. Clean them regularly. They are potent source of transmission of bacterial, fungal and viral infections.
5. Wash your hands twice with a mild soap after using washroom every time.
6. Always use clean towel for wiping off your body.
7. Use clean cotton undergarments. Change them regularly. Always dry them completely in sunlight. Sun rays are natural disinfectants.
8. Change pads during menstruation regularly after every four to six hours. Do not use sanitary pads when you are not menstruating.
9. Wash the genital area with plain water (no soap) after each use of toilet and even after urination.
10. Keep the area between the legs dry. Otherwise skin rashes may occur.
11. It is very important to remember that vagina has its own self-cleaning mechanism. An external cleaning agent like deodorant or soap should not be used inside it.

NUTRITION

Adequate nutritional intake is very important for the adolescent girls. Any nutritional deficiency in this critical phase of life can have an effect future health of a girl and her baby. For example, failure to consume an adequate diet at this time can result in delayed sexual maturation and delayed or retarded physical growth. The growth spurt that occurs in adolescence creates increased demand of energy and nutrients. Adolescence is a time to prepare for the nutritional demands of pregnancy and lactation that girls may experience in later life. The following are some general guidelines that may help you to maintain a balanced and healthy diet:

- Eat three balanced meals a day, with healthy snacks.
- Eat at least one serving of fruits and salads in a day. These contain antioxidants and other bioactive substances known as phytochemicals.
- Coconut water and fresh fruit juice will improve immunity. These also provide vital vitamins. Avoid canned/packaged drinks and juices. These are high in sugar.
- A minimum of two glasses of skimmed milk is necessary.
- Egg or chicken sandwich is a good option after swimming or exercise.
- A milkshake/ limewater is always a better choice as compared to an aerated drink.

- Breakfast is the most important meal. It ensures adequate nutrient supply to brain. It also prevents brain damage due to an overnight fast. Always eat your breakfast and at least one meal with plenty of vegetables. This is healthy and nutritious.
- Always carry a lunch box with you at school. This will give you enough energy.
- A water intake of three- four litres per day clears all toxins from the body. It keeps the skin healthy and glowing.
- A handful of *kala chana* (Bengal gram), sprouts and peanuts make a very good snack during long hours of studies.
- Never exercise on an empty stomach. Eat some fruit. This will do full justice to your exercise session with some simple carbohydrates.
- Avoid foods that are canned or processed. These contain preservatives. These can lead to cancer.
- Fish, chicken, eggs are good sources of protein. These help in growth and repair of our worn out tissues.
- The best way to manage weight is through a balanced diet. Fasting is not good for health. Use of drugs or supplements does not help to lose weight.
- Exercise for five days a week. This will ensure good health and a fit body.
- Increase fiber in the diet. Decrease use of salt.
- Fried, oily foods, cheese and cream take a long time to digest. This cause indigestion. Obesity & high BP may result.
- Walnuts and dried apricots enhance brain function and concentration.
- Eat whenever you are hungry. Do not just eat because everyone around is eating.

WATER: It is an essential component to be included in your diet. Minimum 8-10 glasses of water are recommended for an adolescent girl. Often girls do not drink enough water. They fear if they take water, they have to go to toilet more often. This is a wrong notion. Water will cleanse your system. It will keep your skin healthy. Water is a better choice than the other beverages. It does not contain any sugar and added flavors.

- 60% of our body is made up of water. Drinking enough water maintains the fluid balance of our body.
- It helps in reducing weight. Simply it gives a sense of fullness and you eat less.

- It makes your skin healthier and makes you glow more by flushing out toxins from the body.
- The fluoride present in water helps in preventing tooth decay. It forms a protective coating on the surface of your teeth.
- It helps you to feel refresh and active.
- Drinking more water will also help you in reducing menstrual pain and progression of PCOD.

Some other important information for girls:

- Over the counter cosmetics: Girls at this age start becoming beauty conscious. They start using fairness creams, medicated soaps and other body care products. These may contain toxic chemicals (such as hydroquinone, mercuric iodide etc.). These can harm your skin. These can be carcinogenic also. You should consult your mother/ any skin expert before using any of these products.
- Security: Adolescent girls are more prone to "*Eve Teasing*". This can shake a girl's confidence. You should not afraid of. Instead you have to fight for your right. You should carry safety weapons with you whenever you are going alone such as pepper spray, pen knife, pointed end hairbrush etc. Also keep yourself fit. A good option is to learn self-defense techniques like karate, judo etc.
- Mobile phone use: Today's generation is very fond of technology, especially mobile phones. These can be very useful for girls in terms of security. You can have the facility of emergency calling. You can call someone in case you need any help. These can also help in tracking of exact location.

  But you should restrict yourself from extensive mobile use. These have many bad effects such as sleep disturbances, difficulty in concentration, fatigue and headache etc. Its radiations can be carcinogenic also.

MEASURES TO MINIMIZE THESE BAD EFFECTS

1. Avoid using mobile phones while it has been put up for charging.
2. Don't keep mobile in the breast pocket (electromagnetic radiations can affect your heart).
3. Do not use mobile for longer period. It can alter the activity of your brain.
4. Don't talk with your mobile in a low signal area as it circulates 6-7 times powerful electromagnetic waves.
5. Switch ears every 2-3 minutes in a long conversation.

6. Keep cell phones as far as possible. Handbags and briefcases are better than the pockets.
7. Don't use the mobile phones during thunderstorm and while driving.

END NOTE: It has also been seen that some girls become more creative during menses. Some may start painting/ drawing. Others may like to write. They may indulge in some hobbies. It is in fact possible to convert these 4-5 days of menstrual period to some productive outputs. Some girls may like to sleep more during menses. Do not feel bad about it. It is OK. You have a right to get rest. So, have no fear of menses. Face these courageously. You all are brave girls.

Chapter - 2

Dealing with Menstrual cramps/ Painful menses

—A. Chaudhuri, LK Dhaliwal, AJ Singh

Adolescence refers to the phase of human development encompassing the transition from childhood to adulthood. In terms of age it lies between 10 to 19 years. This period is very crucial since these are formative years in the life of an individual when the pubertal development as well as the psychological and behavioural changes take place. The reproductive health of the adolescent girls is an important area of focus at present. Menstrual problems are a major cause of morbidity among the adolescent girls. More than 90% of girls presenting for primary care suffer from some menstrual pain. Furthermore, one third to one half of these patients report moderate or severe symptoms. Pain is a common complaint of menstruating adolescents. It is often disregarded by many of them who consider pain to be a normal part of the menstrual cycle. Thus, many women fail to report their pain to the physicians. The consequences of untreated menstrual pain range from lost work and school hours to family and personal disruption among female student community. Furthermore, the girls who suffer from menstrual cramps, have lower school marks and more school adjustment problems than their normal counterparts.

The medical term for excessively painful periods is dysmenorrhoea. The term dysmenorrhoea is derived from the Greek words *dys,* meaning difficult/ painful/abnormal, *meno,* meaning month, and *rrhea,* meaning flow. In spite of the frequency and severity of dysmenorrhoea, most women specially in rural areas do not seek medical treatment for this condition as they lack knowledge of and experience with effective treatment. Moreover in Indian culture, girls are not expected to discuss their menstrual problems openly. Sometimes, they even don't share it with their mothers. But the scenario is quite different among the urban adolescents among whom indiscriminate use of over the counter pain killers is being reported. Previous studies so far, have emphasized mainly on the medicinal management of painful menses which has definite side effects after long term use. Home remedies and behavioural therapy for management of menstrual cramps have not received the desired attention and in this context, the cultural aspects have also been more or less ignored by the researchers. Considering the above situation, a study was done by the authors in Chandigarh, India to estimate the prevalence of primary dysmenorrhoea among the school girls and to measure the effect of exercise and hot water bottle on the occurrence and severity of primary dysmenorrhoea among the school girls of Chandigarh.

The study showed that prevalence of dysmenorrhoea in the study population was 58.52%. Backache (62.5%) & general aches and pains (31.2%) were among the first two common physical distresses; of the psychological effects mood swing (73.4%), irritability (70.3%), fatigue (70.3%) were more frequently reported. But only 11(8.6%) out of 128 suffering girls had consulted a doctor. We devised a trial of two intervention packages- exercise & hot water bottle use. According to the result of randomized control trial, there was an increase in the number of girls who were cured of menstrual pain and distress, after practising exercises or using hot water bottle. In the exercise group 28.3% girls became completely cured of pain at the end of 3rd month compared to 37.33% in the hot water bottle group. In each group more than 85% of the subjects had some form of relief.

Thus, both exercise & hot water bottle proved to be successful in home based management of primary dysmenorrhoea. Encouraged by these results, we have developed the training manual used by us in the study in the form of this booklet.

Menstrual cramps are the part of every woman's existence. The pain commonly starts during the adolescent period and continues till the women gives birth to a child. These cramps are sharp pains in a woman's lower abdomen. The pains usually begin with a woman's menstrual period and could continue for two to three days into her cycle. Although some pain during menstruation is normal, excessive pain is not. Menstrual pain can range in severity from a mild ache to severe pain that interferes with normal activity. Symptoms are frequently associated with time lost from school, work, or other activities. In spite of the frequency and severity of dysmenorrhoea, most women do not seek medical treatment for this condition, as in Indian culture, consultations for gynecological problems are seldom acceptable.

Why pain occurs?

The cause of pain in dysmenorrhoea can be understood only after having a general idea about the types of dysmenorrhoea – primary & secondary.

Primary dysmenorrhoea (spasmodic) refers to menstrual pain in healthy women. The pain is not related to any problem with the uterus or pelvic organs. It is caused by prostaglandins, which are chemicals produced by a woman's body. These chemicals are responsible for many of the symptoms associated with menstrual pain. The tissue lining a woman's uterus produces prostaglandins, which stimulate the uterine muscles causing them to contract. Contracting uterine muscles cause menstrual cramps. Women who have high levels of prostaglandins experience more intense uterine contractions, and therefore more intense pain.

It typically occurs in the first few years after menarche and affects up to 50% of postpubescent females. Characterized by fluctuating, spasmodic menstrual cramps, sometimes referred to as "labour-like" pains that begin only a few hours before or with the onset of menstrual flow. The symptoms of primary dysmenorrhoea last only for 2–3 days. The pains are most intense on the first or second day of the menstrual flow, or more precisely the first 24–36 hours, consistent with the time of maximal prostaglandin release into the menstrual fluid. The pain appears in the central part of lower abdomen and then radiates to both sides of lower abdomen, the lower back area, and into the inner aspects of the thighs. Frequently associated symptoms include diarrhea, nausea and vomiting, fatigue, light-headedness, headache, dizziness and, rarely, syncope and fever. Symptoms are more or less similar in all menstrual periods. On physical examination or ultrasonography no pelvic pathology is found.

Primary dysmenorrhoea can be caused by the following:

- Strong uterine contractions xcviii
- Anxiety and stress
- Blood and tissue being discharged through a narrow cervix
- Displaced uterus
- Lack of exercise

Secondary dysmenorrhoea (congestive) is menstrual pain that is attributed to an underlying disease or structural abnormality either within or outside the uterus. This condition is most often observed in women aged 30-45 years .The pain is dull, situated in the lower abdomen & lower back, without any radiation. It usually appears 3-5 days prior to the onset of period and relieves with the start of bleeding. The onset & duration of pain depends on the pathology producing the pain. There is no systemic discomfort unlike primary dysmenorrhoea, but there may be associated symptoms of pelvic pathology. The cause of secondary dysmenorrhoea can be detected on pelvic examination or ultrasongraphy.

Secondary dysmenorrhoea can be caused by the following:

- Endometriosis (inflammation of the lining of the uterus)
- Blood and tissue being discharged through a narrow cervix
- Uterine fibroid or ovarian cyst (tumours)
- Infections of the uterus
- Pelvic inflammatory disease
- Intrauterine device (used for contraception)
- Abnormal pregnancy, such as ectopic pregnancy

Any symptom associated with the above disorders will be present along with the menstrual pain. For example, a uterine fibroid may present with a lump in abdomen, ectopic pregnancy may present with heavy bleeding with shock etc.

Why training manual is developed for primary dysmenorrhoea?

From the above discussion on the types of dysmenorrhoea it should be clear that primary dysmenorrhoea is basically caused by the release of prostaglandins but in case of secondary dysmenorrhoea an underlying pelvic pathology is the actual cause.

The release of prostaglandins in primary dysmenorrhoea can be prevented to some extent by adopting some behavioural therapies like exercise .On the other hand, secondary dysmenorrhoea can be managed only by treating the underlying pelvic pathology; a visit to a gynaecologist is necessary in this case. Hence this exercise manual applies to those suffering from primary dysmenorrhoea, so that they can get rid of their problem by simple self-care. But one must understand that the exercises will not give instant results. One has to practice them regularly in the correct methods to have noticeable improvement after 2-3 months. To understand the mechanism of exercise therapy for control of pain in primary dysmenorrhoea it is essential to have a basic idea of the structure of female reproductive system and the physiology of menstrual cycle.

Structure of Female Reproductive System (Fig 1)

It is associated with a fundamental process of conception of foetus (pregnancy) & its consequent delivery (childbirth). However, when a woman is not conceiving, her egg (ovum) gets expelled from the body every month by a regular flow of blood from the genital region, which is medically known as menstruation.The following schematic representation of the internal genitalia helps to understand the above descriptions in a clearer way;

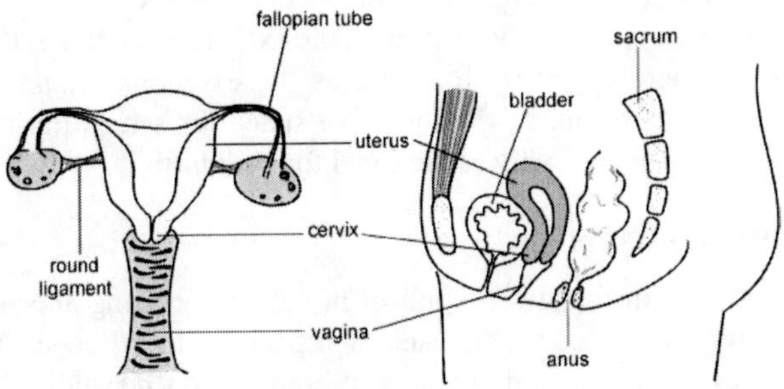

Fig 1: The female reproductive system

The internal genitalia (present inside the body) comprises of:

1. **Uterus:** Situated inside the lower abdomen, it is a hollow bag like organ with a cavity measuring around 6.5-7cm. The uterus is lined by 3 layers; from inside out the layers are – mucosa (known as endometrium), striated muscles (myometrium) & serosa (perimetrium). In the phases before & after menstruation, the striated muscle plays little or no role but the smooth muscle of the uterus and vagina is active and contracts periodically to expel the shedded endometrium along with the unfertilized ovum. These uterine and vaginal contractions are normally not consciously recognised. They only become obvious if they reach painful, spasmodic levels (dysmenorrhoeic pain), lasting for many minutes and producing uterine pressures greater than 60 mm Hg.

   The uterus has 3 parts; from above downwards - body, isthmus & cervix. The body is attached to fallopian tubes one on each side. The isthmus is the part in between the body and the cervix. The cervix is a cylindrical canal measuring 2.5cm and ending into the vagina. Function of the uterus: 1. Hold the baby till delivery. 2. Shed off the endometrium with menstrual blood.

2. **Tubes & ovaries:** The fallopian or uterine tubes are paired structures, measuring about 10 cm and are attached to the upper & outer wall of the uterus. The tubes help in the transport of unfertilized egg from ovary to uterus so that it can be shed during menstruation. The ovaries are two in number present inside the lower abdomen. These communicates with the uterus via the tubes on either side. Either of the ovaries produces and releases an egg on every month, which is either fertilized or expelled with menstruation.

3. **Vagina:** It constitutes a fibromuscular canal communicating the uterine cavity with the exterior at the external genitalia of the female reproductive system. It serves as the excretory channel for the menstrual blood, as the receptive space for semen during sexual intercourse and lastly as the canal for childbirth.

The Menstrual Cycle

Menstruation in females is cyclical in nature occurring approximately every 28 days. Nature considers each menstrual cycle for conception of a foetus. The cycle is broken down into different phases depending upon the chief activity of tat phase. Day 1 of the cycle is the start of menstrual bleeding which continues through to day 5. Day 5- 14 is called the proliferation phase as the uterine lining grows and prepares itself to receive the egg. Day 13 is considered the ovulation phase. Day 14 to Day 28 are known as the luteal or secretory phase; the corpus luteum is formed in this phase which secretes the hormone progesterone, to support the endometrium till menstruation occurs in the next cycle.

The female menstrual cycle is earmarked by its regular, periodic hormonal fluctuations. All changes in the female reproductive system is largely influenced by hormones such as estrogen, progesterone, and luteinizing hormone, which are the most widely discussed and known biochemicals influencing female reproduction. Each hormone is secreted in a timely fashion and works in coordination with each other. The day 1 - 5 of the menstrual cycle is identified by menstruation, the sloughing off of the uterine lining,. Days 5- 14, known as the proliferative or pre-ovulatory phase is earmarked by the thickening of the uterine lining with engorged blood vessels. During the pre-ovulatory phase, estrogen, released by the developing follicle, influences the thickening of the uterus lining. Although estrogen also contributes to the process of endometrial thickening, progesterone is primarily responsible for the endometrial thickening.

The ovulatory phase overlaps slightly with the pre-ovulatory phase. This normally occurs on day thirteen of the cycle. During ovulation, the egg (dominant follicle) gets released from the ovary. Estrogen is secreted within the developing follicle. Under the influence of this estrogen, the follicle continues to mature as the endometrial lining thickens. However, during ovulation this mature follicle is ruptured to release the ovum. The left behind cells ,lining the follicle begin to form the corpus luteum which serve to secrete mainly progesterone .This progesterone encourages the endometrial lining to be edematous and engorged. This stage is also known as the late luteal phase. The late luteal phase occurs simultaneous to the secretory phase in the endometrial cycle. All of this is done in preparation for fertilization and to support fetal development. If fertilization has not occurred on or about the twenty-fourth day of the cycle, the corpus luteum will degenerate and menstruation will commence in approximately four days, day twenty-eight where menses is marked by vaginal bleeding from the sloughing off of the endometrial lining.

When the corpus luteum degenerates in the late luteal phase, the progesterone level falls and brings about the elevation of prostaglandin levels. This elevated level of prostaglandins causes the pain of primary dysmenorrhoea just before or at the onset of next menstrual cycle.However, if ovulation does not occur in a cycle (anovulatory cycle) then the corpus luteum is not formed at all and there is no progesterone secretion. Prostaglandin, whose concentration usually rises in relation to the falling level of progesterone from corpus luteum, remains normal in level. Thus anovulatory (eggless) cycles are painless.

Good Menstrual Practices to Relieve Pain

Certain modifications of the lifestyle can help in prevention and management of the menstrual pain & subsequent complications.

A. Dietary modifications

1. Eat light but frequent meals, particularly during the menstruation when there is nausea and loss of appetite associated with pain.
2. Drink warm beverages like milk, tea. civ
3. Vitamin B(whole grains, fruits, vegetables), Vitamin E, Essential Fatty Acids (omega 3 fatty acids in marine fishes), Iron (dates, jaggery), and Magnesium help to control pain and other symptoms associated with dysmenorrhoea.

ADD more complex carbohydrates to diet (whole grains, fruits, and vegetables).

AVOID salt, sugar, cake, pastry, fast food, coffee, cold drinks (may increase pain)

B. Lifestyle changes

Few changes in the lifestyle can lead to a reduction in the intensity of menstrual pain probably by some psychosocial mechanism,

1. **AVOID** excessive mental stress at home or at workplace or schools.
2. **RELAX** & try to spend more free time in company with friends & family.
3. **PRACTISE** meditation routinely.
4. **WALK** or do light exercise regularly.

5. **AVOID** lifting heavy weights esp. during menstruation (may lead to prolapse)
6. **AVOID** smoking actively or passively.

C. Menstrual Hygiene

1. Take bath daily & keep your private parts clean.
2. Wear cotton undergarments & wash these every day; synthetic undergarments lead to accumulation of sweats which may result in fungal infections. cv
3. Use sanitary napkins during menses; dispose these hygienically. If homemade rags are used, wash these properly, rinse in dettol & dry in sunlight, before reusing.

Be sure to **SEE YOUR DOCTOR** immediately **IF,**

- you experience menstrual pain and a fever.
- your vaginal discharge increases in amount & becomes foul-smelling.
- your pain is significantly more than the previous episodes.
- your period is over one week late.

Exercises to Prevent Dysmenorrhea

Many myths continue to circulate about exercise during menstruation, but it seems in general to be beneficial.

Mechanism of action of the exercises:

1. Exercise may be a way to reduce the pain of menstrual cramps through the brain's production of endorphins, the body's own painkillers. These natural painkillers will fight against prostaglandins, which produces pain.
2. Menstrual pain stems from increased contraction of the uterine muscle innervated by sympathetic nervous system. Stress tends to enhance sympathetic activity, thus leading to menstrual pain. Exercise is a widely accepted way for reducing stress.
3. Exercise also leads to increased blood flow to the pelvic organs & helps in reducing the ischaemic pain during menstruation (due to lack of blood supply).

Time:

The following simple exercises should be ideally practiced regularly two times every day of the month 10-20 minutes each time (except during menses).

Exercise 1. Abdominal Breathing

Lie face up with legs and knees bent; now perform abdominal breathing about 10 times. This can be done by focussing on inflating and deflating the abdomen while breathing, without using much of your chest.

Exercise 2. Curl Ups

Lie on back; now bring your knees to touch your chin as much as possible; straighten back the legs. Repeat it for 10 times. Do not worry if your knees do not touch your chin. Try to bring it as close as you can.

Exercise 3. Heel Raising Exercise

Stand straight while holding the back of a chair (the chair should be stable & sturdy); lift one heel off the floor, then the other heel in the same manner and stand on your toes for 10 seconds with both heels raised. Resume normal standing position again. Repeat 20 times. (Pix 3a & 3b)

Exercise 4. Knee Bends

Stand straight while holding the back of a chair; now do 5 deep knee bends, each lasting for 15 seconds.

Exercise 5. Knee Bends with roll of cloth

Stand with both knee bent and feet together. Put a roll of cloth (small towel or dupatta into a ball) in the back of both the knees. Try to hold it in that position for 1 minute, while doing knee bend. Initially you can support your hands on the back of a chair, but gradually try to do it without any support.

Tips to remember

1. At the beginning, it may not be possible to complete all the steps in 20 minutes;

   Don't give up! By gradual practice you will be able to perform effortlessly just as any routine activity like brushing of teeth or eating a meal.

2. Initially, one may be reluctant to practise the exercises twice a day as the results are not instant. **Have patience!** Do not expect immediate relief; it will take time. After 2-3 months you will feel a noticeable improvement in pain.

3. **Remember** that relaxation of the muscles are as important as contraction during exercise. **Give a gap** of 2 minutes after each step.

4. **Do not** hold breath while doing the exercises, breathe normally.

5. **Follow** the instructions of your trainer about the exercise. If you are confused at any step contact your trainer.
6. **Do not** practice the exercises during menstruation; it may lead to heavy bleeding.

Records of exercises

To assess the amount of pain relieved by practice of exercises, one needs to maintain a record of the following events in a menstrual diary for 3 consecutive months. A menstrual diary is a monthly calendar with dates from 1st to 30th or 31st of each month. The following figure represents a menstrual diary.

Identification no:………..contact no:…………….. Month:…………..

1	2	3	4	5
6	7	8	9	10
11	12	13	14	15
16	17	18	19	20
21	22	23	24	25
26	27	28	29	30
31				

Events to be recorded

1. Days of menstruation are to be circled with red ink.
2. Days on which exercise was performed are to be circled with blue ink; the time of exercises should be mentioned with the dates.

Use of Hot Water Bottle during Menstrual Cramps

It is believed that heat decreases the congestion in the lower abdomen, occurring during menstruation & causing pain. Heat also dilates the blood vessels of uterus and relieves the ischemic pain by increasing the blood supply.

Steps:

1. Fill up a hot water bottle with hot water (the bottle should be made of rubber, ISI marked, available in medicine shops). cxi
2. Expel the air carefully before putting the cap tightly; check for water leakage.
3. Check the temperature & wrap the hot bottle in a towel before application.
4. Apply the bottle to the lower abdomen, below the umbilicus, for 15 – 20 minutes at a time during painful periods.
5. Take warm showers or baths during the days of menstruation.

Be sure to SEE YOUR DOCTOR immediately IF,

- Your pain is significantly more than the previous episodes.
- You experience a heavy menstrual bleeding
- Your period is over one week late.

Use of hot water bottle in dysmenorrhoea: a success story

A few days back, I came across a really interesting incident or should I call it a coincidence, that I would like to share with the medical fraternity. As a part of my research job I resolved to find a non pharmacological intervention for painful menstruation, a major cause of morbidity among the adolescent girls. I was giving a small talk to school girls on the impact of pain during menstruation and use of hot water bottle as a means of prevention, in Chandigarh. After finishing my talk, I asked students to share with me whether they really wanted to use the hot water bottle as suggested by me. I found a single girl of around 14years of age raising her hand; she was reluctant to give any reasons for her action. Later on, however, she shared her experiences and feelings with me, which seemed to me as a replica of the same problems I tried to explain them a few minutes before. The real life experience of the girl came as handy as a live demonstration.

Pratima has had her first period at an age of ten years and since then the monthly pain and backhache has become her companion. Every month before her menses she goes into a state of depression, apprehending her forthcoming suffering. She however, tries her best to divert her mind by watching TV. But nothing could solve the problem. She is anxious, feels like crying out to the world; she can't concentrate on her studies and even avoids social activities. To top it all, she feels so weak that she can not even get up from her bed during "those days".

What came as a shock to me was the fact that she was never been taken to a doctor for consultation, in spite of her four years of agony. Her parents (father is a fashion designer and mother is a manager in some company) are educated enough to at least understand the implication of any pain .Does it really need much sense to understand the impact the pain is having on their daughter's life? May be the busy schedule of the parents have kept them away from sensing their daughter's problem. The girl spends most of her time with her grand mom who gave her a valuable piece of advice "*dard to sabko hoti hain; hamne bhi yeh dard saha thha, shadi ke baad theek ho jayegi. Aage jake bachhe hone ka dard kaise sahegi? baad main mushkil hogi, isi liye abhi se aadat daal lo*". (Everybody experiences pain; we have also had it during our times. If you can't tolerate this pain now, how will you bear with the pain of child birth? It is better if you are habituated with the pain from now onwards).

Pratima believes her so much so that she faithfully undergoes the suffering every month, crying in pain to herself - "*andar hi andar roti rehti hoon*" (I keep crying to myself).

If Pratima is going to follow her *dadi*'s advice, then it means she has miles to suffer before she is ultimately married off, that is probably another 10 years, if not more. It is the same old story of Indian culture & tradition, where the girls are not allowed to discuss their *womanly* problems even with a doctor. She is expected to be tolerant towards her all sorts of discomforts- physical or emotional probably as a preparation for the future when she has to balance the role of a wife, a mother, a daughter in law while working outside for the sake of supporting her family.

After talking to Pratima about her problems, I promised her that I will talk to her mother about it and try to solve her problem. A day after, I called up her mother on mobile and informed her about the agony her daughter was going through every month. She appeared quite indifferent at first and commented- " *mujhe bhi aisa dard hota thha period ke time; lekin woh to apne aap hi thik ho gaya thha*" (I also experienced similar pain during my periods; but it was cured spontaneously). It took really long to convince her about the fact that she should consult a gynaecologist for Pratima's menstrual pain. At the end of our conversation she however agreed to come to PGIMER for the consultation. On my next visit to Pratima's school, I told her the date I have already fixed up for her consultation. Luckily enough, at that time I was having my clinical OPD (Out Patient Department) postings and I could help in getting her gynaecological consultation and afterwards an ultrasound done. The report of the ultrasound turned out to be normal and thus the fear of secondary dysmenorrhoea was almost ruled out. By this time Pratima's mother was quite impressed about the doctors of PGIMER, and told me holding my hand - " *agar aap doctor hoke itne sab kar sakte ho meri beti ke liye; mera to mummy hone ki nate yeh farz banta hain ki main aapki advice sunhu*" (If you people, even being doctors can spare so much time for my daughter; then being a mother it is my duty to listen to your advice for her). I took this opportunity to explain her about the effectiveness of using hot water bottle during menstrual pains and requested her to help her daughter in using it. After around one week, Pratima's mother called up to thank me because of my advice of hot water bottle, which has worked like wonders for her. She has used it for around 2-3 days during her last period and her pain was much decreased. Let us hope that in near future Pratima gets rid of all her sufferings during her menstruation.

Pain is a common complaint of menstruating women. It is often disregarded by many of these women who consider pain to be a normal part of the menstrual cycle. Thus, many women fail to report their pain to the physicians who treat them. The consequences of untreated primary dysmenorrhoea range from lost work and school hours to family and personal disruption among female student community. Despite the fact that half the world menstruates, most people overlook the serious repercussions of the morbidity it causes. Most people don't know that it is a problem. Others find the subject embarrassing. Even those who do understand think there are more pressing problems at hand. In ancient Rome, Pliny the Elder wrote that contact with menstrual blood "turns new wine sour, crops touched by it become barren, grafts die, the edge of steel and the gleam of ivory are dulled." Today, Pliny seems ridiculous, but discrimination and ignorance remain.

References

1. Andersch B, Milsom I. An epidemiologic study of young women with dysmenorrhea. Am J Obstet Gynecol 1982;144:655–60.
2. William F. McCool. Pain in women's health: A multi-Faceted approach toward understanding. Journal of Midwifery & Women's Health 2004;49(6): 473-81.
3. Campbell MA. Use of medication by adolescents for the management of menstrual discomfort. Arch Pediatr Adolesc Med ;. 1997; 151:: 905–13.
4. Banikarim C, Kelder S.H.Prevalence and Impact of Dysmenorrhea on Hispanic Female Adolescents, Arch Pediatr Adolesc Med. 2000; 154:1226-9.
5. Daley AJ. Exercise and primary dysmenorrhoea : a comprehensive and critical review of literature. Sports medicine. august,2008;38(8):659-70.
6. Durain D. Primary dysmenorrhea: Assessment and management update Journal of Midwifery & Women's Health 2004; 49(6):520-8.
7. Golomb L, Warren A, Michelle P. Primary dysmenorrhea and physical activity, Sports medicine. June 1998;30(6): 906-9.
8. Abbaspour Z, Rostami M. The effect of exercise in primary dysmenorrhoea. J Res Health Sci. 2006; 6(1):26-31.
9. Metheny W, Smith R. The relationship among exercise, stress and primary dysmenorrhoea. . Behave J Med. 1989;12:569-86.
10. Ganon L. The potential of exercise in the alleviation of menstrual disorders and menopausal symptom. Women & health. 1986;14(2):105-7.
11. Hubbeli JW. Specific and non specific exercise for relief of dysmenorrhoea. Res Q. 1949;20:378-86.
12. Izzo A, Labriola D. Dysmenorrhoea and sports activities in adolescents. Clinical and experimental obstetrics & gynecology. 1991;18(2):109-16.
13. Menaker JS. Management of primary dysmenorrhea. Obstet Gynecol 1962 Jul;20:66-71.
14. Proctor ML, Murphy PA, Pattison HM, Suckling J, Farquhar CM. Behavioural interventions for primary and secondary dysmenorrhoea. Cochrane database of systematic reviews (Online). 2007(3): CD002248.
15. Akin MD. Use of continous low level topical heat in the treatment of dysmenorrhoea. Obstetrics and gynecology. 2001;97:343-9. cxvi

16. On AY, Colakoglu Z, Hepguler S, Aksit R. Local heat effect on sympathetic skin responses after pain of electrical stimulus. Arch Phys Med Rehabil 1997; 78:1196-9.
17. Singh AJ. Place of menstruation in the reproductive lives of women of rural North India. Indian Journal of Community Medicine. 2006; 31:10-4.
18. Chaudhuri A, Singh AJ. Promoting health of school girls – empowering them by training them in non pharmacological management of primary dysmenorrhoea.In: *Health Promotion in 21st Century India*. Singh AJ.New Delhi, Jaypee Brothers Medical Publishers Ltd. (in press)

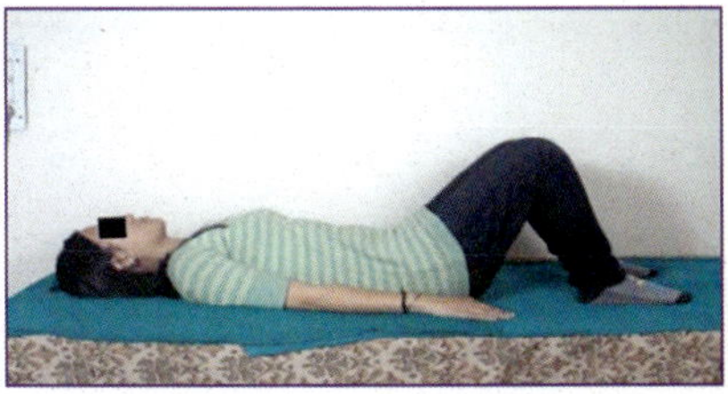

Pix 1. Abdominal breathing exercise.

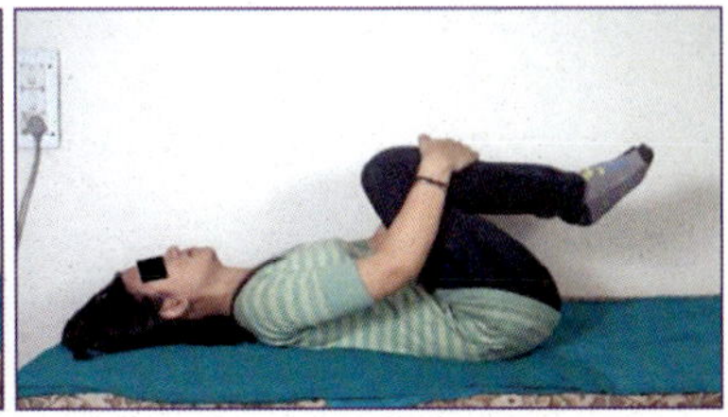

Pix 2. Curl ups.

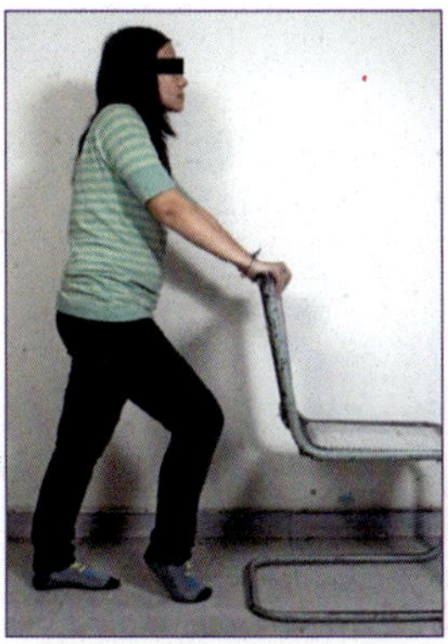

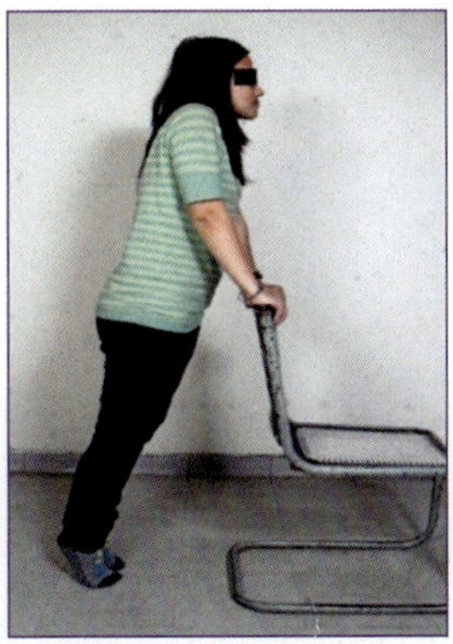

Pix 3 a & b. Raising one / both the heels up.

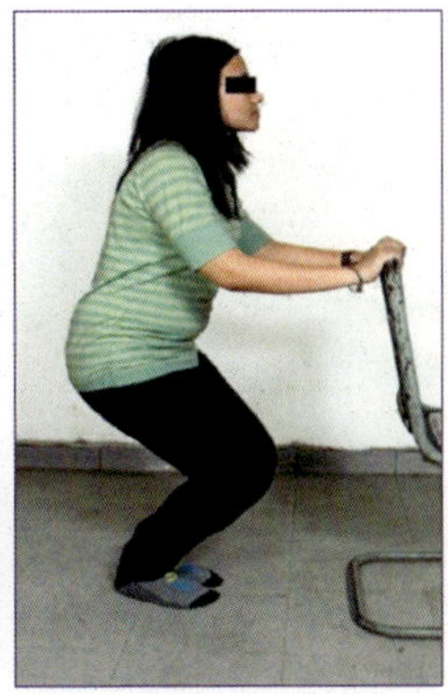

Pix 4. Knee bends.

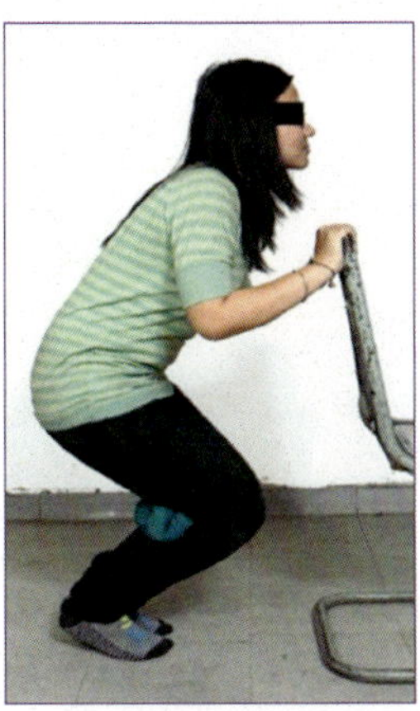

Pix 5.Knee bend with a roll of cloth

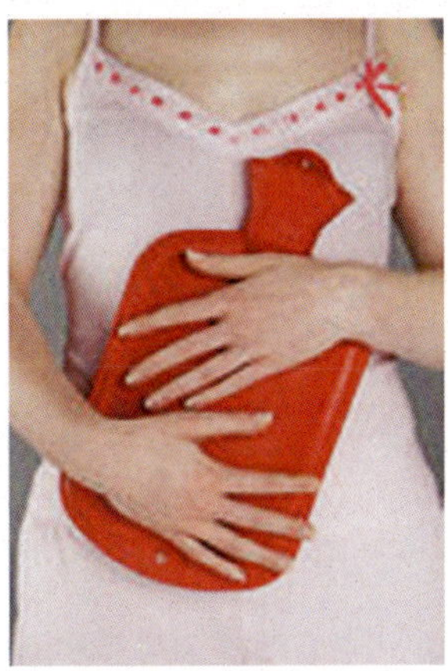

Pix 6. Correct position of hot water bottle

Chapter - 3

A Woman's Guide to Deal with Polycystic Ovary Syndrome (PCOS)

— Ishwarpreet Kaur, Dr. Amarjeet Singh, Dr. Vanita Suri

This material on polycystic ovary syndrome / polycystic ovary disease (PCOS / PCOD) is an initiative towards providing answers to all your questions related with this condition. Through it we aim to impart complete knowledge about PCOS which is scientific, accurate and trustworthy.

This work is outcome of research on PCOS / PCOD. We chose to study this medical condition as it has become one of the most common endocrine and gynaecological problem of the OPDs in Chandigarh. Many unmarried and married females have been suffering silently from this condition. Through our research study we wanted to see whether lifestyle modification can help in managing this condition.

During the course of the PhD work on this condition we learnt a lot about the plight of these females. The emotional and psychological agony they face. After listening to them, it became evident how ignorant the girls were about this problem and how they have been unnecessarily suffering till now. A quite often they have been exploited by the quacks. The whole experience has changed the way we think about the condition. We now understand their problems in much detail and empathise with the affected girls. We felt the need to empower the females with knowledge so that they can be more aware about the issues involved. This will surely help them to be in more control over their condition and also participate in deciding about the course of their treatment.

Through this document readers can hope to learn about what PCOS/PCOD is all about. What causes it? How it is diagnosed? What signs and symptoms are experienced with this condition? We have also shared some of the feeling and verbatim of the patients. How and what it feels to be labelled as PCOS/ PCOD? It also highlights on the treatment options available for this condition. How simple lifestyle changes can correct this condition. We have shared some of the success stories of our patients.

It's important for every female with this condition to know her body and how the disease affects her hormones. Despite the increasing prevalence, masses are not aware of implications of this condition. Due to ignorance they keep trying a variety of remedies, often ineffective. There is a need to increase the awareness in society regarding the condition and importance of healthy lifestyle in the management of this syndrome. There is a lot of confusion regarding its diagnosis and treatment protocol for this condition. The health professionals also need to be updated with the latest advancements in the PCOS management.

The education about the condition will not only empower you with knowledge but will also help you cope with it in a better way. It will help you to make informed decisions about your condition and stop the endless worrying about the unknown which had earlier haunted you. The text is written in simple language for better understanding and thereby giving you the power to have control over your body, emotions and above all PCOS

> ***Gynae & sexual health is a whole community issue – when a woman suffers in silence, so does her family and partner. We need to raise awareness so we can speak openly & are more accepting.***
>
> - Kath Mazzella OAM, founder GAIN Inc.

My struggle with PCOS- a case study

"Polycystic Ovary Syndrome (PCOS), I first heard this word for the first time five years back from my doctor. I was 17 years old then. Actually I visited a gynaecologist as my periods were delayed; I didn't have my period in about 3 months. After seeing ultrasound and hormonal reports she confirmed the diagnosis and said, "It's PCOS". At that time I didn't bother much about it. I thought I will take the prescribed medicines and everything will be fine soon. But that was not to be. I had underestimated this health condition. I never knew that it will have such a big impact on my mind, body and life.

My periods have been very irregular. When I take the medicine I get my periods. Otherwise no show! When my friends discuss about their periods, I feel very embarrassed. I fear if they will know that I don't get my periods they will make fun of me. Because of this I never share my problem with anyone. Not even my close friends. I don't trust anyone. I think they will not keep it as a secret. They are sure to tell others. Only my family knows about it.

Still there are many things which I am apprehensive to share even with my mother and sister. I have this constant feeling of tension, fear and anxiety.

At times the stress is so much that I am unable to sleep properly at night. I often get real scary dreams.

With age the focus of my fears and worry has changed. Initially when it all started my constant concern was regarding excess hair growth and weight. My friend would taunt and say "*teri ladke jaise daadi muche aa gai hai*" (you have grown a beard and moustache like a boy). I would feel very upset. I even cried alone in my room. I would fear that I am becoming more like a man. I hated seeing myself in mirror. I was tired of the weekly visits to parlour to get my hair removed. I started avoiding going out with friends to parties. I skipped family functions. I secluded myself. I had practically no social life. To keep myself happy I would watch T.V. I found comfort in eating. All this resulted in further weight gain.

I have been suffering from within for last five years.

I am 22 years old now. Not much has changed; I am still overweight, have to make constant visits to doctor and parlour for threading and waxing. I still feel bad about these issues. The only thing which has indeed changed is the focus of my tension. Now I am much more concerned about marriage and possibility of infertility. I feel no one will marry me. Even if I get married I won't be able to have a baby. What will happen to me in my future?

Everyone till now just taunts and advises me to be active and eat less. Due to this I have constant fights with everyone. It's been so long; but no one has tried to understand neither me nor my concerns. I still don't know why I have this problem and what it is all about. No one in my family or my friends have PCOS. I keep wondering - Why only I have it? Will I ever get freedom from this disease state? I have many questions in my mind. Even my doctor has never explained me anything about it. I also tried searching PCOS related information on internet. But every site I visited had something different to say regarding the treatment. More I keep looking for information more I get confused. I wish someone could answer all my questions and solve my problems?"

Above text describes / captures the plight of many young ladies labelled as PCOS.

This booklet on PCOS is an initiative towards providing answers to various questions and apprehensions related with this condition as outlined in above case-study. Through it we aim to educate the affected girls and women about PCOS. Our focus is to provide scientific, accurate and trustworthy information. This will not only empower them with knowledge but will also help them cope with it in a better way. It will help them to make informed decisions about their condition. A comprehensive understanding of the condition will help avoid unnecessary confusion and worry regarding all aspects of the disease and treatment. The booklet is written in simple language for better understanding. It will help the readers have control over their health and conquer PCOS.

Polycystic Ovarian Syndrome (PCOS) -Demystified

PCOS has now become a common problem seen among adolescent girls and young women in gynecology OPDs. It is the most common hormonal disturbance affecting 1 out of 10 women worldwide.

This condition is mainly related to the endocrine system. This affects the reproductive system through hormonal disturbance. The endocrine system secretes hormones, which control the overall functioning of our body. Hormones are powerful chemical messengers. They are produced by endocrine glands in our body and travel in bloodstream to all the organs. These then affect many different processes of the body, including – growth and development, metabolism, reproduction & sexual function, even our mood. One example of hormonal disease is diabetes. Nowadays we see many people get diabetes. This is due to disturbances in insulin hormone. It controls glucose (sugar) metabolism in our body.

Similarly, an imbalance in women's hormones causes PCOS. The most affected are the hormones secreted by ovaries (oestrogens, androgens and progesterone). These hormones control the release of eggs from ovaries, hair growth, and other conditions. Therefore the imbalance in ovarian hormone can make menstrual cycle (periods) irregular. Also release of eggs from ovaries can be disturbed. In married women this can cause problems in getting pregnant.

Signs – symptoms and diagnosis of PCOS

PCOS affects women in different ways. The signs and symptoms experienced by affected women vary. Everyone may not have all the symptoms. Some women have few symptoms while others have many. The severity of symptoms also varies from mild to severe from individual to individual.

Some of the most common signs – symptoms of PCOS include:

- Irregular periods or no periods at all. This affects about 7 in 10 women with PCOS.
- Hirsutism or the extra hair on your face or other parts of body (seen in 70% of cases)
- Acne; Oily skin
- Acanthosis nigricans or patches of dark skin on the back of your neck and other areas

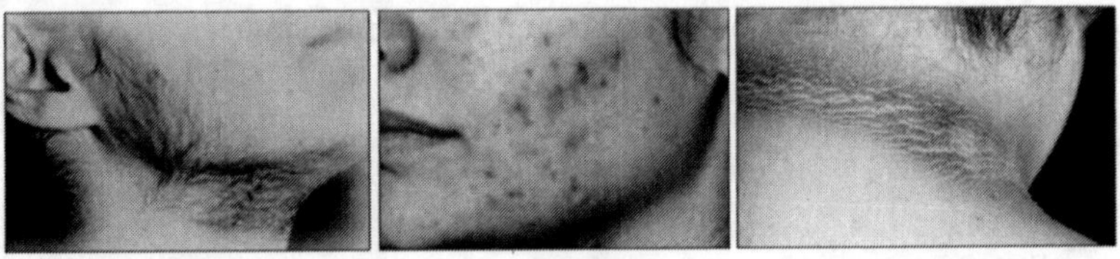

Hirsutism ***Acne*** ***Acanthosisnigricans***

Pix 1 – Symptoms of PCOS/PCOD

- Weight gain and/or trouble losing weight. About 40%-70% of women with PCOS are very overweight or obese. Abdominal or belly fat is more.
- Difficulty in getting pregnant, because of irregular or no release of eggs. In around 75% of the patients' infertility is reported
- Polycystic ovaries: the ultrasound of majority of PCOS women will show polycystic ovaries. The word 'poly' means many.
- Generally every month an egg is developed and ruptures out of the ovary. But due to high level of male hormones in the PCOS the egg begins to develop but fails to rupture (come out of the ovary). As a result they appear as bumps (cyst) on the surface of ovary.

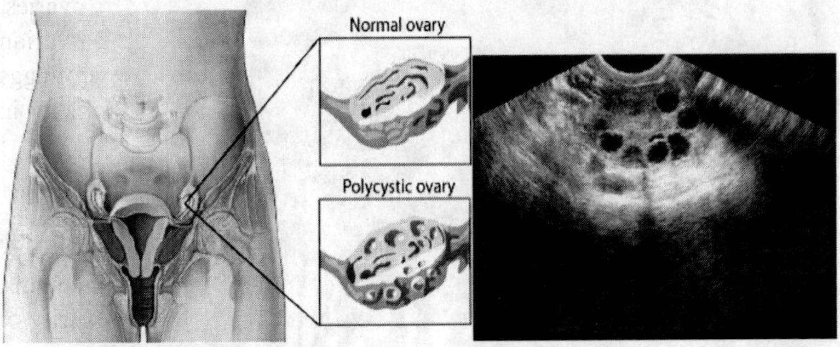

Pix 2 – Normal and polycystic ovaries + USG

- High Androgens or male hormones (e.g. testosterone)
- Insulin (a hormone) is found to be higher in women with PCOS. This can result in insulin resistance. It is common in both obese and lean women with PCOS, affecting up to 70% of the PCOS population
- Anxiety; depression; Mood swings; Fatigue
- Sleep apnea — brief spells where breathing stops during sleep.

Weight gain and insulin resistance with PCOS can worsen the symptoms. It can further lead to diabetes and heart related diseases.

PCOS SIGNS & SYMPTOMS

Visible signs = Irregular periods, Weight gain, Abdominal or belly fat, Facial hair, Acne, Thinning of hair, Dark spots on skin, Infertility

Internal signs = Ovarian cysts, Insulin resistance, Anovulatory period, High androgens

General symptoms = Fatigue, Anxiety, Mood swings, Rage, Depression, Insomnia

Figure 1 - PCOS signs & symptoms

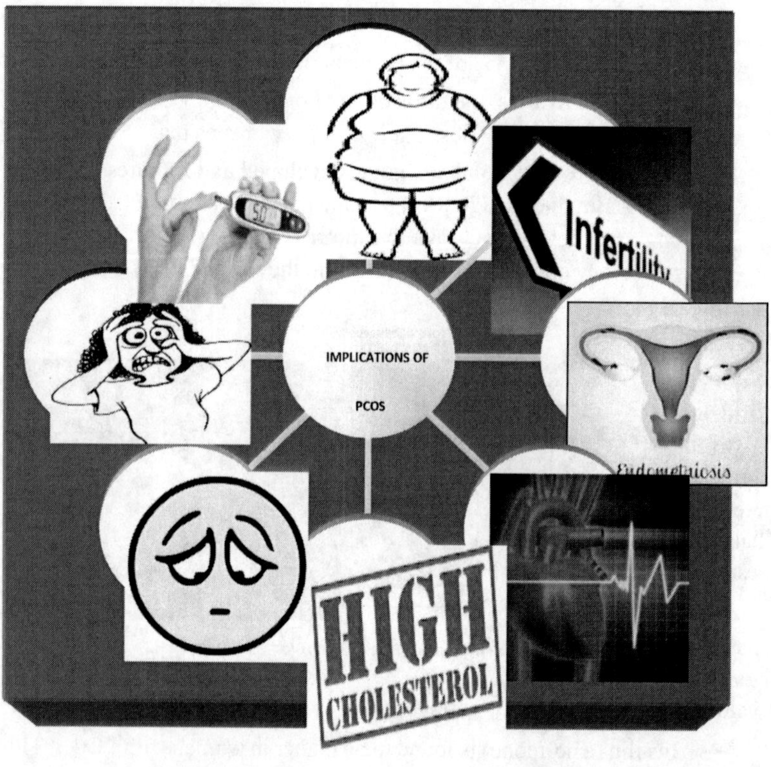

Figure 2: Implications related to PCOS/PCOD.

Implications of PCOS

It is common to see that girls who are diagnosed as PCOS do not take this condition seriously. After few years it can result in many other health complications. This includes infertility, insulin resistance, diabetes, high cholesterol, heart disease, endometriosis, metabolic syndrome, etc.Not just physical but it can also play emotional havoc. Weight might continue to increase. Excessive fat on body can make PCOS women feel image conscious. Other than this hair growth and acne can also increase concern regarding self-image, beauty and looks. Inability to conceive is another reason that can cause constant concern. All this can raise stress levels. This may even result in anxiety and depression.

Women with PCOS appear to have higher rates of:

- Miscarriage
- Gestational diabetes
- Pregnancy-induced high blood pressure (preeclampsia)
- Premature delivery

Human body: Reproductive and Endocrine system

Girls with PCOS generally face the problem of irregular periods. They are curious to know how they are different from other girls (without PCOS). What exactly is going wrong in their bodies which makes the periods so irregular.

Aetiology of PCOS

No one knows how exactly this condition develops but it is believed to be due to hormonal imbalance. The name PCOS is misleading as it makes one believe that the condition is an ovarian condition. Though ovaries are also involved but the truth is that PCOS is an endocrine condition that affects the entire body. A constant state of high hormonal levels over a period of time can interfere with the normal functioning of the ovaries in females. The hormones that are involved the most in this condition include luteinizing hormone (LH), oestrogen, male hormones (androgens) and insulin.

To understand how the imbalance of these hormones can develop into the characteristic symptoms of PCOS, it is first important to understand about the human body, endocrine and reproductive system, and normal menstruation cycle.

For more clarity and better understanding of the PCOS it is also important to know the meaning of important terms, their role and relation with PCOS. It will help in understanding what goes wrong and how the body function changes with PCOS.

HUMAN BODY

The human body refers to the entire structure of a human being. It comprises of a head, neck, trunk, arms and hands, legs and feet. Each and every part of the body is composed of various types of cells. These cells and extracellular materials are organized into tissues, organs, and systems.

Body systems: Our bodies consist of a number of biological systems that carry out specific functions necessary for everyday living. The different systems in the body are: Musculoskeletal, Digestive, Respiratory, Circulatory, Lymphatic, Nervous, Reproductive, Endocrine, Excretory and Integumentary.

The two main systems related to PCOS are the endocrine and the reproductive system.

ENDOCRINE SYSTEM -This system is also known as the control centers of our body. It regulates body function using hormones. It tells our body cells what to do. Without them the cells would not know when and what to do. For example, bones won't grow till they receive a message to do so. It won't even come to know when it's time to begin puberty.

The endocrine system of females has glands of different sizes and shapes. These are located in different parts of the body. The names of the glands are Hypothalamus, Pituitary, Pineal, thyroid, Thymus, Adrenal, Pancreas, and Ovaries [**Fig. 3**].

PITUITARY GLAND
(Master gland) secretes many hormones some of which affect other glands

HYPOTHALAMUS
Controls secretion of hormones by the pituitary gland

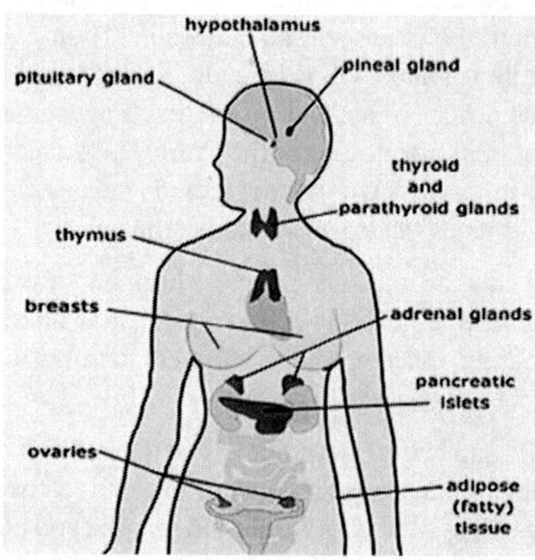

OVARIES
Control ovulation and secondary sexual characteristics

PANCREAS
Regulate the level of sugar in blood

Figure 3 - Endocrine System

Table 1 - Endocrine system involved in PCOS/PCOD

Gland	*Hormone*	*Function*
Pituitary gland	follicle-stimulating hormone (FSH)	■ stimulates maturation of egg follicles in females
	luteinizing hormone (LH)	■ stimulates rupture of mature egg follicles, and ■ production of progesterone and androgens in females
Ovaries	oestrogens	■ stimulate development of female sex organs and secondary sex characteristics, ■ maturation of egg follicles, and ■ contraction of the uterine muscles
	progesterone	■ stimulates /activates secretion of substances from the lining of the uterus (endometrium) in preparation for egg implantation in the uterine wall
	testosterone	■ stimulates development of male sex characteristics including facial hair growth
Pancreas	insulin	■ Largest endocrine gland (found in your belly) ■ Helps glucose / sugar enter the cells of your body from blood; glucose is needed by cells to function ■ Its malfunctioning results in diabetes

Diseases of the endocrine system can result from two reasons; viz over or under secretion of hormones and inability of target organs to respond to hormonal messages. These glands ensure that hormones are released in just the right amounts at just the right time. If there's a problem with this system, a person's body might not grow or work the way it's supposed to. The doctors who treat the conditions related to endocrine system are called endocrinologists.You might be surprised to know that the "master gland", i.e. the pituitary gland, is about the size of a pea (beneath your brain). It secretes hormones that control other glands and body functions.

FEMALE REPRODUCTIVE SYSTEM

The reproductive system allows organisms to reproduce or give birth to young ones. The inside (internal) female reproductive system includes the following parts:

(i) *Ovaries:* These are small, oval-shaped glands that are located on both side of the uterus. It produces eggs and hormones.

(ii) *Fallopian tubes:* These are attached to the upper part of the uterus and act as tunnels for the ova (egg cells) to travel from the ovaries to the uterus. Fertilization of an egg by a sperm, normally occurs in the fallopian tubes. The fertilized egg then moves to the uterus, where it implants into the lining of the uterine wall.

(iii) *Endometrium:* It is the lining of the uterus. The fertilized egg gets embedded in it.

(iv) *Uterus (womb):* It is a hollow, pear-shaped organ where fetus develops. It is divided into two parts. Corpus is the main body of the uterus. It can expand to hold the growing baby. Cervix is the lower part that opens into the vagina.

(v) *Vagina (birth canal):* It joins the cervix to the outside of the body. It is a channel which allows sperms to enter through and menstrual blood flows out [Fig. 4].

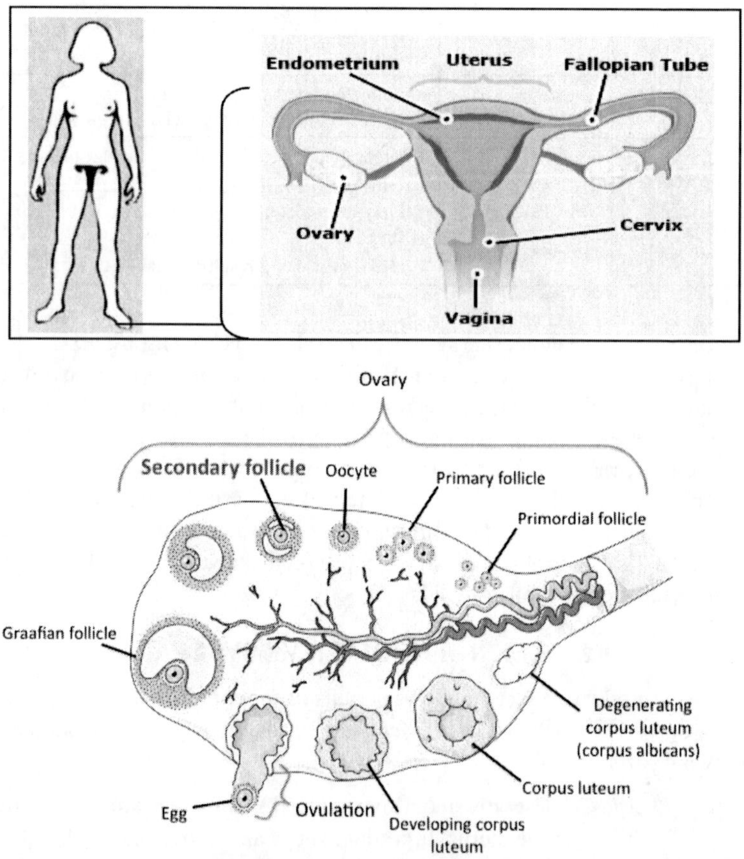

Figure 4: Female reproductive organs.

The female reproductive system is designed to perform various functions.

- Produces egg cells necessary for reproduction, called the ova / oocytes. These are produced by the ovaries.
- Transports the ova to the site of fertilization.
- Conception (fertilization of an egg by a sperm) in the fallopian tubes.
- Fertilized egg implants into the walls of the uterus (initial stages of pregnancy).
- If fertilization and/or implantation do not take place then menstrual cycle begins (the monthly bleeding, i.e. shedding of the uterine lining).
- It also produces female sex hormones that maintain the reproductive cycle.

KEY TERMS

OOCYTE = immature egg

FOLLICLE = a fluid-filled sac that contains an immature egg. Follicles are found in the ovaries. Each follicle contains an immature egg.

OVULATION = Release or liberation of the egg

CORPUS LEUTEUM = ruptured follicle after ovulation. The follicle that releases an egg turns into a corpus leuteum

Fun facts

- The human body contains nearly 100 trillion cells.
- There are at least 10 times as many bacteria in the human body as cells.
- The average adult takes over 20,000 breaths a day.
- Each day, the kidneys process about 200 quarts (50 gallons) of blood to filter out about 2 quarst of waste and water
- Adults excrete about a quarter and a half (1.42 liters) of urine each day.
- The human brain contains about 100 billion nerve cells
- Water makes up more than 50 percent of the average adult's body weight

How Many Eggs Does a Woman Have?

- At birth, there are approximately 1 million to 2 million eggs in the ovaries; by the time of puberty, only about 300,000 remain. Of these, only about 500 will be ovulated during a woman's reproductive lifetime. Any remaining eggs gradually die out at menopause.

The most anatomically correct 'vagina pants' you're ever likely to see

A British art student has created underwear showing intricately labelled diagrams of the female reproductive system. It's time to wear your biology textbook on your body, says Claire Cohen

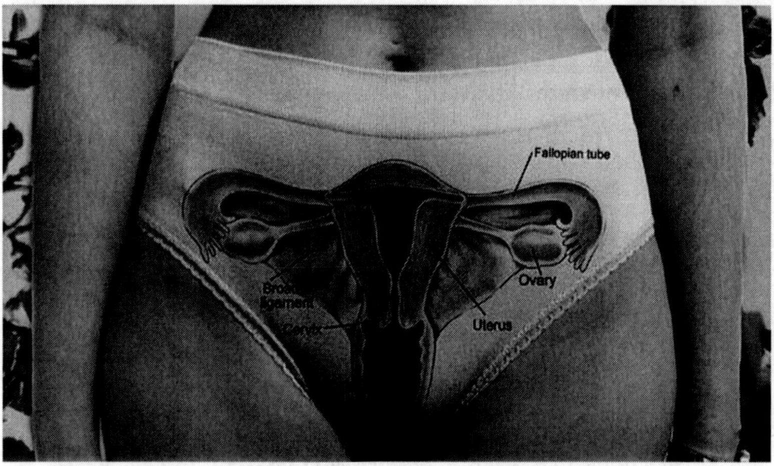

Ref- [the-body-system-study-sheet

Cause of hormonal imbalance in PCOS women

Exactly what causes hormonal imbalance that finally results in PCOS is still not known. Many factors are considered to play a role in its occurrence.

- Heredity; if PCOS is in family, you have more chances to have it.
- Unhealthy diet (processed foods with low fiber, high carbohydrates and fats).
- Adulterated foods (presence of pesticides, chemicals, hormones like oxytocin and growth hormones in food)
- Lack of physical activity and more sitting hours
- Increased intestinal permeability / leaky gut
- Stress

- Obesity
- Disturbed sleep / circadian rhythm

Probable reason for increasing prevalence of PCOS

1. In earlier times women were confined to the household tasks. They were supposed to play with dolls and stay indoors. It was only men's responsibility to earn bread and butter for the family. This way the work burden was segregated between the two. However, recently this old gender stereotype has changed. Women are now more educated and empowered.

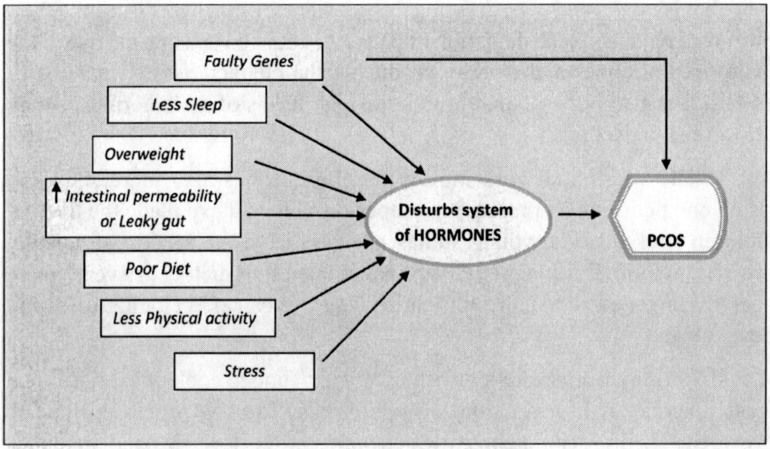

Figure 5. Aetiology of PCOS.

Figure 5 shows that many factors alter the hormonal balance to cause PCOS.

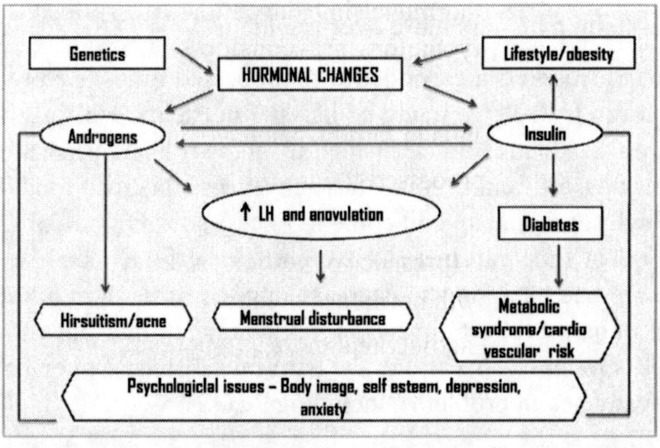

Figure 6. How hormonal imbalance results in PCOS symptoms.

Their duty is not just limited now to taking care of family but also to maintain a professional career. This change is catching up not only because of gender equality or their interest but also to support the family monetarily. Though females are also supporting the family financially their husbands may not help them with the household work. Many men still think it's only the job of females. As a result of this the women's work burden has increased drastically. It has led to stressful life.

2. The women are now very much into male bastion. This kind of work change may also affect hormones. Normally a female has the correct balance of both the female and male sex hormones in their body. As the girls are doing more boyish tasks and even dressing up like them, this may be disturbing their hormonal balance. Such deviation of behavior could be causing the rise in the male sex hormones and thereby producing the characteristic symptoms of PCOS. It is also possible that prolonged high levels of male hormones may affect the mindset further.

3. The stress and work burden on children has also increased. The rising competition and pressure to outperform others have made the lives of children stressful. The young adolescent girls have the additional societal pressure to look slim and pretty. This makes them start dieting at a very young age. Missing meals and unhealthy eating behavior can affect their growth and development.

4. Working women are left with hardly any time to cook or exercise. The food generally is brought from outside or easy to cook processed food is prepared. The household chores which were earlier done by hand are either done by domestic help or by machines. Also, the advancement in technology and the trend of mobiles and internet has further made women lives less physically active. Even the children are far less active now. They are hardly playing any outdoor games. All their free time goes in playing mobile games, chatting on phones or working on laptops. As a result the kids at such young age are becoming more and more overweight.

5. Even the markets are flooded with processed food. The processing of whole fresh foods depletes many of its vital nutrients. Not just this, many additives are also added. These are which are not very healthy like high sodium, sugars, trans fats, artificial colours, taste enhances, etc. Such foods have very low fiber, high sugar, salt and oil content. Excess consumption of these foods over a period of time can increase weight. These foods can also cause an increase in the bad bacteria and decrease in good bacteria in intestines. The overgrowth of harmful bacteria can harm the lining of intestines and result in change of its structure. This allows the harmful substances to enter the blood and cause many health problems, including PCOS.

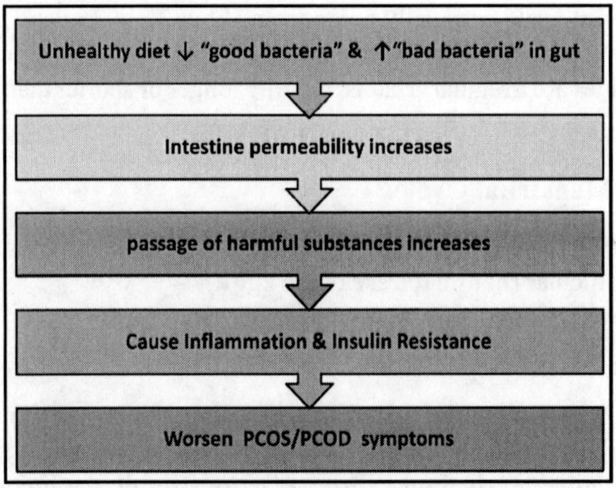

Figure 7 – DOGMA theory.

6. Another problem is the rising use of plastic in our daily life. Earlier our food was stored in steel, aluminum, glass or earthen ware containers. Now everything is replaced by plastic. Everything we eat or drink is stored in plastic container or packet. Perfluorinated chemicals (PFCs) found in food packaging material has shown to affect women's fertility. Even bisphenol A (BPA), a chemical in our environment, is a known oestrogenic "hormone disrupter".

"Back to nature" is the clarion call for PCOS girls/women.

Menstrual cycle and ovulation: the main focus area of PCOS

Due to hormone imbalance in PCOS cases the ovaries do not get the right hormonal signal. As a result the ovaries may not release egg (ovulate) every month. It can result in irregular or no period. Let's see how normal menstrual cycle occurs. Knowledge about this will help in better understanding of the how things actually change in PCOS, resulting in irregular periods.

Normal ovulation process and menstrual cycle

The normal menstrual cycle or menstruation helps to prepare the body for pregnancy. If pregnancy fails to occur the lining of the uterus (endometrium) sheds and causes bleeding. It lasts 3 to 7 days. Blood loss during a cycle is about 15 to 70gm. During normal menstruation cycle the brain (pituitary gland), ovaries, and uterus follow a series of events. Menstruation occurs every month throughout a woman's reproductive life, except during pregnancy. It starts during puberty (at menarche) and stops permanently at menopause. The hormones involved are the FSH and LH of pituitary gland; and progesterone and oestrogen made by ovaries.

Menstrual cycles normally range from about 25 to 36 days. Only 10 to 15% of women have cycles that are exactly 28 days. Also, in at least 20% of women, cycles are irregular. That is, they are longer or shorter than the normal range.

Stages of Menstrual Cycle

The cycle has three phases:

1. Follicular (before release of the egg)
2. Ovulatory/Ovulation (egg release)
3. Luteal (after egg release)

At the beginning of the first phase, the lining of uterus (endometrium) is thick to support pregnancy. If egg is not fertilized (no pregnancy), oestrogen and progesterone levels drop in 3rd week. As a result, the lining of uterus shed, and bleeding starts.

1. Follicular phase (lasts about 13 or 14 days)

This phase begins on the first day of menstrual bleeding (day 1). Day 1 is by definition the day period starts. During this phase the follicles develop in the ovaries.

The following events occur during this phase:

- Brain releases 2 hormones - follicle stimulating hormone ***(FSH)*** and luteinizing hormone ***(LH)***
- These hormones reach ovaries through blood.
- They cause the ovary to develop 15-20 follicles (immature eggs) and also ***increase the*** production of the female hormone ***oestrogens***.

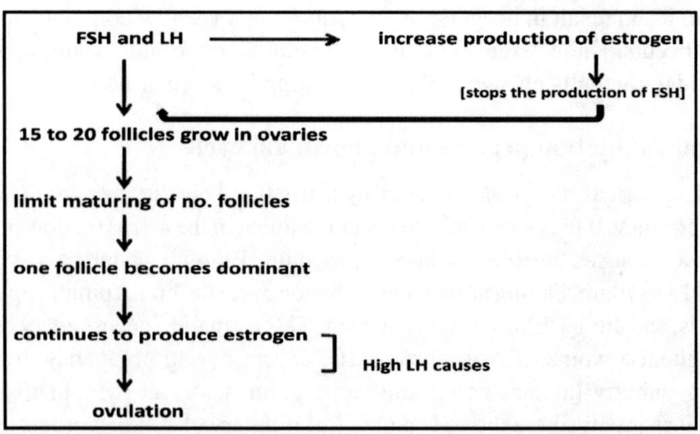

Figure 8. Effect of LH and FSH levels in ovulation.

- As ***oestrogens*** levels ***rise*** it ***stops*** the production of ***FSH;*** this balance of hormones helps limit the number of follicles that mature. It also thickens the uterus lining and stimulates pituitary to release a large amount of LH.
- Finally, one of the follicles becomes dominant. The main follicle continues to produce oestrogens.

2. Ovulatory phase or **ovulation (Day 14)**

Ovulation is the when an egg is released from the ovaries. It is one of the phases in the female menstrual cycle. It starts about 14 days after the follicular phase started. The ovulatory phase usually lasts 16 to 32 hours. It ends when the egg is released [about 10 to 12 hours after the rise in the level of luteinizing hormone]. The egg can be fertilized for only up to about 12 hours after its release.This release of the egg is called ovulation.

During this phase, the following events occur:

- The sharp increase in LH causes the egg to be released from the ovary.
- As the egg is released from the ovary it travels through the fallopian tubes.
- There is an increase in the amount and thickness of mucus produced by the cervix (lower part of the uterus). If a woman has intercourse during this time, the thick mucus captures the man's sperm, nourishes it, and helps it to move towards the egg for fertilization / pregnancy.

3. Luteal phase

This phase begins after ovulation. It lasts about 14 days (unless fertilization occurs) and ends just before a menstrual period.

The luteal phase involves the following processes:-

After ovulation, the ovary produces both oestrogen and progesterone

These hormones prepare the uterus for possible pregnancy

- If intercourse has taken place and a man's sperm has fertilized the egg (conception), the fertilized egg will travel through the fallopian tube to implant in the uterus. The woman is now considered pregnant.
- If the egg is not fertilized it passes through the uterus and lining of the uterus breaks down and sheds, and the next menstrual period begins

Role of LH and FSH in normal menstrual cycle and ovulation

Figure 9 shows a regular menstrual cycle with normal ovulation taking place.

In a regular cycle the LH is always less than the FSH hormone. It is only once the LH hormone level rises sharply (surges) and that's when ovulation occurs. Thereafter the hormones are secreted normally and cycle continues.

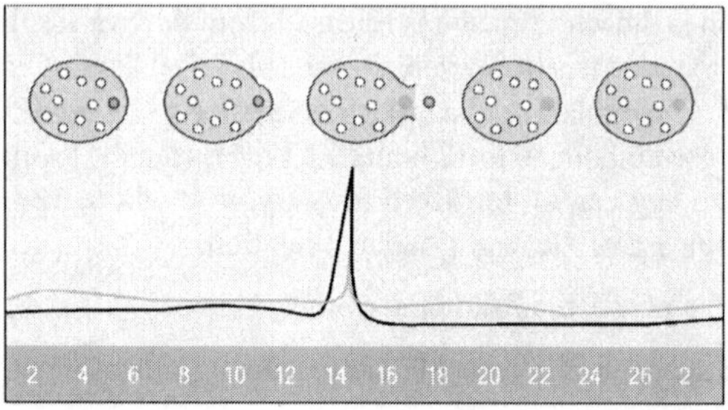

Follicles in the Ovary Pituitary Hormones FSH (light) LH (dark) Cycle Day

Figure 9- Regular Menstrual Cycle with ovulation.

This was the normal cycle. Now the question is what happens when it goes awry? To know more read on!! cxxxviii

Menstrual cycle in PCOS

In women with PCOS the levels of oestrogen, progesterone, LH, and FSH become imbalanced. As a result of none of the follicles are capable of growing to a size that would result in ovulation. Such a condition over long period of time can result in infertility. Figure 10 shows a PCOS cycle with no ovulation.

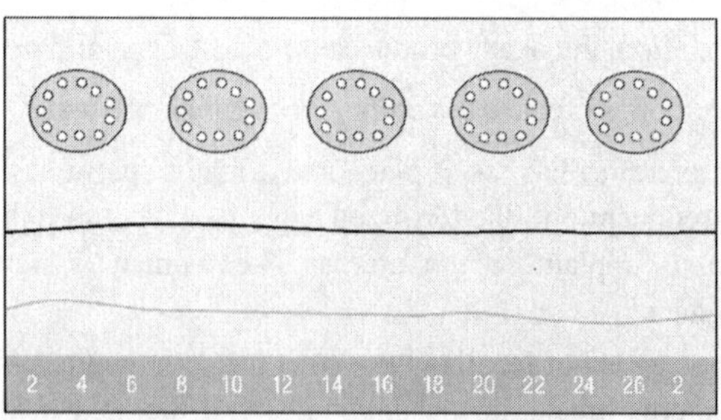

Follicles in the Ovary Pituitary Hormones LH (dark) FSH (light) Cycle Day

Figure 10. PCOS cycle with no ovulation.

This results due to high levels of LH when the menstrual cycle starts. The levels of LH are higher than FSH levels. Because the LH levels are already quite high, there is no LH surge (rapid rise). Without this LH surge, ovulation does not occur. As a result some follicles may remain as cysts and are diagnosed as poly - cystic ovaries in ultrasound.

Without ovulation the hormone progesterone is not made. Without it menstrual cycle becomes irregular or absent. High levels of LH and insulin increase production of male hormones like testosterone, androstenedione, dehydroepiandrosterone (DHEA), and DHEA sulfate (DHEA-S)]. This prevents ovulation and produce symptoms like excess hair growth, acne, etc.

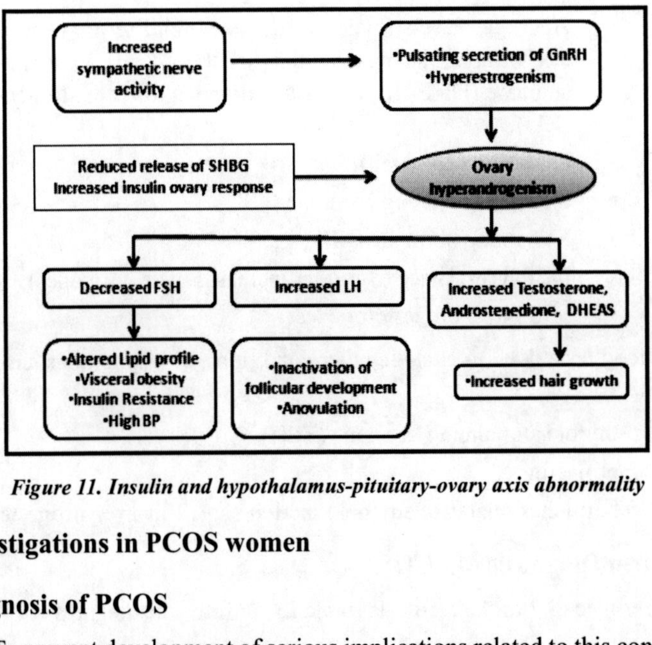

Figure 11. Insulin and hypothalamus-pituitary-ovary axis abnormality

Investigations in PCOS women

Diagnosis of PCOS

To prevent development of serious implications related to this condition the first step is to have proper diagnosis. This must be followed by appropriate treatment. Timely and regular follow up visits to the doctor. Just by looking at the signs and symptoms a doctor cannot confirm the diagnosis of PCOS. For this few tests are needed. These will also help rule out other disease with similar symptoms. This includes blood tests and ultrasound scan. The following steps are followed to find out if you have PCOS or if something else is causing the symptoms.

(i) **Medical history.** A doctor (gynaecologist or endocrinologist) generally asks about the patient's menstrual periods, weight changes, other symptoms, past health, family's health, allergies, and other issues.

(ii) **Physical exam.** This includes measuring the blood pressure, weight, height, waist size and checking physical signs such as acne, hair growth, and darkened skin.

(iii) **Ultrasound (USG)** - The sound waves are used to take pictures of your pelvic area to look at ovaries and check for cysts or other abnormalities. The test should be done between day 2-5 of periods. For accurate diagnosis 2-3 ultrasounds are required. In case of adolescents Magnetic Resonance Imaging (MRI) scan is more accurate to diagnose poly cystic ovaries.

(iv) **Blood tests.** The level of few hormones is tested in the blood to confirm the diagnosis of PCOS. These include:

- Androgen levels (male hormones) – total serum testosterone, sex hormone binding–globulin (SHBG), dehydroepiandrosterone sulphate (DHEAS), androstenedione and free androgen index (FAI).
- Estradiol (oestrogen)
- follicle stimulating hormone (FSH)
- luteinizing hormone (LH)
- Insulin resistance (it further increases male hormones)
- Mid-luteal progesterone test

Blood tests done to exclude other conditions with symptoms similar to PCOS:

- thyroid stimulating hormone (TSH)
- prolactin
- hormones related to adrenal function e.g. 17-hydroxyprogesterone

Confirm Diagnosis of PCOS

Presence of 2 of the 3 criteria (table 2) confirms the diagnosis of PCOS

Table 2 - PCOS diagnosis Rotterdam criteria 2003 (2 of 3 criteria needed)

(a)	Polycystic ovaries
(b)	Clinical and/or biochemical signs of hyperandrogensim
(c)	Oligo and/or anovulation

Table 3 - Laboratory evaluation

(a) Polycystic ovaries = Ultrasound scan (multi-follicles, 12 or more, throughout the ovary measuring 2–9 mm in diameter and/or increased ovarian volume higher than 10 ml in at least one ovary)

(b) Clinical signs of hyperandrogensim (high level of male hormones) = Hirsutism, hair loss, acne

Biochemical signs = Higher LH/FSH ratio (2:1)

High testosterone (>60 ng/100 ml.)

High DHEAs (Normal levels= 40 to 410 ug/dl)

Low SHBG (Normal levels= 0.4 to 3.5 ug DHT/100 ml

(c) Oligo and/or anovulation

Menstrual irregularity (<21 days period cycle or >35days cycle)

Anovulation (lack of ovulation) - Serum Progesterone on Day 21 of regular cycle. In case of irregular cycle obtain Serum Progesterone 7 days before anticipated menses onset (<4 ng/ml suggests ovulation did not occur)

Life with PCOS & Emotional Health

What it feels being a girl or woman?

The word 'woman' is synonymous to 'strength'. We the women should realize that we are the procreators. We even carry the word 'men' in our label = women. So, we are more than 'men'. We are truly the owner of this world. Even in the Vedas woman is given the supreme status and is called the "*jagat jannani*".

Women are the epitome of beauty and sophistication. Nature has made us caring, calm, sincere, and protective. Diligence and responsibility comes naturally to women. They are very attached their family. They make all sorts of adjustments and sacrifice for the family.

If one is asked 'what it means to be a girl or woman' everyone will give their own perspective and explain it differently. One can say that, 'woman and poetry are two sides of the same coin'. Both are difficult to comprehend. One needs a different level of intelligence to understand and to draw any inference about them.

To settle the matter we asked some girls, "How do you feel being a woman?" We got very interesting replies. A few are shared below:

- "Have never thought about what it feels to be a woman. There has never been any need or situation where had to think about it. Nature has made me like this. Being a girl comes so naturally to me that I have never felt the need to think about it."
- "I was born a girl. I was not given a choice that's why I have never thought about it."

- "Until I get my period, I forget I am a girl."
- "I feel I am unique and superior to others. I have the qualities and capability to complete every task I undertake."
- "I am very happy the way I am born. Being a girl has its own advantages. Society accepts you even when you behave in a boyish way or dress like a man. While a boy behaving in a girlish manner looks awkward and people make fun of it. Having menses every month is a blessing as nature has given the responsibility only to women to give life to a new being. It is a natural phenomenon. Woman is caring by nature. Though women are not very strong physically yet they are mentally very strong. It was important to have some difference in men and women as otherwise the world would have not been the same. The way a girl expresses her feelings is different from boys. I wish to have daughters only."
- "*Hum mein mai hunn hi kaha... where I stand.*" A female is so busy looking after her family life that she has no time and energy to think about herself. Her family is her priority.
- "It's a "*syapa*", "*bakwas*" being a woman. One has to mould according to the wishes of others. A woman can't do what one feels like doing. She is always conscious and concerned about her image in society."
- "There are lot many restrictions on woman. I would like to put the same restrictions on men. Especially after marriage the girl is burdened by responsibilities. I have been brought up like a boy till the age of 25 years. I have to behave more girly after marriage. It doesn't look good if I continue to behave like a boy. A typical girl like behaviour and mannerism is expected from me. I also wish monthly periods *ki jagah kuch aur tarikey* se reproductive cycle chalta."
- "Being a girl is a mix of both emotions. Depending on situations, sometimes you have to be soft and humble while at other times you have to be ruff-tuff."
- "It feels nice to be a woman. I get to wear beautiful dresses and jewellery. And also I enjoy talking and gossiping."
- "Girls are image conscious. Particularly concerned about what family and relatives will think of them."
- "It feels great to have a nice figure. I am tall, slim, and very particular about fitness. I do almost all the things by myself. I get stronger every passing day."

- "Women are busier and thus have no time to think. While men have all the free time and that's why they are more involved in wrong activities."
- "I feel proud and superior being a girl. Girls are like pretty, sophisticated dolls. They have been blessed with the power to give birth. God has made girls very family oriented. They are given more respect, importance and are protected. They are more virtuous. They can't see others suffering."
- "Women are great at multitasking. They are mentally very strong and less aggressive than men. They are bold and beautiful. They have far better features than males. *At least log palat kar to dekhte hai.* I take it as a compliment. It's a confidence booster."

How PCOS affects this feeling

PCOS is a condition in which the hormonal balance of the body is disrupted. Normally the females produce high amount of female hormones (progesterone and oestrogen) and very less male hormones (androgens). Women with PCOS show a greater production of male hormones. This is called hyper-androgenism. The high concentration of androgens has a great effect on the female's body. Girls gain weight. There is male pattern of hair growth. Facial hairs become more visible. Periods become irregular. Release of eggs from ovaries get disturbed (anovulation). They also have acne (more on face). Naturally, against the background of above comments shared by females these physiological changes in the body would also have an effect on their behaviour and feelings. The type and severity of the symptoms will affect the degree / intensity of feeling of PCOS patients. Generally almost all females are concerned about their menstrual cycle. Though initially at menarche they are troubled by the changes in their lives and routine associated with the onset of menses, they get used to it eventually. So much so that they feel something is wrong with them when ever their periods falter.

As against the above mentioned PCOS related issues in girls. Married PCOS women have other concerns. They fear about infertility. This is because with PCOS there is disturbance in release of eggs from ovaries. Hence pregnancy does not occur. In the prevailing atmosphere in our society we equate being a woman with having a baby. Without a child a female is considered incomplete. **Thus, PCOS endangers the very essence of being a woman**.

How it affects their relation with family and peers

The hormonal turmoil in women with PCOS causes constant concern resulting in frustration and anger. It is generally their family members on whom they vent out their anger. This leads to more tensions and misunderstanding in the family. During this phase actually the family members should support them and help them in every possible way. The women with PCOS often make fewer friends. They hardly share their feeling with them. They try and pretend to be very normal with them. Yet at times they lose their cool and have arguments with their colleagues.

Again the effect of PCOS on the person's family and social life will depend on the type, severity of the symptoms and the stage of life when the symptoms appear. Majority of women and our society give more value to appearance and facial beauty, whether we admit or not. The things which are not visible to others and can be hidden have less impact on a woman's social life. For example, if an unmarried girl has irregular menses then it might hardly prevent her from socializing. However, if the same problem is in the married girl and she is facing difficulty having a baby this might affect her family and social life. The excessive hair growth, acne and weight gain generally haunts their mind almost all the time. They do not feel happy about their body. Rather they feel bad about it. They have to struggle very hard to manage their symptoms. These kinds of constant concerns increase their stress and anger. They experience mood swings, anxiety and at times depression. They feel different from other girls. At times the feeling of inferiority sets in. They avoid going out and socializing. They feel misfit in their own bodies. Also, females of any age who have more hair or acne on face will probably have a huge impact on their life.

Impact of PCOS on emotional health

Being labelled as the one suffering from PCOS can surface a variety of feeling and emotions in an individual. Some people might experience many intense emotions while others might have a few. There are no set feelings or any specific order in which they occur.Few of the feeling that generate in majority of females on diagnosis include grief, shock, fear, disbelief, anger, sadness, anxiety, frustration, acceptance, determination, etc.

Research has also found that PCOS patient are at greater risk of having depression and anxiety in comparison to normal women. In one such study depression was reported in 34% women with PCOS in comparison to 7% of in normal women. Similarly, 45% of PCOS had anxiety, compared to 18% in normal women. The more time taken to diagnose the condition or seek treatment the chances of anxiety and depression increases.

Factor influencing the emotional reactions

The emotional reaction to the condition is influenced by many factors, e.g.:-

- Time taken for diagnosis

- Awareness and knowledge of the disease
- Type, number and intensity of symptoms experienced
- Overall health of the patient
- Current lifestyle and quality of life
- Treatment options and their outcomes
- Patient's personality and their social, economical and cultural background
- Confidence and faith in doctor
- Family support and empathy (understanding of what you are going through)

Effect of the emotions on PCOS women

The symptoms of PCOS can cause worry about body image. This can make them feel embarrassed, frustrated and stressed out. All these things can impact their quality of life in many ways:

(i) Physical – worrying constantly disrupts sleep pattern, eating and activity.

(ii) Psychological – reducing the zeal and motivation to perform daily activities, lower self-esteem, increased feeling of worthlessness and hopelessness. The negative emotions if overlooked and left untreated for long can result in depression and anxiety.

(iii) Social – stress and anger generally result in arguments. This can affect relationships. Affected females may avoid meeting relatives and friends.

Ways to maintain emotional health

There are simple ways in which anxiousness and stress can be reduced. These can help patients to improve their quality of life.

- Gaining more knowledge and understanding of PCOS and its complications
- Seeking medical help as soon as possible to treat and manage symptoms
- Learning how stress affects physical and emotional health
- Enhancing knowledge about the techniques to control emotions
- Finding the sense of purposc of life. Understanding that each of us have a unique coping style
- Making healthy changes to improve the way of living.
- Getting help and support from family and friends.

Management of PCOS cases

How can it be tackled?

There is no cure for PCOS. But its symptoms can be treated. Thus, the main goal of PCOS treatment involves management of the symptom and preventing complications. The treatment for managing PCOS varies. It depends on from the kind of symptoms a patient has, whether or not patient want to become pregnant, and also on the age. Treatment includes both pharmacological and non-pharmacological strategies.

Irregular periods

(a) Weight Loss

- Even 5-10% of weight loss has been reported to restore regular period cycle. This is achieved as loss of weight lowers male hormones, and also reduces insulin and LH levels. There by correcting the hormonal imbalance. Compared to other treatment options weight loss through natural means has no side effect.

(b) Oral Contraceptive Pill (OCPs)

- These contain both estrogen and progestin (female hormones) to correct hormonal balance.
- These are given if the patient does not intend to conceive or even if the woman is not sexually active.
- For adolescents a low dose of OCPs is used for short period (up to 7 days)
- Regular periods with OCP do not mean that the PCOS is cured. The periods will again become irregular when the OCP is stopped. These pills restore periods by reducing the male hormone (testosterone).

Advantages – these medicines also reduces hair growth and acne. By inducing monthly periods it also protects women from the risk of endometriosis and cancer.

Side effects – Some women develop nausea, breast tenderness, bloating, mood change, irregular bleeding after beginning the pill. But these symptoms usually resolve after two or three months.

The pill is safe and effective, however it slightly increases the risk of blood clots in the legs or lungs in women who smoke, have high blood pressure, are obese or old. Oral contraceptive pills with higher oestrogen (Diane/Brenda/Juliet) may increase insulin resistance.

(c) Cyclic Progestin

- A hormone called progestin (Provera) is generally given for 10 to 14 days every one to three months. It induces periods in almost all women with PCOS. It reduces the risk of uterine cancer. But it does not prevent pregnancy. It reduces LH and oestrogen, improves SHBG, and suppresses free testosterone level.

(d) Metformin

(i) It restores menstrual cyclicity in 68-95% of patients treated for as short of a time as four to six months.

(ii) It improves the effectiveness of insulin hormone. It may be recommended for women who cannot / do not want to take birth control pills. In this case metformin is given along with progestin.

(iii) It is also given in cases of high levels of insulin/insulin resistance / diabetes.

(iv) In adolescents if glucose intolerance is not established by OGTT, metformin should not be given.

Side effects –Some women experience temporary gastrointestinal side effects (nausea, abdominal bloating, vomiting and loss of appetite). It should not be given to elderly women or those with liver or kidney failure.

Hirsuitism (hair growth) and acne

(a) Weight loss

- It lowers the male hormones, reduces obesity and insulin resistance and thus reduces hair growth and acne

(b) OCPs

- In adult women who do not intend to conceive, a low-dose OCPs can be given. OCPs decrease the body's production of male hormones. If after six months of this treatment no improvement is seen, anti-androgen drugs should be added.
- These should be stopped 6 months before planned pregnancy.

(c) Anti-androgens

- Cyproterone acetate, drospirenone, desogestrel, Spironolactone, Ketoconazole, Flutamide, Finasteride are some of the antiandrogens. These can also help clear up skin and prevent hair fall.

(d) Other options include:

- Vaniqa (van-ik-uh) cream to reduce facial hair

- Tweezing and waxing
- Laser hair removal or electrolysis to remove hair by dermatologist

Acne

- Oral contraceptives and anti-androgens can also reduce acne. Other prescription skin treatments (e.g., medicated lotions) or oral antibiotics may be recommended in some cases.

Anovulation/Infertility

If a woman does not ovulate or is unable to conceive because of it then ovulation induction is done. This includes:-

(a) Weight loss

- Women who are unable to become pregnant are advised to lose weight. Even a 5-10% of weight loss may help the woman to get normal ovulation. It also improves results of other infertility treatments.

(b) Clomifene citrate

- Clomifene citrate (clomid or Serophene) is the medication which is most commonly used to treat anovulation. This stimulates the ovaries to release one or more eggs.

(c) Metformin taken with clomiphene

- Metformin may be added if clomiphene alone fails. The combination may help women with PCOS ovulate on lower doses of medication.

(d) Gonadotropins

- These are given as injection and are more expensive increase the risk of multiple births.
- Human chorionic gonadotropin (hCG) is a hormone similar in structure to luteinizing hormone (LH). LH is secreted just before ovulation occurs, whereas hCG is released during pregnancy. hCG along with clomifene citrate is more effective in ovulation. This medicine is only to be administered at certain points in the cycle (around the time of ovulation).
- Human menopausal gonadotropin (hMG) is a very powerful treatment in causing ovulation. It consists of a combination of LH and FSH.
- Follicle-stimulating hormone (FSH) injections have now used as a replacement for hMG.

(e) Laparoscopic Ovarian Drilling

This is done when a woman does not respond to fertility medicines. The doctor makes a very small cut above or below the navel (belly button) and inserts a small tool that acts like a telescope into the abdomen (stomach). This is called laparoscopy. The doctor then punctures the ovary with a small needle carrying an electric current to destroy small cysts in ovary. This surgery can lower male hormone levels and help with ovulation. But, the effects may only last a few months.

(f) Assisted Reproductive Technology

IVF offers the best chance of becoming pregnant but it is very costly.

Lifestyle modification an integral part of PCOS treatment

A major societal transformation has taken place in the recent years. With these changes the old gender stereotype has also changed. Women are no longer confined to the home jobs. Their duty is not just limited to taking care of family but also to maintain a professional career. They are more educated and empowered. Contributing to all the fields of society, they are working and performing even better than men in every possible task. This increased work burden on women has not just raised stress levels but has also affected their family life.

Role of Insulin Resistance

Insulin resistance may lead to overweight and slow weight loss.

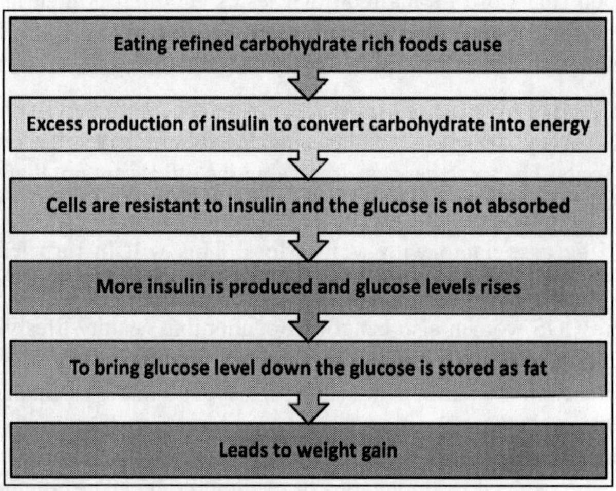

Fig.12 - Role of IR in PCOS/PCOD

Lifestyle modification is the key treatment to improve quality of life of PCOS cases. Diet modification, increased physical activity, stress management can do wonders. This can help in control of weight and hormones. Many studies have proved the efficacy of a high protein and complex carbohydrate diets along with aerobic exercises in improving this condition. Weight loss even of 5% has shown improvement in ovulatory function, reduced testosterone and insulin levels [14]. Stress reduction through yoga and meditation can help maintain emotional health.

What is lifestyle and why it is important?

The term lifestyle covers different dimensions including nutrition, exercise, self-care, cigarette smoking, alcohol / substance use, social support, and stress control. Lifestyle modification is highly recommended by all doctors across the world as a treatment for PCOS/PCOD. Increased physical exercises in combination with healthy, balanced diet consisting of regular, calorie-restricted meals are advised. As excess body weight worsens the underlying hormonal disturbances and the clinical symptoms in women with PCOS. Weight loss is always proposed in such cases.

A high protein and low carbohydrate diet is recommended. This may aid in increased weight loss due to the increased satiating power of protein compared with carbohydrate or fat and may reduce insulin resistance through maintenance of lean body mass with weight loss.

Here proper nutrition doesn't mean starving yourself or dieting rigorously. All you have to do is eat in moderation and eat healthy balance diet, rich in whole grains, raw vegetables and fruits. Avoid processed, refined foods or "junk" food (the word means food that tastes good but is high in calories having little nutritional value). Don't treat your tummy as a bin. You will never add bad things to your plants but you keep adding the wastes to your system.

If you keep pouring waste and chemicals to plants they will soon dry and not bear fruits. The same happens to you but the effects are not that visible.

Lifestyle intervention is anticipated to help PCOS cases. A reduction in BMI will be associated with weight loss. This will in turn lead to an improvement in the reproductive and metabolic features of PCOS cases.

Lean PCOS women also benefit from adopting healthy lifestyle. Basic healthy changes in lifestyle can give good results in managing PCOS symptoms. The imbalance in the hormone levels brings about number of changes in the reproductive and other physiological systems of a woman. This 'change' needs to be tackled through adopting healthy lifestyle. Stress a common symptom in PCOS can be reduced by doing yoga or meditation. It can be combined with some light regular exercise. Involvement in religious activities may also help. Making lifestyle changes is an easy way to get rid of many problems associated with PCOS. It is very simple to practice. Maintaining a healthy lifestyle can have an enormous impact on health. Controlling weight and managing stress are additional life style factors that contribute to optimal health.

Weight loss can be very effective in lessening many of the health conditions associated with PCOS, such as high blood pressure and diabetes. Sometimes weight loss alone can restore hormone levels to normal, causing many of the symptoms to disappear or become less severe.

Exercise is a great way to help combat the weight gain that often accompanies PCOS as well as a way to reduce bloating, another symptom these girls sometimes experience. It's time to be 'back to nature'. Follow what your great-great ancestors did. Follow the nature's path and more than half of your troubles will be gone. All you need to do is change your lifestyle from unhealthy to healthy. Always remember doctors or dieticians can only office advice. But it's you who have to actually follow them. No one make you healthy. You have to earn it through commitment and effort.

PHYSICAL ACTIVITY- the key to CONQUER PCOS

For restore overall wellbeing, physical activity is a must. It really works as a medicine. For this reason, we are often been advised by our elders to stay physically more active. Compared to us our forefathers, in the past, were physically very active. The majority of their day would be spent in fields ploughing, tilling land or looking after their harvest. All the work was done by hands. They would walk miles by foot. There were hardly any machines or means of transport. Even women would do every household work by hand and would also help in fields.

With time and technological advancement the way we live now has changed drastically. Majority of the work is done by machines. We have machines for almost everything. The amount of physical work done these days has radically reduced. We can compare their and our level of activity with a simple example of a household task. Let's see the amount of work done in making "chapatti", then and now. Earlier people would work in the field to grow their own crops (this involved preparing the soil, sowing, manuring, irrigating, and harvesting). Once the crops were harvested, the wheat was hand pounded to remove the outer husk. It was then washed and dried in sun. Next it was grinded on stone grinders by hand and then the *chapattis* were made from the flour on the *chulla*. They would cut their own firewood and use it as a fuel to cook *chapattis*. Today, all we have to do is to get the packaged wheat flour from the market and prepare chapattis on the gas stove with the click of a lighter (even that we get done by maids).

We are definitely leading a far more comfortable life. But this lifestyle is making us sicker. The number and rate of diseases are increasing. One way to control this situation is by increasing our level of activity.

Meaning of Physical Activity and Exercise

Physical activity means any movement by the body that utilizes energy. It includes the daily life activities, household chores, occupational work,

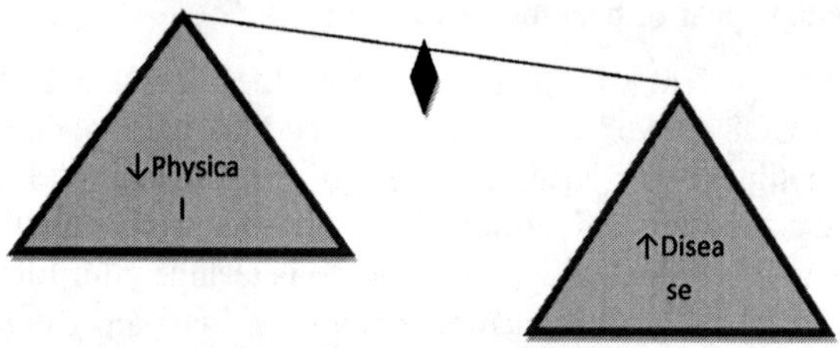

Figure 13. More occurrences of diseases with less activity.

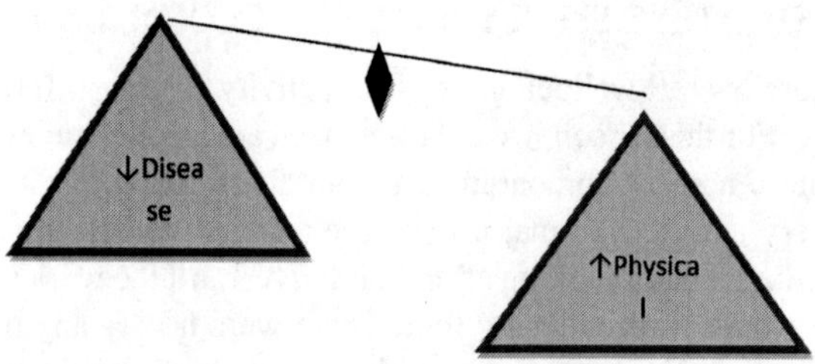

Figure 14. No or Less occurrences of diseases with more physical activity.

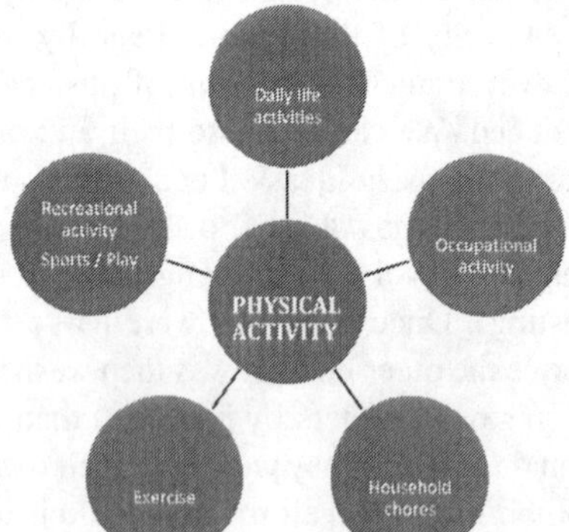
Daily life
activities
Recreational
activity
Sports / Play
Occupational
activity
PHYSICAL
ACTIVITY
Exercise
Household
chores

Figure 15. Types of Physical Activity.

recreational activities, exercises or play or sports and dance. An activity that is performed in a planned, structured and repetitive manner is termed as exercise. It is done purposely for maintaining or improving the fitness and health.

Benefit of doing exercise or being more physically active with PCOS. Physical activity helps in more than one way in PCOS women. The proven benefits include:

- Greater ease in performing everyday tasks and reducing the risk of injury. Regular physical activity and exercises increases muscle strength, flexibility, range of motion, enhance balance and posture. Better mobility and balance lowers the risk of falling. Strengthened muscles protect joints from injury.
- The women with PCOS are at a greater risk of having obesity, diabetes, heart conditions, metabolic syndrome, cancer, etc. More physical activity reduces the risks of developing these non-communicable diseases.
- Physical activity helps reduce weight. This happens due to increase in muscle mass with more activity. The more the muscles in body, greater is the metabolism, i.e. more calories are used by the body. This prevents or reduces overweight and obesity, which is common among PCOS women.
- Women with PCOS have greater chance of having insulin resistance resulting in diabetes. Regular exercise can keep blood sugar low by making body more sensitive to insulin.
- Regular exercise lowers cholesterol level and keeps blood pressure in control. (thereby preventing heart diseases).
- It has been seen that more active people have less chance of having cancers like colon and breast.
- Physical activity and exercise tones muscles and strengthen bones. It also minimizes the loss of muscle tissue associated with aging. Strengthened bones mean greater bone density and less risk of osteoporosis.
- Exercise makes the heart and lungs work harder. This improves their efficiency. One can work longer without getting any fatigue.
- Physical exercise also prevents constipation (important to maintain gut health)
- It boosts energy and enhances mood and overall sense of well being. It helps keeps thinking, learning, and judgment skills sharp. It also reduces the risk of anxiety and depression.

- It improves quality of sleep and helps sleep better.
- Slimmer, fitter and toned body improves looks and boosts self confidence.
- Regular physical activity helps maintain hormonal balance. It reduces hair growth on body / prevents darkening of skin - a common feature of PCOS.
- Weight loss (as less as 5-10%) has shown to improve overall symptoms of PCOS and reduce the chances of infertility.

Types of physical activity

Physical fitness includes four basic components, i.e. cardiovascular fitness, flexibility, muscular strength, and muscular endurance. For complete fitness it is important to include all these components by performing different types of physical activity.

Three main types of activity are:

(i) Aerobic – These activities moves large muscle groups like chest, arms and legs. They have the greatest impact on weight reduction and makes heart and lungs stronger. This is because these activities make breathing harder, use more oxygen and increase heart rate. To see whether you are performing these activities correctly try to speak. You should be able to speak few words but not able to have long chat or sing. Examples include brisk walking, cycling, swimming, skipping rope, playing tennis, etc.

(ii) Anaerobic – These are also known as strength or resistance training activities. These activities involve moving muscles against resistance. They will tone, strengthen the muscles and improve endurance. They also help body to utilize insulin more efficiently. Examples are push ups, pull ups, sit ups, lunges, lifting weights, climbing stairs, using resistance bands digging in the garden and bicep curls. Filled water bottles or cans can be used instead of dumbbells.

(iii) Flexibility – these exercises stretch and lengthen body muscles. They improve flexibility and range of motion. Examples are stretching exercises, yoga, etc.

Intensity of activity - Intensity refers to the rate at which the activity is performed and how hard the body has to work to do the activity.

The intensity of these exercises varies from light, moderate to high. clvii

(i) Light intensity activities are the common daily activities. These do not require much effort nor do they increase heart rate. Examples are shopping, cooking, standing, ironing, playing a musical instrument, slow walk, doing the laundry, house cleaning, child care, golf, recreational table tennis, etc.

(ii) Moderate intensity activities make heart, lungs, and muscles work harder than light intensity activities do. These raise the heart rate and cause sweating. One way to tell is that you'll be able to talk, but not sing. Examples of activities that require moderate effort are brisk walking, weeding and gardening, carrying a load, cycling, tennis, dancing, Weight lifting, mopping floor, volley ball, badminton, dancing, Skating, Rowing.

A moderate amount of physical activity uses around 150 calories of energy per day /1,000 calories per week. Some of these are listed below:

Table 4: Physical activity & calories

Common Chores	Sporting Activities
Mopping floor / washing floors or windows for 45–60 minutes	Walking 3km in 35 minutes
Gardening for 30–45 minutes	Aerobic dance for 30 minutes
Stair climbing for 15 minutes	Basketball 15–20 minutes
Washing a car for 45–60 minutes	Jumping rope for 15 minutes
	Running 2.5km in 15 minutes
	Playing volleyball for 45–60 minutes
	Playing football for 45 minutes
	Basketball for 30 minutes
	Swimming laps for 20 minutes
	Water aerobics for 30 minutes

(iii) High or vigorous intensity activities make heart, lungs, and muscles work hardest. A person doing vigorous-intensity activity can't say more than a few words without stopping for a breath. These activities make breathing fast, and increase heart rate. During these activities an individual can't speak more than a few words without pausing for a breath. Examples are: jogging, running, walking with a load uphill, jumping rope, swimming, cutting wood, weight lifting (heavy loads), cycling uphill, heavy digging in garden, scrubbing floor, swimming, soccer, basketball, tennis, very fast walking.

Amount of activity to be done each week

As per WHO, the recommended amount of physical activity for adults is moderate intensity physical activity for 30 minutes, five days in week.

This adds up to 150 minutes/week. Else 75 minutes of vigorous-intensity aerobic activity in a week can be done. It's not necessary to do all the activity at once. Activity can be divided and different activities can be performed. But make sure to perform the activity for at least 10 minutes, e.g., A 30 minute walk can be split into three 10-minute walks.

Apart from this an adults should also do muscle-strengthening / resistance training activities on 2 or more days per week.

For *more health benefits and weight loss*, moderate intensity activity for 300 minutes each week or vigorous activity for 150 minutes is required. After *weight loss* to prevent regain moderate- intensity exercise (60–90 minutes daily) is advised.Due to individual variation one may need to do more physical activity then this.

Barriers that may arise and techniques to overcome to stay active

"When it comes to eating right and exercising, there is no 'I'll start tomorrow.' Tomorrow is a disease."– *V.L. Allineare*

People who are completely inactive cite various reasons for their inactivity. It is vital to overcome the barriers that prevent keeping up with the exercise routine. If facing any problem then try to solve it. Every problem has a solution, just find yours! Don't find excuses and lose to your problems. Don't let these stop you. Instead "outsmart" your problems by changing your mind set and overcome the barriers.

BARRIER = "I don't have time."

SOLUTION = Physical activity does take time, but if you weigh its benefits you will realize that taking out only half an hour from your routine is not that difficult. Being Active increases fitness and decreases chances of getting sick. Sparing few minutes from daily schedule on exercise means sparing the time and money wasted on doctor's visits. It is rightly quoted by *Edward Stanley that, "Those who think they have no time for bodily exercise will sooner or later have to find time for illness"*.

If you don't have enough time to spare then chose to perform vigorous activity instead of light or moderate. High intensity workout for short time can bring same result spent on long moderate intensity exercises.

Make your new healthy habit a priority. Whenever you can, fit in physical activity. Try taking the stairs or getting off the bus a stop early, if it is safe to do so. Set aside one grocery shopping day a week; make healthy meals. Instead of having one long exercise session, you can perform several short bursts exercises (5 -10 min) which will not disrupt your day.

Include activity in your routine work. Many activities can be performed while watching T.V. for example riding an exercise bicycle, performing stretching exercises, using hand weights, etc. Walk with a co-worker at lunch or try standing or walking after every half an hour. You can incorporate the IDEA commercial catch phrase "walk when you talk" in your daily life.

BARRIER = "Healthy habits cost too much"

SOLUTION = It's not necessary to take up membership of a costly gym or purchase expensive sport equipments. Simple walking/jogging won't cost you a penny.

Start a walking group. Walk in a park/school track/ mall. *"There are really only two requirements when it comes to exercise. One is that you do it. The other is that you continue to do it."* – ***The New Glucose Revolution for Diabetes***

BARRIER = "I can't make this change alone."

SOLUTION = Take help from your family members. Ask your friend, family or co-worker to join you in your activity regime. If no one is ready to join you, then join a gym or dance class and make friends there. This way you won't feel alone.

BARRIER = "I feel self-conscious working out in front of others"

SOLUTION = Until you feel confident you can exercise at home. You can do stationary cycling, skipping, yoga exercises, dancing, etc. You can do workout in the privacy of your room using exercise DVD. You can be active with friends who make you feel less conscious

BARRIER = "I forget or do not remember to exercise"

SOLUTION = Use technology to help you remember. Place reminder on your phones. There are many fitness apps that can be downloaded in phones and can help you with this. You can even keep your exercising shoes near door, which reminds you of exercise. Ask your family members to remind you to follow your exercise plan.

Never give an excuse like -…I do lot of activity like cooking, washing, mopping the floor. I think it's enough and do not need to do any extra activity."

Table 5: Common excuses / barriers to exercise

"I don't like physical activity."	You might have old memories or notion of physical activity as lifting weights in a gym or doing sit ups or running in high school, sweating, puffing, and panting.There is good news; you can be active doing activities that appeal to you. Explore options you never thought before, and do what you enjoy. This can

(Contd...)

	include dancing, walking, gardening, or taking fun fitness classes. The more you will exercise the more you develop liking for it.
"I'm not motivated."	Think about your most important reasons for being healthy. For example, do you want to lose weight and look better? Would you like to be able to wear your favourite dresses which you are not able to due to weight gain? Would you like to stop worrying about your PCOS complications or conception problems? Think about these things when you want to quit. Try different activities and exercising at new places to prevent boredom.
"I don't have the energy to be more active"	*Don't worry about lack of energy. Start slowly and once you become a little more active, you will have more energy and daily tasks will seem easier.*

A new way of dealing with PCOS patients in OPDs MPBT Room, our experiences & success stories

When patients come to OPD for consultation they also need somebody to listen to. Quality of doctor patient interaction is very crucial in deciding the outcome. Patient satisfaction is important in any health care system. The patient-centered approach in field of medicine is grounded on the idea that the patient is his/her own best resource to solving problems. Even in the case of Polycystic ovarian syndrome (PCOS) this approach holds true, as maintain a healthy lifestyle is the most influential factor in its treatment. Patients with this condition not only need medical help but also reassurance, support, detailed counselling and, of course, a patient listener. This helps them cope better with the issues related to their health.

But research shows that most women express dissatisfaction with their treatment and the way they are counseled in hospitals. They feel there is not enough being done for them. In medical institutions were OPDs are quite crowded. Much of the time of gyne specialists is wasted in explaining routine aspect of care to the patients. Thus they have to sacrifice the care due to complicated cases. Establishment of a patient counselling room in OPD will help in saving the time of doctors. Counselor could take on the responsibility of providing an open and comfortable atmosphere to the patient which allows expressing their problems freely. This type of counseling is heavily focused on the patient's development as a person and their self-perceptions and power to change. Patients should be advised to use simple lifestyle changes in their routine so as to get rid of the symptoms. Maintaining a healthy lifestyle can have an enormous impact on health. Apart from this, at this point of time family support and husband support is also very important. Controlling weight and managing stress are additional life style factors that contribute to optimal health.

Against this background a Multipurpose Behaviour Therapy (MPBT) room has been successfully established and operated in Obstetrics and Gynaecology (OBG) OPD of PGIMER. The patients are referred to this room for counseling after the clinical check up by doctors.Here the counselor takes on the responsibility of providing an open and comfortable atmosphere to the patient which allows expressing her problems freely. This type of counseling is heavily focused on the patient's development as a person and her self-perceptions and power to change. Approach of de-medicalization is also important. Patients should be advised to use home remedies and simple lifestyle changes in their routine so as to get rid of the symptoms. Maintaining a healthy lifestyle can have an enormous impact on health. Apart from this, at this point of time family support and husband support is also very important. Controlling weight and managing stress are additional life style factors that contribute to optimal health.

The advantage of this kind of counselling is that it is not boring and is actually very interactive. Instead of just passive listening to the advice of the health care professional, it allows patients to speak and vent out their feelings. It progresses in a gradual and subtle way, unlike the traditional brusque and mechanical manner.

One such interaction, with a 24 year old girl diagnosed with PCOS, in the MPBT room is discussed in the following paragraphs. This girl had round - thick set sort of face. She was a little stout and plump. Her periods have always been late, ever since she attained menarche. Her ultrasound showed multiple small follicles in ovaries. Her blood investigations confirmed higher testosterone levels and LH: FSH ratio more than 2. She had taken laser therapy for hirsutism in the past. This time she came for lifestyle counselling. Before advising her healthy changes we asked about her past and present lifestyle habits. While taking about her activity level she said she had no time to exercise due to her studies, but as a child she was active in sports like basketball, football, etc. She emphasised that she disliked all girlish games and was tom-boyish since her early days. She shared that she is very protective about her girlfriends. She doesn't even let them carry their luggage bags. As we were explaining the role of elevated male hormone in such kind of behaviour, without any hesitation she added that she is bisexual.

As our talk moved towards food and her eating habits, a big smile came on her face. She affirmed that she loves her food. In the mean while another fat mother and daughter duo came. We called them in to join our discussion, as this girl too was a PCOS patient. The girl continued expressing her love for food and keenly shared her knowledge about all the eateries of Chandigarh. Listening to this the mother of the new patient enquired, "From where can I get the best *dosa* in the city". She didn't even take a second to reply, "there is a food joint in Sec 26 where they serve lip-smacking '*palak dosa'*." She further added, "you might be thinking how can a *dosa* with *palak* stuffing taste good, but trust me it was the yummiest I have ever eaten".

I. Case study 1 of PCOS patient

Poonam, a 21 year old woman, had been a very active child. She loved playing outdoor games. In her teens, as she took admission in medical stream she stopped doing all sort of sports. At that time she never gave importance to her diet and fitness. She was simply engrossed in her studies. At the age of 14 years her periods started (menarche). Initially she had very regular periods. It was only after the age of 19 years that her menstrual periods started to get delayed. At this time she ignored her problem thinking it to be normal. But, after few months her periods stopped altogether. From 60 kg she went on to weigh 85 kg and developed severe acne. She panicked and decided to see a gynaecologist. The doctor diagnosed her with PCOS and prescribed oral contraceptive pills. She took the treatment, but whenever she would stop taking the pills the periods would be irregular again.

She changed her doctor. The new gynaecologist advised her to lose weight. With great enthusiasm she started with a crash diet and joined a gym. As she could not keep up to the drastic change in lifestyle she soon gave up. Disheartened and frustrated she was back to her normal routine. In her next visit to her doctor she discussed how she failed on keeping up with her regime and didn't lose any weight.

The doctor then gave some pretty sound advice to her. She explained, "PCOD is a result of unhealthy lifestyle and you had been following it for long time. When you did not get this problem in a day then how can you expect it to be cured overnight? To treat your condition you have to be patient and gradually incorporate a healthy lifestyle in your routine. It will yield good results. But it takes time."

She then took to walking and yoga. She did *suryanamaskars* in morning and went for walk in evenings as it suited her routine. She stopped eating processed foods and had only home cooked food. She took 6 small meals instead of her three large meals. Her mother supported her by keeping a strict watch over her eating and ensured that she did her exercise daily. She slowly started losing weight and in 6 months she lost 8.5 Kg. Her periods are regular now and her skin is much clearer!" This case study highlights a single thing that PCOS, a malady that seems to be a by-product of modern life, can be effectively managed. Self care has a major role to play here. Good results can be obtained without using medicines.

II. Case study 2 of PCOS patient

A patient aged 19yrs, hailing from Punjab, visited the gynaecology OPD for irregular periods and excess weight. A chirpy BBA student pursuing her training in Chandigarh was 72kg. Though never being diagnosed with PCOS she had been put on OCP's many times by doctors from her town. In spite of this her problem has not been cured. She was not satisfied with her previous treatment to an extent that she called the doctor *'a dangar doctor'*. She feels she does not need to take medicine and can be cured by losing excess weight. Her mother is her inspiration.

Her mother was diagnosed with B.P. In past and was put on medication. She was obese at that time. She refused to take any medicine and was determined to cure herself though natural means. She started doing yoga everyday and also started running 5 kms a day. Soon her flab reduced and her B.P. was normal. She incorporated this schedule in her lifestyle permanently. She even started eating healthy and avoided fried foods completely. Now she looks slim, fit, active and younger. Her daughter proudly says "my mother looks like my sister". Their relatives and friends now tease the patient's father that he has got another daughter now.

Following her mother's footsteps now she also do a lot of yoga and exercise. She claims to have lost 7 kgs in past few months. But thinks her weight loss is very difficult. She says "*koi mera weight kam kar ke dikhaye to mannu usse. Mai itni exercise karti hun fir bhi patli nai Ho pa rahi hun.*"

As I examined her she had dark pigmentation behind her neck, a clinical sign of insulin resistance (IR). I explained her that it's the IR that is making her weight loss difficult with exercise difficult. I told her she should also correct her dietary habits. As per her she eats healthy. Also previously a diet chart was given to her by a dietician but she never followed it. She felt it was too difficult for her to follow.

When I started taking her dietary recall, it was clear that she was eating a lot of junk food everyday and her portion size were also large. Her previous day evening snacks included daliya, 2 tikkis, 4-5 spring rolls followed by 3 parathas and curd at night. She justified her eating and said to compensate it I walked for an hour.

I then explained her that even if she had walked for 5hours still she won't have been able to burn all those calories she had taken. She was astonished to know that.

As it was her first visit I advised her only few changes in her diet so that she gets used to it. In her next visit will review her diet again and incorporated some more changes. Looking forward to the next meeting!"

Frequently asked questions

Does PCOS mean I have cysts on my ovaries?

The term polycystic ovaries actually mean many cysts in the ovaries. But that's not the truth. The term polycystic is misleading as usually the enlarged ovaries are not cysts but atretic follicles (an ovarian follicle in an undeveloped state). They are called cysts because they look like them. Even if you do have these so called cysts (atretic follicles) you do not need to get them removed as they're not harmful.

Why do I get acne and/or extra hair on my body?

This happens because your body is making too much testosterone. All women make testosterone, but if you have PCOS, your ovaries make a little bit more. Skin cells and hair follicles are extremely sensitive to testosterone and any excess of it can cause the Acne and extra hair growth.

Why do I have dark spots or patches on my skin?

Generally girls with PCOS have higher insulin levels in their blood. This high level of insulin can at times results in dark patches of skin on the back of your neck, under your arms, and in your groin area (inside upper thighs).

Can PCOS affect my ability to have children?

Women with PCOS have a normal uterus and healthy eggs. Many women with PCOS have trouble getting pregnant, but some women may have no trouble at all. If you're concerned about your ability to get pregnant, talk to your doctor about all the available medical options to lower your insulin levels and to help ovulation every month. Many women go on to have children, with or without treatment.

What can I do about having PCOS?

The most vital treatment is to follow healthy lifestyle that includes healthy eating, daily exercise and managing stress.

There are various medical options available which can help manage your symptoms. You can discuss with your doctor in detail about them.

What will happen to me?

As the every women show different symptoms, so it's hard to tell how you will get affected by it. It all depends on the symptoms you get and whether you take treatment for it or no.

How your hormones are affected will change your symptoms like getting pregnant, putting on or losing weight, or going through the menopause.

If you don't follow a healthy lifestyle regime there is a possibility of you having diabetes or heart related conditions.

Can losing weight help in treating PCOS?

Lot of women with PCOS find just losing weight can help their symptoms. Some studies have shown that losing weight may help PCOS women to start releasing eggs (ovulating). This might help you get pregnant. Losing weight can only help if you are overweight. Do not try to lose weight if you're already at a healthy weight.

What else do I need to know?

It is important to follow a healthy lifestyle even after relief in symptoms. You should go to doctor for regular follow ups. Take your medicines regularly. You should try to keep your weight in healthy limits as you are more prone to diabetes. You should get yourself tested periodically for blood glucose and insulin resistance.

What if I worry about having PCOS?

You are not alone to have such thoughts. Almost everyone diagnosed with a health condition feels the same. You should not feel sad or frustrated because of PCOS. Look at the positive side that at least there is treatment for this condition.

It is important for you to know that you are not alone. Many girls of your age too have this condition. You must always clear your doubts and concerns with your doctor. A doctor can make you feel comfortable. Always remember to follow lifestyle regime regularly even if you fail to achieve desired results. Achieving weight loss is a little difficult with PCOS due to hormonal imbalance. As per research many PCOS women feel better after talking to counsellors or chatting with friends with similar condition.

Phase I – Follow this workout for first 3 months

Month 1 – Do each exercise 5 times and hold till the count of 5

Month 2 – Do each exercise 5 times and hold till the count of 10

Month 3 – Do each exercise 5 times and hold till the count of 15

(Contd...)

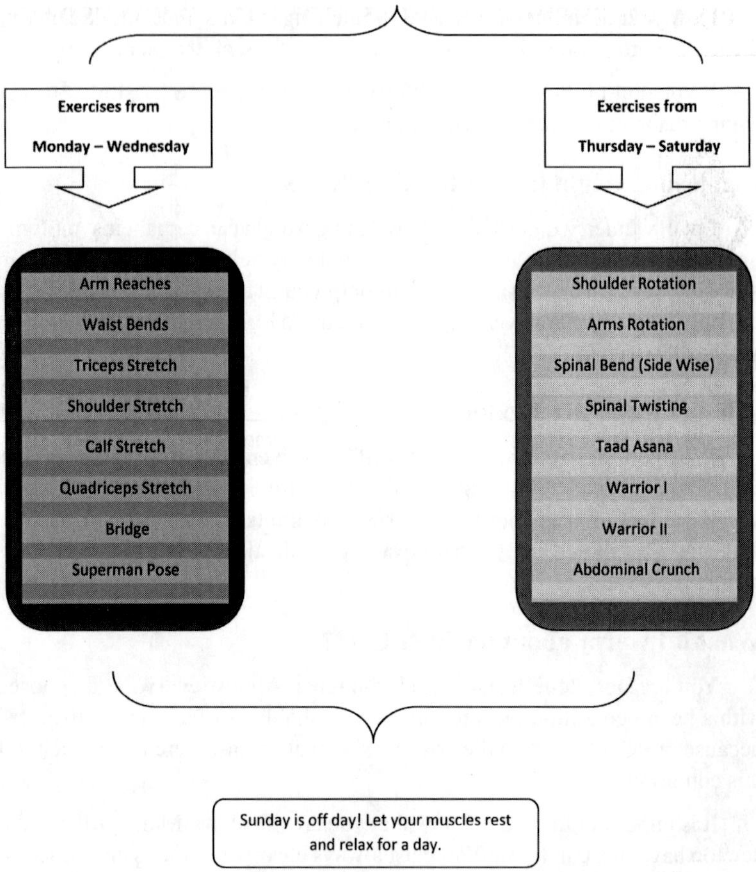

Figure 16: Plan of workout.

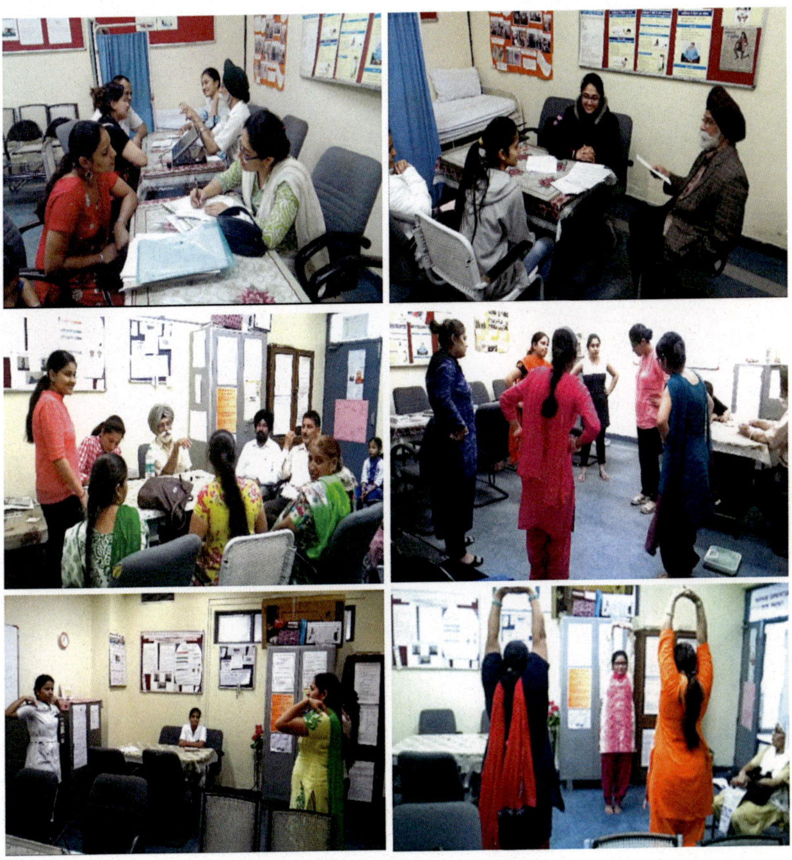

Pictures 1 – 6: MPBT room ambience.

PIX 7- 47: EXERCISES FROM MONDAY – WEDNESDAY

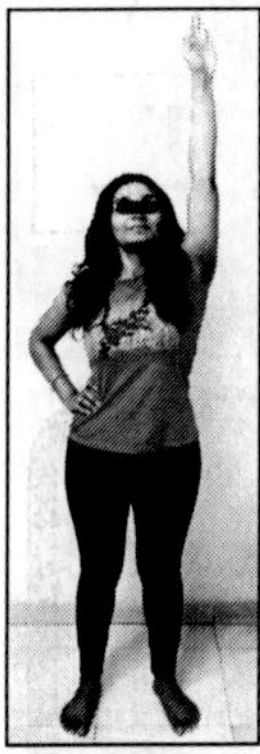

ARM REACH

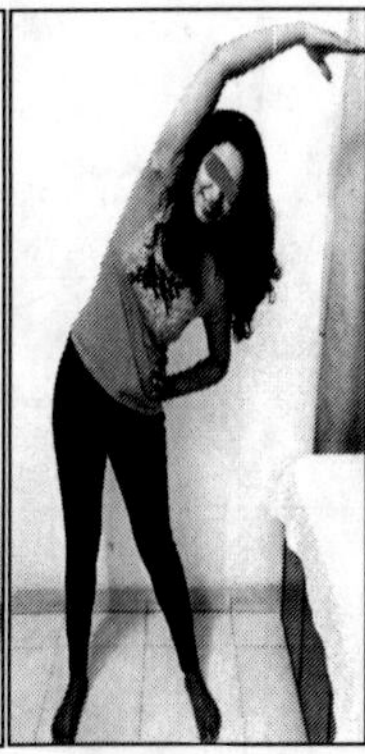

WAIST BEND

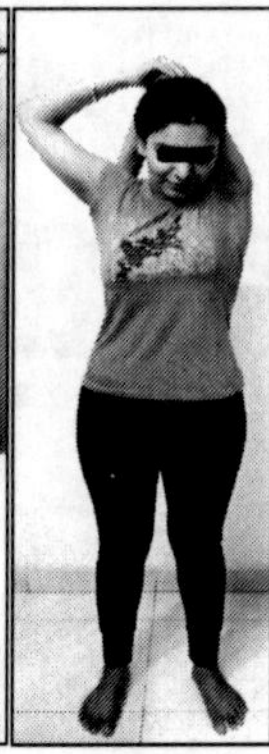

TRICEPS STRECH

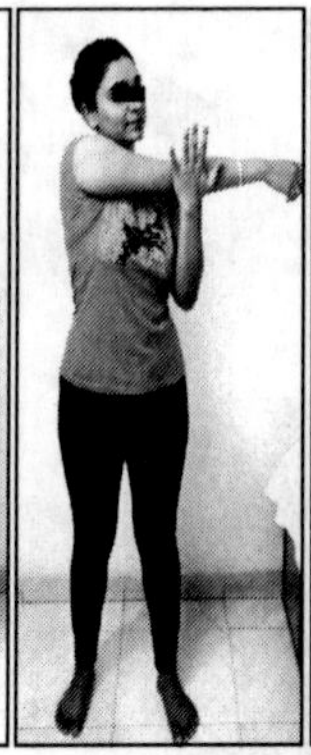

SHOULDER STRETCH

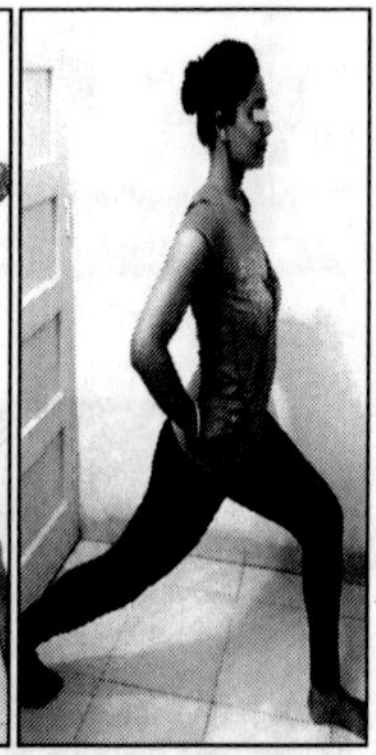

CALF STRETCH

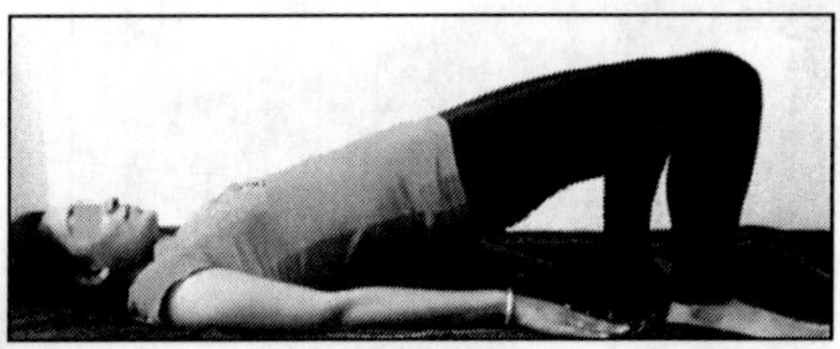

BRIDGE

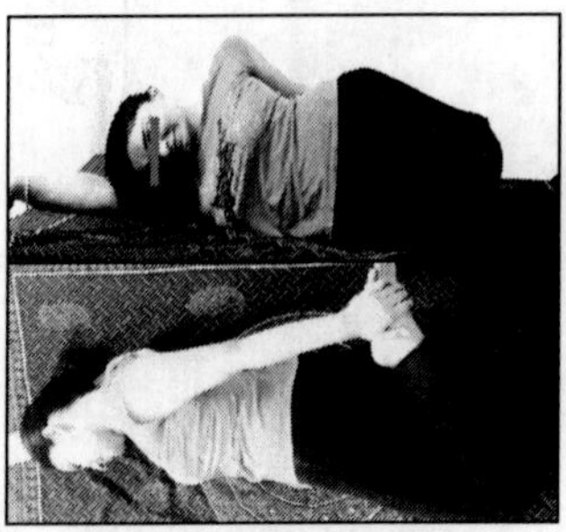

QUADRICEPS STRETCH

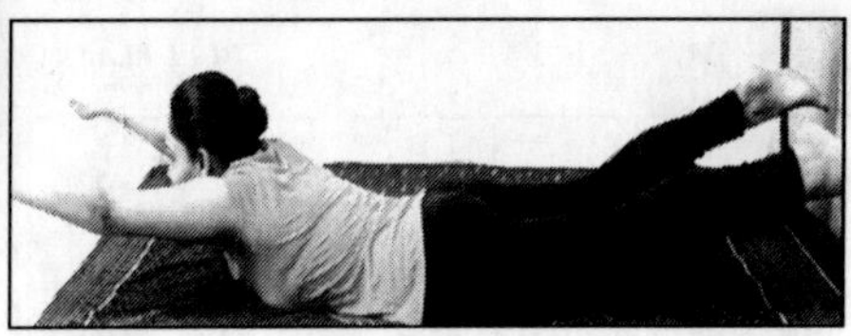

SUPERMAN POSE

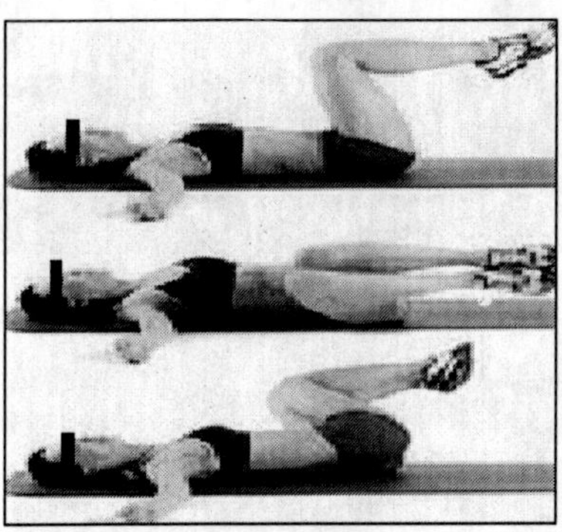

HIP CROSS OVER

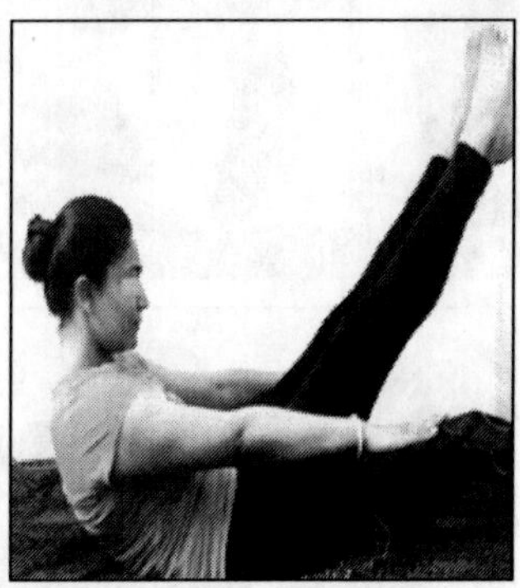

LEG RAISE

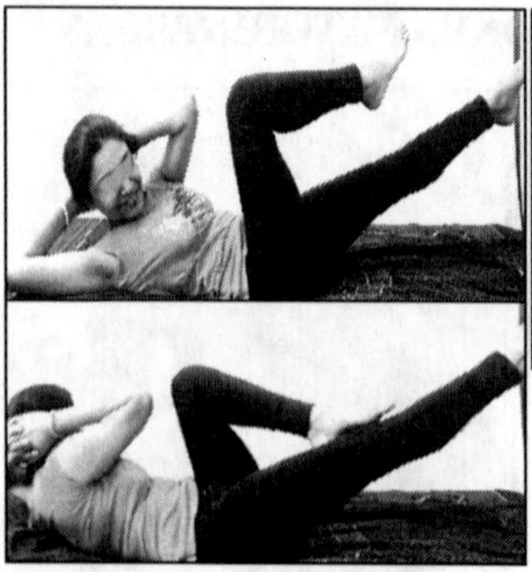

LEG CYCLING EXERCISE

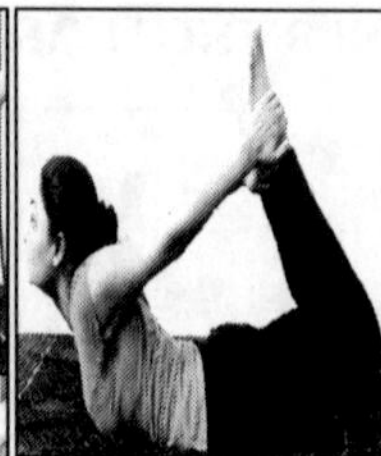

BOW POSE

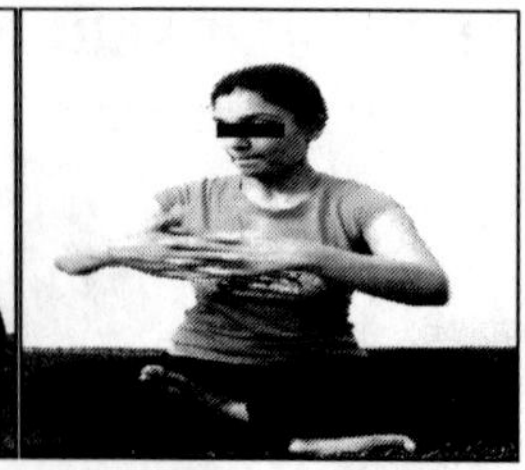

SITTING TORSO STRETCH

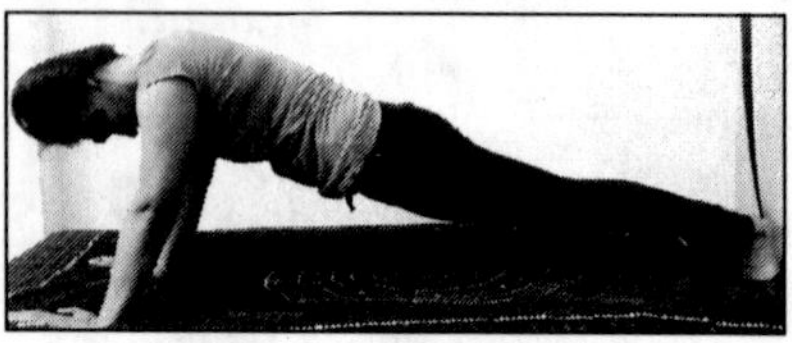

FULL PLANKS

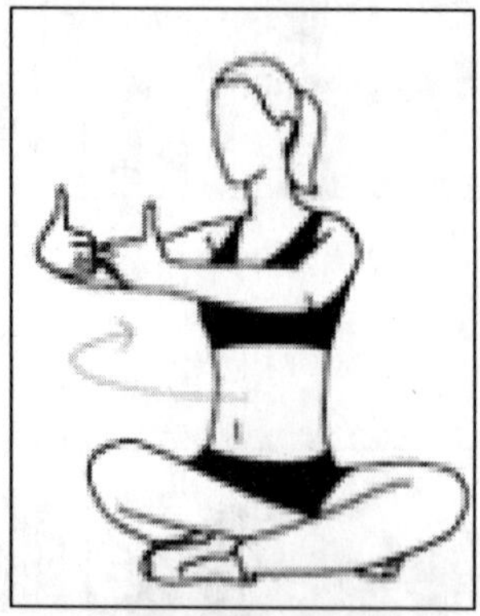

SURYANAMASKAR

FULL PLANKS

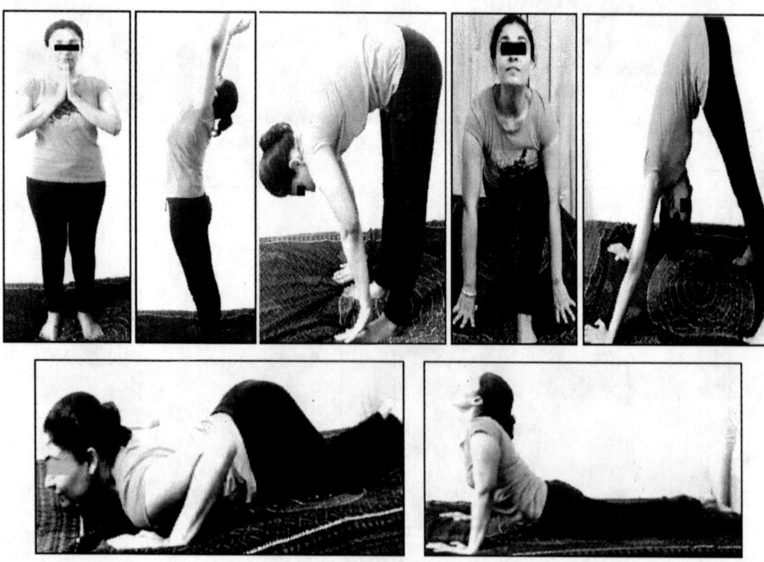

EXERCISES FROM THURSDAY – SATURDAY

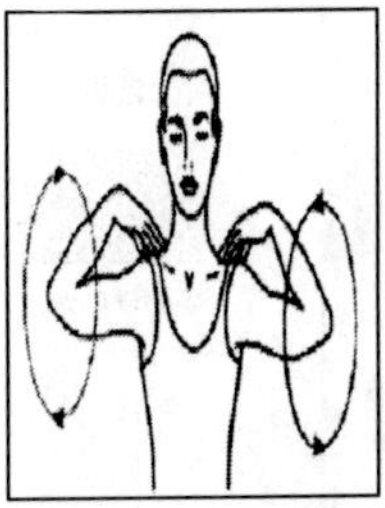

Shoulder Rotation

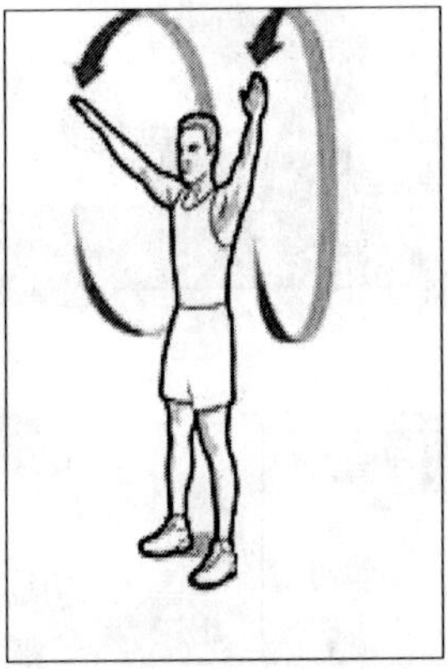

Arms Rotation

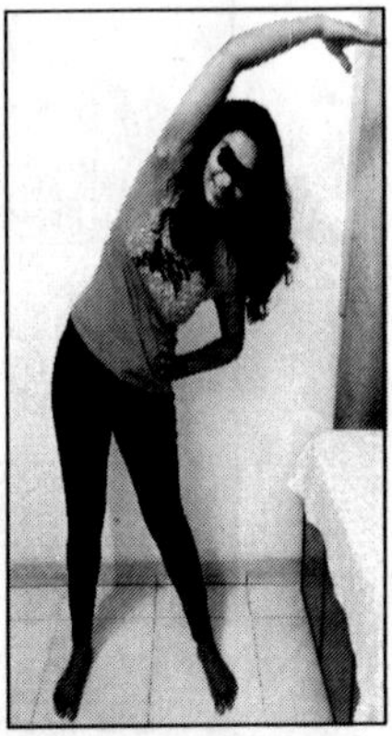

Spinal Bend (Side Wise)

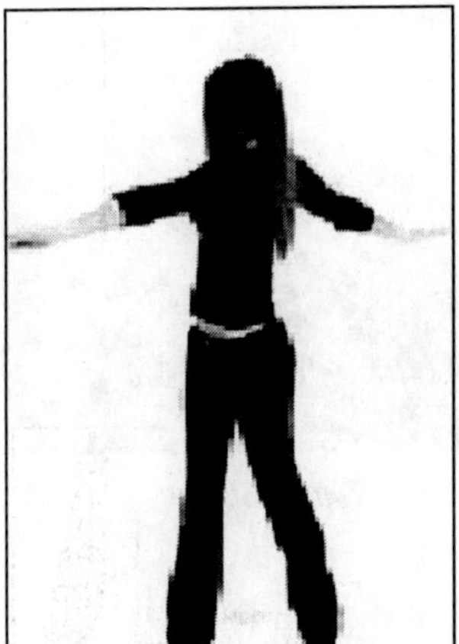

Spinal Twisting

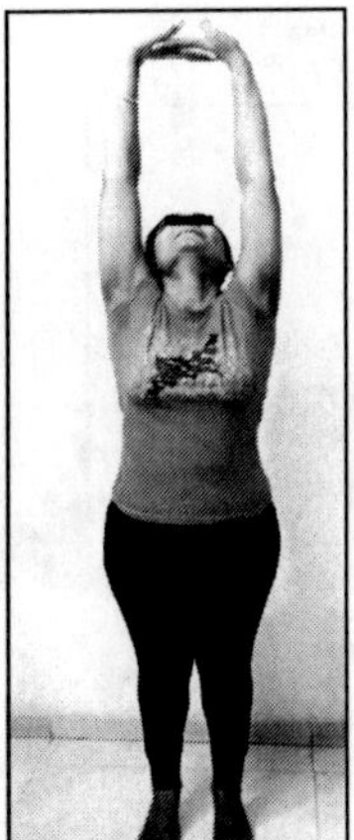

Taad Asana

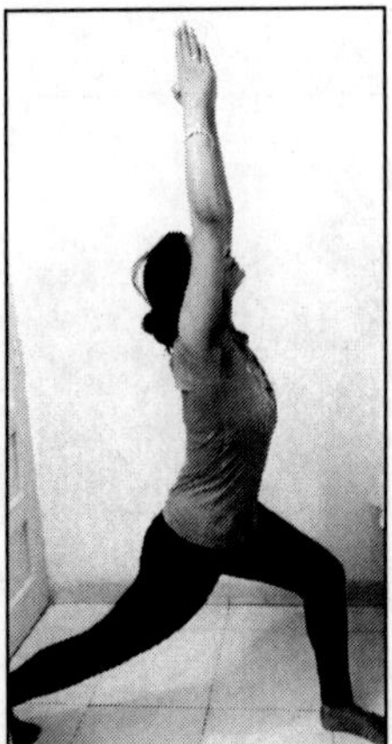

Warrior I

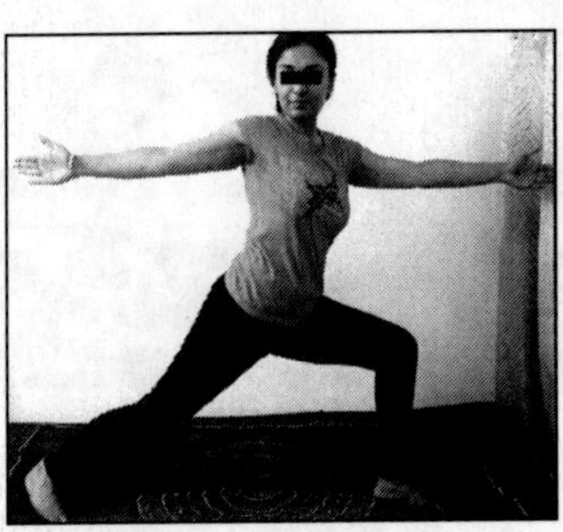

Warrior II

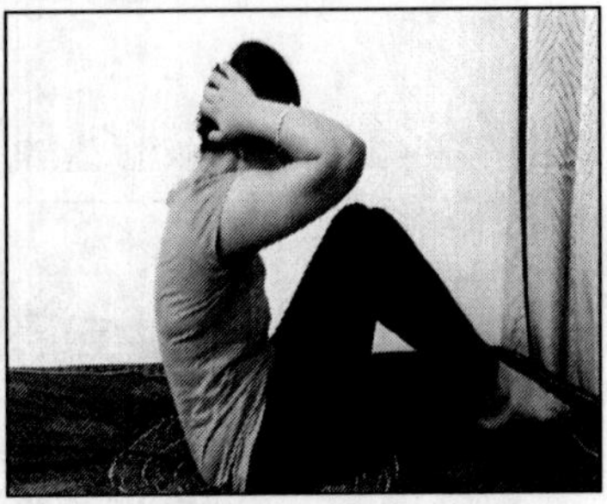

Abdominal Crunch

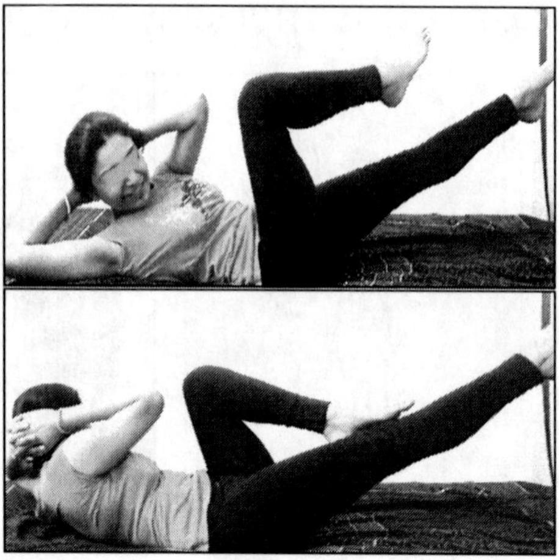

Leg Cycling

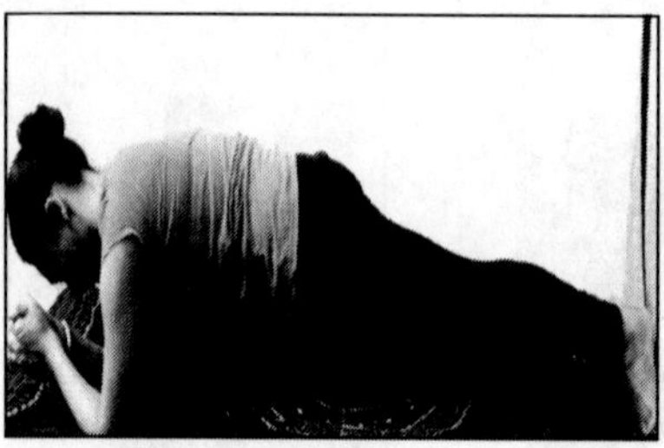

Elbow Plank

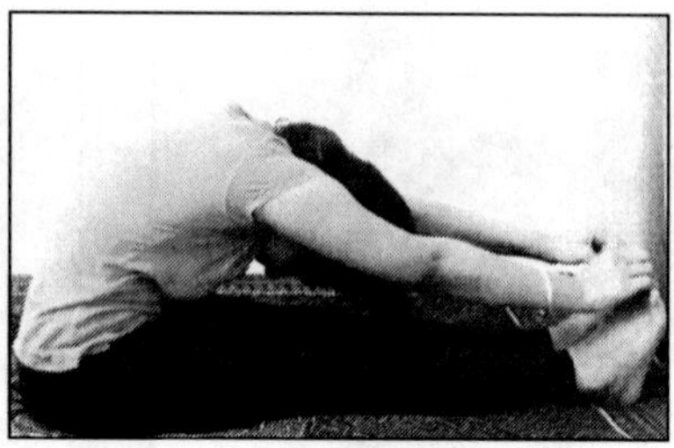

Roll Plank

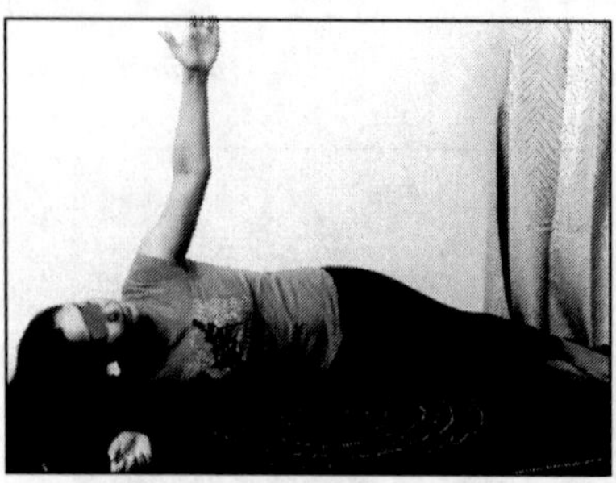

Side Plank

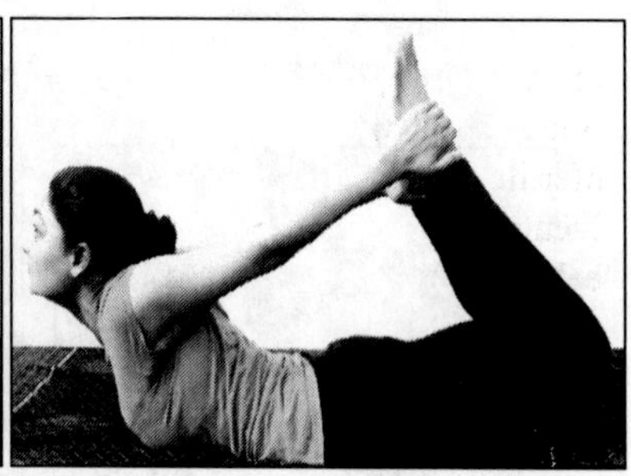

Bow Pose

Chapter - 4

Infertility Management in OPD Setting

—Davinder Kaur, Vanita Suri, Rupinder Kaur, AJ Singh, LK Dhaliwal

Introduction

Children are gift of god. Quite true! Everybody says that. After 1-2 years of marriage when couple bears a child, it is time for celebration for the family. But this may or may not happen in the real life. What about those couples who fail to bear a child? They are denied of this happiness, festivities and celebrations. Such couples try hard to conceive. Since infertility is still associated with stigma in our society, it is like a curse for women in particular. To get rid of this stigma couples are ready to go to every possible extent. They even fall prey to faith healers or quacks. Many infertile couples are misguided by advertisements. They are willing to spend any amount of money to get a child. But they may be in for disappointment. As is rightly said money can't buy everything. All efforts may go in vain.

Until proper diagnosis is made about underlying problem, correct infertility treatment may not be possible. Even if correct diagnosis is made but is not followed by proper treatment then every effort would be useless. In some infertile cases, treatment is of no use as underlying problem is not remediable. Eventually the woman may not be able to conceive. This may result in intense feeling of frustration, failure and sadness.

In our society quite often, the wife is blamed for infertility though the husband may be having azoospermia (i.e. 0 sperms). If she fails to conceive after marriage everyone taunts female for being childless due to some fault in her. She even becomes vulnerable to mental / physical violence, threats of abandonment, divorce, social exclusion and denial of access to adequate treatment. The problem may be in both husband and wife. Worldwide 1 couple out of 10 fails to conceive (10%). In about 40% cases of infertility the defect is in males, in 40% the defect is in females. In remaining 20% cases both have some defect.

It has been seen that because of stigma and discrimination associated with infertility in our society, couples do not share their problem with family or doctors. Ultimately they fall into hands of local healers and quacks. They become so much obsessed with idea of having a child that they are easily misguided by them. It is a common mistake which drains them emotionally, physically as well as financially. Couples need to be cautious about such faith healers and quacks, who boast about treating all conditions like sexual dysfunction, infertility.

Infertility is clinically defined as the failure of a couple to conceive after having regular sexual intercourse for a period of one year. Epidemiologically, this period is of two years. This is reduced to 6 months for women 35 years and older.

It is also important to know here that nearly 30% couples labelled as 'infertile' conceive spontaneously without any treatment during the course of investigations only. Thus, it emerges that 'infertility' is only a label. It is a relative description, not an absolute one. Thus, even if a woman conceives after 13 months of trying, the couple will, by definition, have been labeled as infertile. Many cases of infertility are treatable. First of all, it is important to understand that preparing one's mind and body for pregnancy is critical for a successful outcome.

Recently married couples are often seen to be anxious for pregnancy, mainly due to family pressure. Such couples are advised not to take undue stress about conception. They need to try for at least 2 years before seeking treatment. Young females should keep themselves busy, go for outings and stop thinking about pregnancy all the time. This time should be spent for understanding each other and gradually getting ready physically, mentally and emotionally to bear a child.

Two case studies

1. 'A newly married couple with wife aged 21 and husband aged 24 had been coming in infertility clinic in PGI, Chandigarh from last 2 months. They were married just 4 months ago and were anxious about wife not getting pregnant. Wife was graduate and non-working. When enquired about her daily routine it emerged that she had nothing to do at home. She was busy thinking about being infertile all the time. She cried too often. As reported by her *"sara din kya karun..tension hoti ha ki baccha nahin ho raha.. jab man*

hota hai jee bhar ke ro leti hoon.." Her husband was a businessman. He remained busy all the time. This couple was advised to have a carefree attitude and enjoy being together. They were counseled not to be too anxious for a baby. They were told that it was too early to seek treatment. Wife was advised to keep herself busy; look for a job or join her husband's business. The consultant suggested them to take a break from their routine life and go for outing and spend quality time together. Eventually, they conceived within 6 months, without any treatment.'

2. 'An interesting case presented in our infertility clinic 2 months back. It was a case of primary infertility, with wife aged 24 yr and husband 26 yr married for 2 years. After preliminary examination, the history revealed that the couple had a coital frequency of 2-3 times /week and they were avoiding coitus in the first two weeks after the last menstrual period. The lady had a regular menstrual cycle and her cycles were of 26 to 28 days, Instead of doing any invasive techniques only semen analysis and baseline sonography was done. Counseling the fertile period and how the cervix gets closed due to thickened mucus after ovulation was advised. The couple was lucky in the very first cycle and conceived without any medicine. As the couple was young, a conservative approach was adopted. Thus, many times, it is possible to help our patients by simple strategies.'

These case studies show that couples are not at all aware of concept of infertility. Rather this unnecessary stress further delays pregnancy. This case study should be interpreted rightly. In present times, there is an increasing trend among females of getting married at later age. Late marriages and delay in pregnancy tend to increase chances of infertility. Pregnancy should be planned by couple as early as possible after marriage if the female is 25 or above. Real problem is if there is 'no show' even after 2 years of marriage, provided that couple is residing together. Such cases definitely need medical intervention. We should not encourage the idea of delaying 1st pregnancy or getting early pregnancy aborted. Abortion itself or if not done under aseptic conditions can cause infections or adhesions. This may lead to secondary infertility. Hence, the1st child should not be delayed particularly if the wife's age is above 25 yrs. Rather, it should be planned immediately after marriage. In case female is 30 or above she is advised to plan pregnancy as soon as possible. After age of 30, chances of being pregnant gradually decline.

Females should be conscious about regularity of their periods from a young age. They should consult a doctor if their menstrual cycle are irregular. Couples need to understand the idea of fertile period and the need of cohabitation during these days. Occupation of husband can also be a cause for infertility. Working in excessive hot conditions; refinery etc. can exaggerate or cause infertility. Husbands' touring jobs can also create trouble in getting pregnant. There has also been a rise in cases of low or nil sperm count in men. Excessive use of laptops, mobiles, wearing tight undergarments is also blamed for low sperm count in males.

Infertility is a sensitive issue, and often individuals do not feel free to share this with friends or family. Do not feel embarrassed. Infertility is a common problem. Couple can maximize chances of pregnancy by seeking prompt evaluation and treatment. Many young women conceive without difficulty provided they live a healthy lifestyle. Relaxing, going on vacation, or finding positive ways to de-stress can improve overall well-being, but these lifestyle changes won't help if there is some underlying pathology responsible for infertility. It should be immediately treated.

Being unable to conceive a can fill a couple with sadness, grief, anger, despair, and even a sense of personal failure. While it's normal for infertile couples to experience a range of powerful emotions, most people do move through this life crisis successfully and gradually put it into better perspective. For some couples, 'moving on' means letting go their initial dreams of having a baby. Other couples decide to adopt. But in either case, couples do learn that there is life after infertility and find myriad ways to fulfill themselves - with or without children. Majority of couples do survive the infertility crisis, learning in the process new ways of relating to each other, which strengthen their relationship

Unexplained Infertility: The current rate of unexplained infertility is probably about 30% for couples with a female partner under age 35. Generally anticipated per-cycle pregnancy rates for this group are 5% for timed intercourse, 10% for superovulation with intrauterine insemination, and 15% to 25% for assisted reproduction therapies. These rates must be adjusted downward for older women and will be influenced negatively as duration of infertility increases in years to follow.

Possible problems could be that the egg is not released at the optimum time for fertilization; it may not enter the fallopian tube; sperm may not be able to reach the egg; fertilization may fail to occur; transport of the zygote may be disturbed, or implantation fails. It is increasingly recognized that egg quality is also of critical importance. In some cases, both the man and woman may be infertile or sub-fertile, and the couple's infertility arises from the combination of these factors. In other cases, the cause is suspected to be immunological or genetic; it may be that each partner is independently fertile but the couple cannot conceive together without assistance.

What is wrong then if everything is normal?

Unexplained infertility may be a misnomer. In fact, there is often something wrong at a more basic level. For example, it is possible that there is something wrong at the level of the gametes (egg & sperm), their interaction with each other, or their interaction with the female reproductive organs. Unexplained infertility therefore is not a specific diagnosis, but possibly a combination of one or many inefficiencies in the processes of conception.

Information about the chances of conceiving spontaneously may be of great help to the couple. For couples who have been trying for less than a year, the success rate is between 80% and 90%. Couples need to be aware that some time is required to achieve pregnancy. They should not aim for instant success.

Female age and fertility

Often women, over the age of 35, approach the doctor because they are keen to conceive. There is a significant reduction in fertility with advancing female age. In addition to this the likelihood of the other problems including risk of miscarriage increases. There is also a need for genetic counseling as risks of certain abnormalities like Down syndrome increase with age. Today due to social circumstances a number of women aged 40 and above are keen to attempt conception either with partners or using donor sperm. At this age women also face the problem of the oopause.

OOPAUSE: even though we cannot predict the age at which the menopause will occur the average age is 52 years. However, fertility specialists are aware of a 10 years' time period preceding the menopause irrespective of when the menopause occurs that is associated with a significant reduction in fertility and this is called the OOPAUSE. During this time the female patients will initially have regular menstrual cycles, feel well, be able to collect oocytes during an IVF cycle, generate healthy looking embryos, some of which will implant and lead to miscarriages but seldom a live child. This is one of the most frustrating times in woman's life as everything seems normal and yet she cannot conceive.

In addition, the older the woman, the greater is the likelihood of the others problems occurring, including increased risk of miscarriage. There is also a need for genetic counseling as risk of certain abnormalities, e.g., Down syndrome, increases with age. Yet age alone should not be considered a barrier to infertility.

Mechanism of normal conception

Normal conception occurs when a sperm fertilizes the egg (ovum) in a woman's fallopian tube. This process is highly complex and to a large extent, still not completely understood. However, in simple terms, this process requires the production, maturation and release of both male and female gametes (sperm and egg respectively) and their subsequent transport and joining together.

An embryo (the earliest stage of the child) is formed once the ovum has been fertilized and starts to divide. It then migrates back along the tube into the uterus where following repeated cell division it reaches the blastocyst stage. The blastocyst must then escape from its protective covering the zona pellucida. It is called hatching. Thereafter, the embryo burrows into the already hormonally prepared uterine lining, a process called implantation. It is mainly under the embryo control. Endometrium may act as a filter preventing abnormal embryos from implanting. Failure of this mechanism may lead to recurrent miscarriage.

It is vital to understand that in normal healthy fertile couples, not all sperms are fertile and neither are all eggs. After fertilization embryo forms. But once again, not all embryos will survive and travel to the uterus, nor implant, nor will lead to a live baby! Therefore an egg or sperm or embryo represents a chance at reproduction but not a certainty. This selection process is probably part of nature's way of ensuring that only the best reproductive outcome is assured.

It is interesting to note that all these events and changes will have occurred before the women misses her first periods. For a couple to have a better chance of conceiving, the following basic requirements must be fulfilled:

1. NORMAL SPERM

Sperm consists of two parts, the actual cells (spermatozoa) and fluid (seminal plasma). The sperm cells and some fluid are produced in the male's testicles and then pass along the collecting system to be stored in the seminal vesicles. Sperm production only begins at puberty and is under hormonal control. The collecting system, vesicles and prostrate add additional fluid.

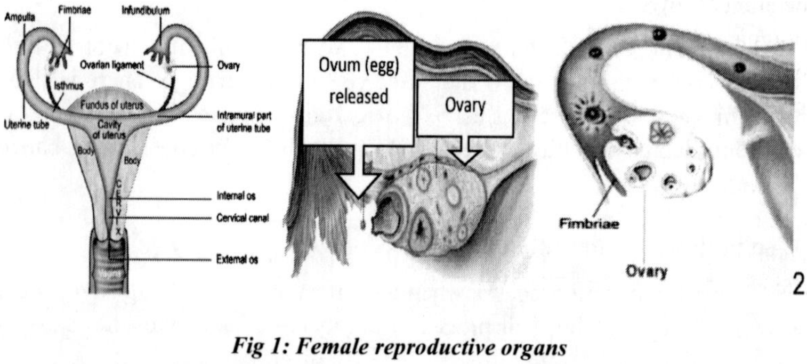

Fig 1: Female reproductive organs

Once the male has as erection and ejaculates, contraction of the seminal vesicles allows sperms to leave the body via the penis. Men are capable of producing sperm right through to old age. Advancing male age appears to affect sperm quality.

NORMAL EGG (OVUM)

Eggs are housed in the ovaries which lie close to the fallopian tubes. Females have a fixed supply of eggs which lasts until they reach early forties. These are used up and cannot be replaced. A normal woman ovulates ~ 400 times in her lifetime. A natural loss of eggs begin in the female while she is still developing in her mother's uterus. She loses more eggs before the onset of puberty than will occur throughout her reproductive life. After puberty, ovulation begins normally under the control of hormones. With time eggs also age. This leads to major reduction in the fertility of older women. Also there is increase in the age related abnormalities of the offspring, and an increased risk of miscarriage. So, one should not delay the first pregnancy.

3. NORMAL PATHWAY

Ovaries: These are a pair of small glands about the size and shape of almonds, located on the left and right sides of the pelvic body cavity lateral to the superior portion of the uterus. Ovaries produce female sex hormones such as estrogens and progesterone as well as eggs. Each month during ovulation, a mature ovum is released. It travels from the ovary to the fallopian tube, where it may be fertilized before reaching the uterus.

Fallopian Tubes: Two muscular tubes extend from the left and right superior corners of the uterus to the edge of the ovaries. These carry the ovum to the uterus.

Uterus (womb): Uterus (*bacchedani*) is a hollow, muscular, pear-shaped organ located posterior and superior to the urinary bladder. It is connected to the two fallopian tubes on its superior end and to the vagina (via the cervix) on its inferior end. It surrounds and supports the developing foetus during pregnancy. The inner lining of the uterus provides support to the embryo. The muscles of the uterus contract during childbirth to push the foetus through the birth canal.

Vagina: The vagina connects the cervix of the uterus to the exterior of the body. It functions as the receptacle for the penis during sexual intercourse and carries sperm to the uterus and fallopian tubes. It also serves as the birth canal by stretching to allow delivery of the foetus during childbirth. During menstruation, the menstrual flow exits the body via the vagina.

Vulva: The vulva is the collective name for the external female genitalia located in the pubic region of the body. It surrounds the external ends of the urethral opening and the vagina. It includes the mons pubis, labia majora, labia minora, and clitoris.

Physiology of female Reproductive System

The Reproductive Cycle

It is the process of producing an ovum and readying the uterus to receive a fertilized ovum to begin pregnancy.

Oogenesis and Ovulation

Under the influence of follicle stimulating hormone (FSH), and luteinizing hormone (LH), the ovaries produce a mature ovum in a process known as ovulation. By about 14 days into the reproductive cycle, an oocyte reaches maturity and is released as an ovum. Although the ovaries begin to mature many oocytes each month, usually only one ovum per cycle is released.

Fertilization

Once the mature ovum is released from the ovary, the fimbriae catch the egg and direct it down the fallopian tube to the uterus. It takes about a week for the ovum to travel to the uterus. If sperm are able to reach and penetrate the ovum, the ovum becomes a fertilized zygote containing a full complement of DNA. After a two-week period of rapid cell division known as the germinal period of development, the zygote forms an embryo. It will then implant itself into the uterine wall and develop there during pregnancy.

Menstruation: While the ovum matures and travels through the fallopian tube, the endometrium grows and develops in preparation for the embryo. If the ovum is not fertilized in time or if it fails to implant into the endometrium, the arteries of the uterus constrict to cut off blood flow to the endometrium. The lack of blood flow causes cell death in the endometrium. Eventual shedding of this is known as menstruation. It begins around day 28 and continues into the first few days of the new reproductive cycle.

The 3 successive phases of the menstrual cycle are described below.

1. *The follicular phase (or the phase of follicular maturation)*

   During the follicular phase, the ovaries secrete hormones: estrogens which prepare the uterus to receive the embryo, should one be conceived.

2. *The ovulation phase*

   Ovulation occurs around 14 days before the onset of menstrual bleeding. Thus, a woman with a 28-day cycle will ovulate around the 14th day of her cycle. However, if she has a longer cycle, ovulation will occur later. During ovulation, the oocyte is extruded from the follicle, whose wall breaks, and is aspirated into the Fallopian tube. The oocyte now starts its migration towards the uterus.

3. *The luteal phase (or preparation of the uterus for the potential implantation of an embryo):* During this phase, the wall of the uterus (called the endometrium) is prepared for implantation of the embryo resulting from the fertilization of the oocyte by a spermatozoon.

   A woman can also tell the time of ovulation by taking her basal body temperature daily. This is taken with a very sensitive thermometer first thing in the morning before the woman gets out of bed. The temperature is then tracked to show changes. In the uterine cycle, a normal temperature will be around 97 – 98. The day of ovulation the temperature spikes down, usually into the 96– 97range and then the next morning it will spike up to normal of around 98.6 and stay in that range until menstruation begins.

Table 1: Assessment of female factor infertility

Factors	*Causes*
Problems with ovulation	• Ovulation is the result of a well synchronized interplay between central nervous system and various hormones, along with the reproductive organs ? Central causes - Disruption of hypothalamic-pituitary-ovarian axis, obesity etc ? Peripheral causes - Systemic diseases, endometriosis, neoplasms, etc. ? Combined causes - polycystic ovaries, disorders of thyroid, adrenal glands etc.
Tubal problem	• Tubal occlusion or dysfunction due to mucosal damage or adhesions ? RTI / STI leading to salpingitis ? Other causes - Genital tuberculosis, post partum / post abortal infections, acute appendicitis, unsafe obstetrical practices
Anatomical & immunological problem	• Congenital anomalies, uterine malformations like incompetent cervix ? Polyps, fibroids etc.
Age factor	• Fertility begins to decline significantly beyond the age of 35 years

History taking: It is very important to cover all the important factors dealing with infertility during history taking, so that maximum causative factors are identified or ruled out. The following flowchart highlights these important points.

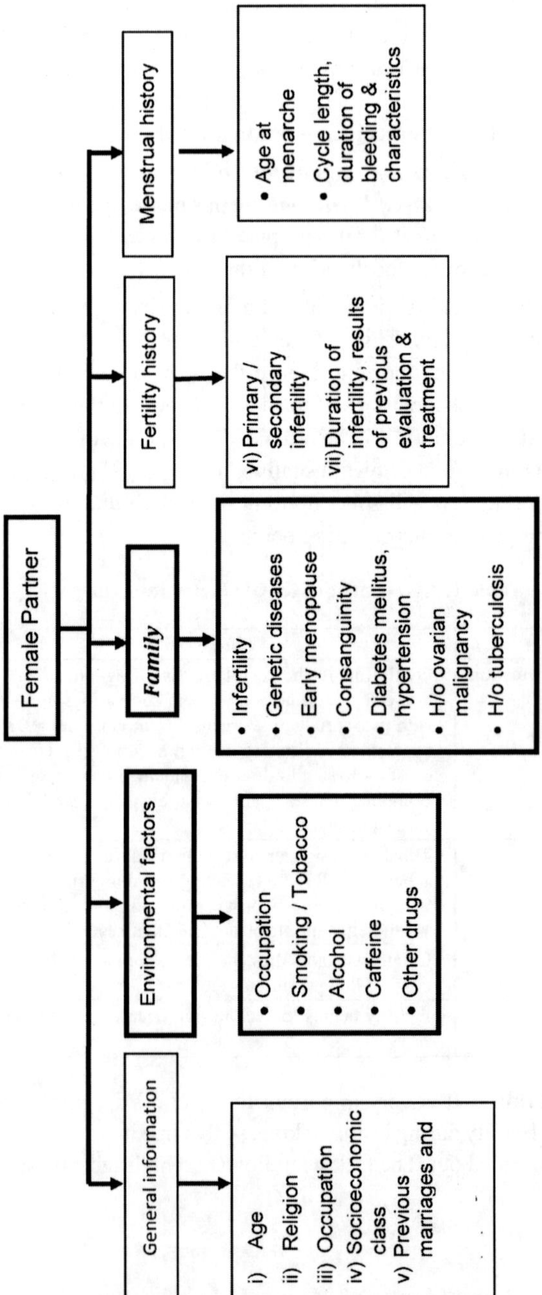

Fig 2: History taking of the female partner

History of the female partner (*Contd...*)

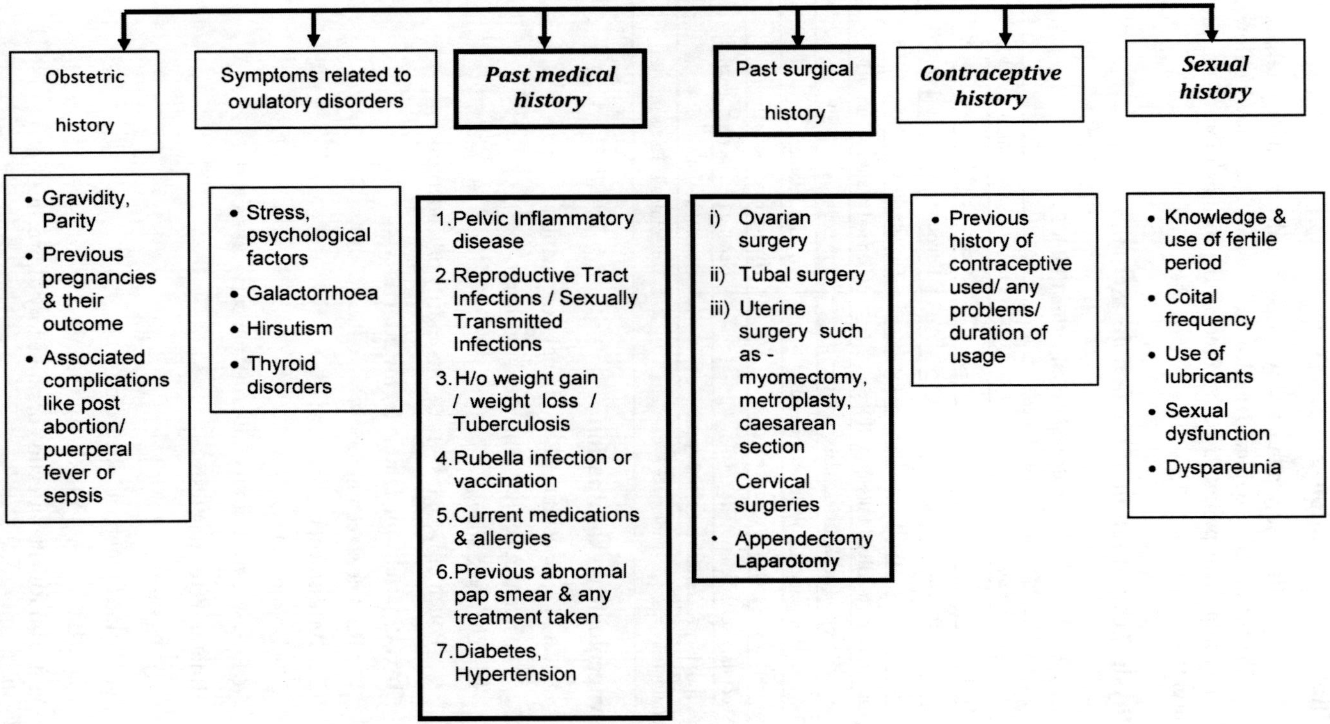

Clinical Examination

This confirms any abnormality suspected during history taking and helps the health care provider to reach at a diagnosis. The following flowchart depicts important points to be covered in the examination of the female partner.

Physical examination of the female partner

General examination (Table 2)

Factors	***Significance***
Height	Genetic e.g. Turners syndrome
Weight / Hirsutism	Endocrinological e.g. PCOS
Body Mass Index (BMI)	Obesity, PCOS
Vital parameters, Blood Pressure (BP)	General health, hypertension
Head & neck – lymph nodes, scars, sinuses	Tuberculosis
Thyroid enlargement, nodule or tenderness	Thyroid disorders
Breast development & any discharge	Hyperprolactinemia
Secondary sexual characters	Genetic / Endocrinological
Respiratory & Cardiovascular System	General health
Abdomen – mass or tenderness / scars	Tuberculosis, Past surgeries

Gynecological examination

Local / Per Speculum / Per Vaginal examination

- Vagina & cervix – abnormal discharge
- Uterus & adnexa
- Pouch of Douglas – mass, nodularity or tenderness

Investigations for female factor infertility —

1. Routine screening test
2. Assessment of ovulation
3. Hormonal tests
4. Assessment of tubal, uterine and cervical factors

Routine screening tests

(i) Pap smear

(ii) Blood group and Rh typing

(iii) HIV, HbsAg, VDRL, Anti HCV

(iv) H/o Rubella infection or no history of vaccination

(v) Screening for STI for all women (Clinical / PS examination and treatment as per National Guidelines on RTI / STI management)

(vi) X ray chest

(vii) Screening for diabetes – Random blood sugar

Assessment of ovulation

The period around ovulation is also known as the fertile period. During this time there are physiological changes taking place in female. These include a slight increase in their basal body temperature (BBT) (at least 0.4°F) due to the thermogenic properties of raised serum progesterone after ovulation. BBT charting can help in assessment of ovulation, but only after it has occurred. It involves taking the temperature (with a special thermometer) at the same time every morning, before getting up and marking this baseline temperature on a chart or graph.

The consistency of cervical mucus also changes during the cycle due to hormonal fluctuations. The woman is considered most fertile when the mucus becomes clear, slippery, and stretchy like raw egg white.Assessment of ovulation can be done more accurately by taking a detailed menstrual history, ultrasonography and hormonal tests as described below.

Menstrual history

Menstrual history is often sufficient to establish a diagnosis of anovulation

- Normally ovulating - Menses are generally regular, predictable and consistent in volume and duration & typically accompanied by a recognizable pattern of premenstrual / menstrual symptoms.
- Anovulatory – Menses are irregular, unpredictable or infrequent, menstrual flow varies in characteristics such as scanty, no flow or excessive flow. Premenstrual symptoms such as mood swings, mastalgia, food cravings, fatigue, sleep problems, headaches, or fluid retention may be absent

Ultrasonography (B): Simple non-invasive method.

Hormonal tests

Patients with the following conditions can be advised hormonal tests additionally and referred to appropriate referral centers for further management. These hormonal tests should ideally be done on day 3 or 4 of menstrual cycle and any abnormality detected by these tests should be treated accordingly.

Table 3: Hormonal tests

Indication	*Hormonal tests*
Menstrual irregularities; Ovulatory disorder Galactorrhoea	Prolactin
Menstrual irregularities	TSH / Thyroid function tests
Secondary amenorrhoea, PCOS Symptoms suggestive of premature ovarian failure	FSH, LH, Estradiol

In PCOS patients it is desirable to do fasting serum insulin, blood glucose and androgen levels.

CAUSES AND MANAGEMENT OF INFERTILITY

At best, the objective of infertility treatment is to restore normal fertility. A pregnancy cannot be guaranteed. Time is a factor of normal fertility. Thus, the reason for making timely investigations is to use this time efficiently rather than wastefully. There are numbers of specific considerations to be made when approaching the problem of infertility.

Problem related to eggs

(a) Absence of ova in ovaries or absence of ovaries themselves.
(b) Failure of maturation or release of eggs.
(c) Apparent lack of quality of eggs.
(d) Polycystic ovaries or PCOS.

Problem related to sperms

(a) Absence of sperms in testicles or absence of testicles themselves.
(b) Failure of normal maturation or release of sperms.
(c) Ejaculation of sperms into the bladder.
(d) Effects of male ageing
(e) Oxidative damage /DNA fragmentation.
(f) Obesity.

Additional causes of infertility

These include:

1. The release of an abnormal egg despite apparently normal ovulation.
2. The inability of the sperm to penetrate and fertilise the eggs.
3. Failure of the egg to divide and grow after fertilisation.
4. Failure of the embryo to hatch.

5. Failure of the embryo to implant into the wall of the uterus.
6. Recurrent loss or losses of early pregnancies/ recurrent miscarriages.

If the ovum is fertilized by a sperm cell, the fertilized embryo will implant itself into the endometrium. Following things can change a woman's ability to have a baby:

- Age
- Stress
- Poor diet
- Athletic training
- Being overweight or underweight
- Smoking
- Excess alcohol use
- Sexually transmitted infections (STIs)
- Health problems that cause hormonal changes, such as PCOS and primary ovarian insufficiency

Some health problems also increase the risk of infertility. So, women should talk to their doctors if they have:

- Irregular periods or no menstrual periods
- Very painful periods
- Endometriosis
- Pelvic inflammatory disease
- More than one miscarriage

Factors relating to female infertility are-

Ovulation Disorders- they involve the inability to release an egg or the egg not being released at the right time in the cycle to facilitate conception. Ovulation disorders can be characterized by absent ovulation (anovulation) resulting in infrequent periods (oligomenorrhoea). These may be due to:

- Hormone imbalances
- Hyperthyroidism
- Hypothyroidism
- Vitamin or Mineral deficiency
- Low body weight
- High body weight
- Chronic illness
- Luteal Phase Defect

The problem with ovulation disorders in women who are trying to conceive is that there are fewer chances to conceive. It also causes a difficult time determining when to try to conceive because of the lack of certainty when ovulation will occur.

Blocked Fallopian Tubes

If tubes are blocked then there is no way that the egg and sperm can meet. It is possible for one or both to become partially or totally blocked. This makes it nearly impossible for a woman to conceive. Several different conditions can cause the fallopian tubes to become partially or fully blocked including:

- A history of ectopic pregnancies
- Endometriosis adhesions
- Infections like TB or Pelvic Inflammatory Disease(PID)
- Inflammation
- Surgical procedures in the abdominal area
- Certain types of fibroids (rarely)

Polycystic Ovarian Syndrome (PCOS)

It is a common cause of ovulation failure. In this many follicles with eggs form in ovary. But these do not mature properly resulting in the woman's inability to ovulate. This happens because the ovaries produce an excessive amount of testosterone and androstenedione (male hormones). There may be hirsutism (excessive hair growth on face), irregular menstrual cycles, obesity and acne.

Obesity

In women, early onset of obesity favours the development of menses irregularities, ovulation problems and infertility. It can also increase risk of miscarriages. It impairs the successful outcomes of ART. This may be due to insulin excess and insulin resistance. These effects of obesity are specifically evident in PCOS.

Endometriosis

In this the endometrium (the lining of the uterus) starts to grow outside of the uterus causing adhesions. These can cause the obstruction of organs and can cause some organs to stick together. It can grow inside of the woman on the ovaries, fallopian tubes, vagina, rectum, lining of the pelvic cavity, outer surfaces of the uterus, bladder, cervix and even the vulva. On very rare occasions, it can grow outside of the abdominal cavity. Bleeding from these sites may occur during menses. The most common symptom of endometriosis is pelvic pain. Other symptoms include mild to extreme pain before, during or after the menstrual period, pain during bowel movements or urination, pain during sex, nausea and vomiting. Sometimes, there are no symptoms at all.

Congenital Anomalies

Malformation of the reproductive organs can, at times, cause difficulty with conception or carrying a pregnancy to term. Signs of this condition are recurrent miscarriages, difficulty with coitus, vaginal tampons not effective in absorbing menstrual blood, and pregnancy despite the use of copper T.

Uterine Fibroids

Rarely uterine fibroids may cause infertility. A fibroid is a tumour that grows from muscle tissue. It is the result of the uterine muscle tissue growing into a mass. They can vary in size. If a fibroid grows too large or gets in the way of the reproductive organs proper functioning, then it can create problems with conception. There is no sure cause of fibroids although oestrogen levels do appear to play a role in their formation. There may be painful and heavy periods, disrupted urination, pressure on the abdomen and constipation. They can be diagnosed through a typical pelvic examination or through an ultrasound.

Management of ovulatory disorders

Ovarian problem due to anovulation or irregular ovulation can be treated by using ovulation inducing agents. These are available as oral and injectable preparations.

- Ovulation induction involves use of medication (ovulation inducing agents) to stimulate development of one or more mature follicles in women who have infertility, irregular cycles or anovulation, to stimulate development of multiple mature follicles in order to increase pregnancy rates (even in normally ovulating women as an adjunct to intrauterine insemination/ ART)
- This has the potential to result in pregnancy if the woman has good quality eggs remaining in her ovaries, and if other causes are not present
- Oral medications are simple to take and inexpensive while injectable drugs (mostly used in ART), are more complex to administer and monitor but give far superior results

Antioestrogens - Clomiphene Citrate (CC)

- Most commonly used oral ovulation inducing agent
- It is safe, easy to administer, low cost and requires minimal monitoring

First line of treatment for WHO group II ovulation disorder (Hypothalamic pituitary dysfunction) and PCOS patients.

- Clomiphene failure - If there is no conception by 3-4 ovulatory cycles. Other causes of infertility must be ruled out
- Clomiphene resistant - If no ovulation with CC 150 mg

Note: A maximum of 150 mg/day should be used and maximum 12 cycles in the lifetime of a woman otherwise it increases the risk of ovarian cancer.

Ovulation induction in PCOS patients

1. Starting dose of Clomiphene citrate is 50 mg daily
2. Ultrasound follicle monitoring is a must in every cycle
3. In Clomiphene citrate resistant cases: Metformin 500 mg BD to 500 mg TDS, is started along with life style modification
4. After 2-3 months of metformin, CC is added
5. Still no ovulation → Lean PCOS - Ovarian drilling
   → Obese PCOS - Low dose Gonadotropins

In PCOS patients there is always the risk of hyperstimulation of ovaries and side effects. In these cases, minimal stimulation protocol is much better and safer.

- Drug related side effects including OHSS are less frequent
- Cost effective, easy administration and with fairly good results
- Can be used in CC responsive cases only
- It is also a good protocol for patients with unexplained infertility with or without intra uterine insemination (IUI)

Assessment of uterine and tubal factors

These can be detected by transvaginal ultra-sonography, saline hysterogram, hysteron-salpingography and endometrial biopsy. However laparoscopy and hysteroscopy are the gold standards for diagnosis.

Endometrial biopsy (EB) –

It is an essential investigation in symptomatic patients to rule out endometrial TB. In India TB is reported in 10 - 32% infertile couple. So, it should be excluded before doing the invasive tests.

Trans vaginal ultrasonography (TVS)

- TVS is a very good tool for pelvic organ assessment

- It is done on day 3 / 4 of menses to assess uterine and tubal pathology
- TVS with saline contrast (sono-hysterogaphy) can also be used

Saline Hysterogram (SHG) or Saline Infusion Sonogram (SIS)

During a pelvic ultrasound, saline is injected through the cervix to outline the uterine cavity, which allows the doctor to see walls of the uterus and cavity at the same time. It is an effective method for diagnosing polyps, fibroids and adhesions.

Hystero-salpingography (HSG): X-ray of uterus and fallopian tubes that involves injection of contrast (dye) through cervix

2. Accurately defines size and shape of uterine cavity and fallopian tubes.
3. Reliable, less invasive and efficient
4. Documentation and record available for future

Indications

- To evaluate the uterine cavity and its malformations
- To assess the patency of fallopian tubes.

Contraindications

- Known allergies or allergic reactions to contrast dye.
- Pregnancy or uterine bleeding at the time of procedure
- Pelvic infection, especially rule out active genital tuberculosis (GTB)

Risks

- Allergic reaction to contrast.
- Vomiting, fainting, abdominal pain / cramping
- Fever or chills, foul-smelling vaginal discharge, endometrial or tubal infection
- Perforation of uterus (rarely)

Results

Normal – Uterine cavity and cervix seen, without defects. Contrast can be seen freely leaking out of the tubes into abdominal cavity

Abnormal results – e.g. obstruction of fallopian tubes, intrauterine adhesions, congenital anomalies of uterus etc,

Laparoscopy

- It is a surgical technique by which operations in the abdomen and pelvis are performed through small incisions (usually 0.5 – 1.5 cm)
- Allows visualization of uterus, tubes, ovaries and pelvis, any abnormalities such as adhesions, endometriosis, fibroids or structural deformities
- Patency of tubes can be assessed by chromo-pertubation i.e. spillage of methylene blue dye injected through cervix from fallopian tubes
- Abnormalities can be corrected by operative laparoscopy in the same sitting

Risk: Trocar injuries to blood vessels, bowel, bladder, electrical burns.

Hysteroscopy

A small fiber optic telescope is inserted into a woman's cervix to examine uterus, cornual end of tubes and diagnose conditions such as submocosal fibroids, scarring, synechiae and polyps.Prophylactic antibiotics should be considered before uterine instrumentation.

Medical and surgical management of endometriosis

- Medical treatment (ovarian suppression) of minimal and mild endometriosis does not enhance fertility in subfertile women and should not be offered
- Minimal or mild endometriosis – Should be offered surgical ablation or resection of endometriosis plus laparoscopic adhesiolysis, only if laparoscopy is being done for diagnosis
- Moderate / severe endometriosis - Surgical treatment and pelvic clearing followed by assisted conception by ovulation induction. If unsuccessful IVF should be offered

Tubal microsurgery and laparoscopic surgery

- Mild tubal disease - Tubal surgery may be more effective than no treatment
- Where expertise is available, it may be considered as a treatment option

Tubal catheterization or cannulation

- Proximal tubal obstruction - Selective salpingography plus tubal catheterization, or hysteroscopic tubal cannulation, may be treatment options because these treatments improve the chance of pregnancy

Treatment of uterine and tubal factors

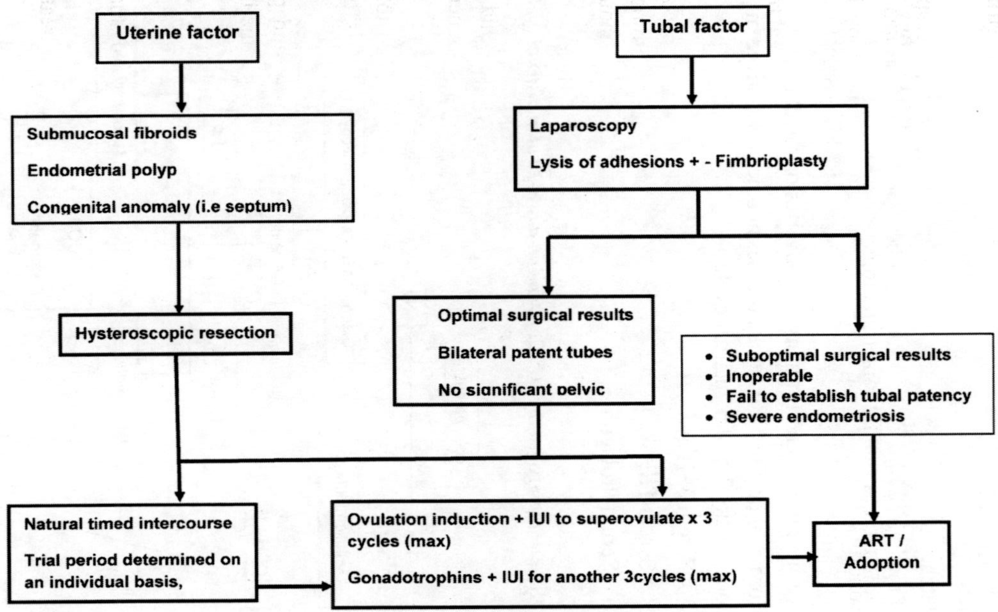

Fig 3: Diagnostic & treatment algorithm of tubal & uterine factors

Management of female partner in a summarized form

History, examination and counseling

Basic investigations and management

- If history suggestive of Tuberculosis -
    - Hb, ESR
    - Chest X-ray
    - Mantoux's test
    - Premenstrual Endometrial biopsy → Histopathology / AFB – Smear/culture
- Baseline ultrasound for uterus and ovaries on day 2 or 3
- Hormonal profile { If irregular menses or other suggestive symptoms, done on day 2-5 of menstrual cycle }
    - Serum FSH and LH
    - Serum TSH
    - Serum Prolactin

Fig 4: Hysterosalpingography (HSG) {Done on day 8-10 of menstrual cycle}

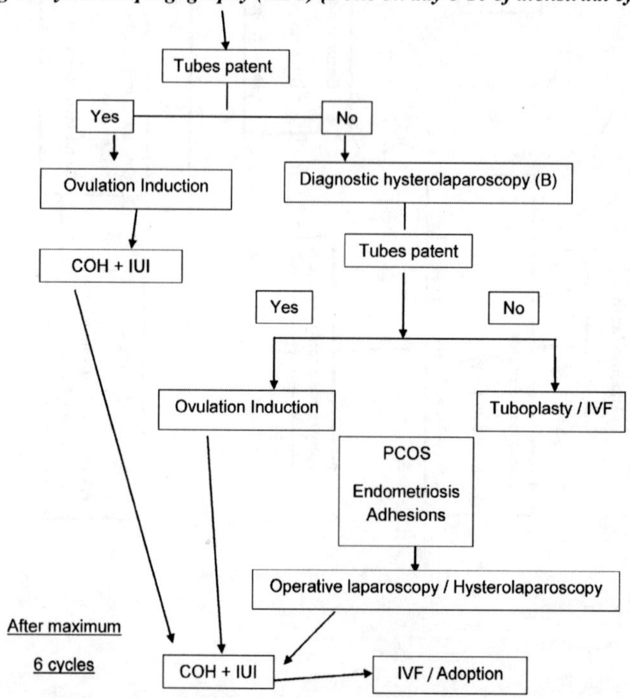

Available treatments options

- While treating couples with unexplained infertility one must reassure them to continue attempting natural conception if the female is < 35
- Medical intervention has a few disadvantages including cost, and increased possibility of a multiple pregnancy and subsequent sequelae.
- Above age 35, it may be prudent to evaluate ovarian reserve by means of an ultrasound to count early ovarian follicles (antral follicles), and measuring serum AMH, cycle day three Estradiol and FSH levels. Results of these tests may result in recommendations to proceed with treatments more aggressive than expectant management

Clomiphene Citrate (CC) and intrauterine insemination or IUI (CC/IUI)

- Empiric treatment with ovulation inducing agents is based on the rationale that increasing the number of eggs available for fertilization in a given cycle, may increase the probability of at least one or more released egg, to produce a viable pregnancy.
- CC/IUI improves pregnancy rates by doubling the couple's chance of getting pregnant per treatment cycle.

Injectable fertility drugs and IUI

- Empiric treatment with injectable drugs, gonadotropins (hMG or FSH) is more aggressive and triples pregnancy rates.
- This is a reasonable next step after three to six cycles of CC/IUI has failed to produce a pregnancy, or unacceptable side effects resulted from treatment with CC/IUI..
- sually three cycles of injectable fertility drugs with IUI is reasonable before moving on to a more aggressive treatment option

In Vitro Fertilization (IVF) is a method in which the woman harvests multiple eggs, which are then combined with the man's sperm in a petri dish. The main thing to realize from this definition is that it is dependent upon time.It gives a very high chance of success after at least 3 IVF cycles (cumulative pregnancy rates of 10 - 45 % depending on the female partner's age).

Unexplained infertility encompasses many possible abnormalities resulting in a less efficient conception process. The standard tests for infertility barely scratch the surface and are really only looking for obvious factors. These do not address the molecular issues.

Since many couples will conceive with less invasive and less costly treatments, empiric treatment with inseminations is the most appropriate plan for 3-6 months before a more aggressive treatment with IVF is recommended.

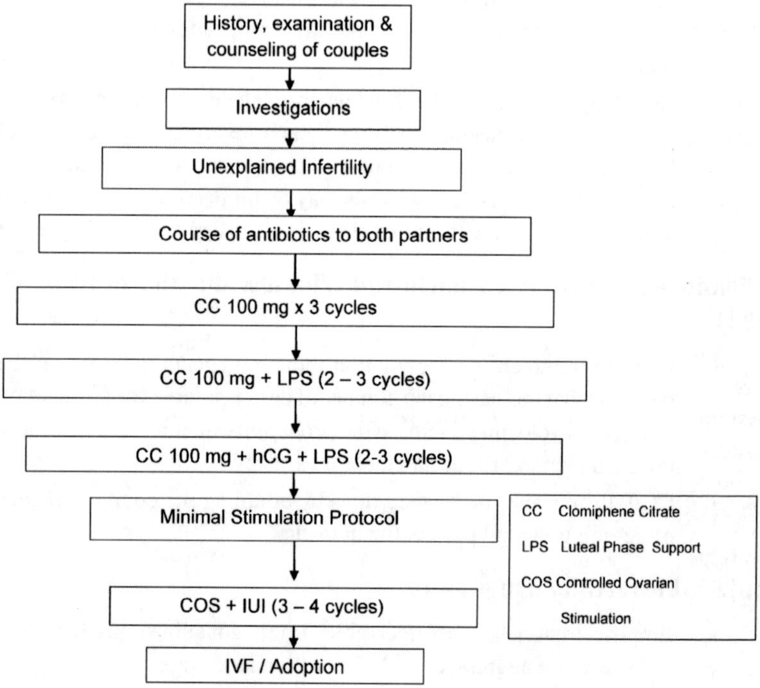

Fig 5: Algorithm for management of unexplained infertility

IVF can be a first-line approach in tubal sterility and when IUI cannot be performed because the number of motile sperms is insufficient, but is usually also the final treatment attempt when other methods have failed. ICSI is a further option, which should be limited to couples: a) with very poor semen parameters; b) previous failed fertilization; c) presence of obstructive or non-obstructive azoospermia in which ICSI is combined with sperm extraction from the epididymis or the testis.

The success rate of various infertility treatments are largely influenced by many factors. The important among these are duration of infertility, age of female partner, history of PID and severe male factor whereas anovulation and unexplained cause of infertility are more favorable. For shorter duration of infertility conception rate is > 20%. The success of IUI is also influenced by etiology of infertility and number of treatment cycles. Probability of becoming pregnant is greatest during first six cycles.

For many couples conception has moved from bedroom to the laboratories. The various treatment options in ART are as:

Controlled ovarian hyperstimulation (COH): It is the medical treatment to induce the development of multiple ovarian follicles to obtain multiple oocytes at follicular aspiration.

ICSI (Intracytoplasmic Sperm Injection): In ICSI, a single sperm is injected into the cytoplasm of the ovum to effect fertilization, before the fertilized ovum is transferred to the uterus of the woman.

Intrauterine Insemination (IUI): Intrauterine Insemination involves the introduction of specially prepared sperm into the uterus of the woman.

IVF-ET (In vitro Fertilization-Embryo Transfer): In vitro Fertilization-Embryo Transfer (IVF-ET) is the fertilization of an ovum outside the body and the transfer of the fertilized ovum to the uterus of a woman.

PESA (Percutaneous Epididymal Sperm Aspiration) and TESA/TESE (Testicular Sperm Aspiration/ Extraction): Percutaneous Epididymal Sperm Aspiration (PESA) and Testicular Sperm Aspiration (TESA) are simplified procedures to recover the sperm for fertilization in patients with obstructive azoospermia.

Beside this number of newer future advances in ART are being developed in western countries.

- Freezing eggs obtained from the woman's ovaries for future use.
- Freezing part of the ovary containing immature eggs, so that when the need arises maturing of the eggs is carried out in the laboratory.
- Improving the culture media used for growing the embryos in the IVF laboratory to reach the blastocyst stage (5 days after fertilization) where the best embryos are selected, one or two embryos transferred to the uterus, consequently chances of pregnancy and success rates are increased without the need for transferring many embryos with risks of multiple pregnancy.

The latest advances in computer technology: has enabled choosing the best sperms for doing intracytoplasmic sperm injection by a method called Keiss method where the computer chooses the best sperms for use avoiding the human error factor thereby improving the success rates.

Splitting cells for using instead of sperms: This method is still under research. It could be possible to use any cell from the man's body, such as skin cell for example, divide it in the lab and each half could be used (which contain half the chromosome number) to inject inside the egg's cytoplasm using intracytoplasmic sperm injection method, this method will solve the infertility problem for men with no sperms in their seminal fluid or testicles.

Stem cell research, Cytoplasm donation, Intra uterine culture of embryos and artificial Uterus are still confined to labarotories.

The success rate of infertility treatment has been a matter of research in many countries. A number of studies have proposed standardized investigation and treatment protocol for infertile couples. Infertility treatment plan depends on the etiology of infertility. Infertility treatment also depends on whether the problem is from the woman's side, the man's side, both sides, or remains unexplained. About 85% to 90% of couples dealing with infertility are treated with low-tech treatments, like medication or surgery, with less than 3% being treated by Assisted Reproductive Technologies, like IVF.

In the last two decades the use of assisted reproductive technologies (ART) has become an inevitable and often indispensable part of gynecological consultation as well as women's lives. On one hand, the increased knowledge and availability of a wide range of ART options has redefined 'traditional' notions of conception and procreation, on the other, the introduction of each new device or technique has served to renew a growing flux in the way reproductive choice is understood.

Moreover, the success rate of any ART procedure is below 30% under the best of circumstances. There are an estimated 250 IVF clinics in India today. At present neither guidelines nor legislation are in place in regard to the practice of ART centers in India.

Most IVF patients want to know about the clinic's pregnancy rate, though pregnancy depends on so many variables that average numbers mean little. In the absence of a central registry monitoring IVF clinics, patients must believe what the doctor tells them.

In fact, infertile couples face a lot of uncertainty about the treatment outcome. They are usually quite apprehensive about their future. They need proper counselling. So, there is a need of further studies in this field to search determinants of successful outcome of treatment in infertile couples for their guidance.

Important issues in counseling of infertile couple

Infertility is a common condition affecting approximately one in six couple (15%). In case of infertility neither partner should ever consider it as "my fault", "her fault" or "his fault". No one should be blamed. In approximately 15% couples there is more than one causative factor of infertility. Unfortunately, it may not be possible to find the cause in them. Their infertility is unexplained. Even so, treatment is available.

Infertility is a medical condition that affects all aspects of life. Every step a couple takes to have a child can add to their emotional, financial and physical strain, along with family and social pressure. Greater awareness needs to be spread and couples cautioned about faith healers and quacks, who boast about treating all conditions like sexual dysfunction, infertility; which can cause more harm to them. Effective guidance and support along with communication of information, linked with effective treatment is a key in management of infertility. Even when treatment is not available at outreach service delivery settings, prevention information, guidance and emotional support can be of tremendous help.

Goals of counseling depend on the life situation of the couples and treatment desired. One should attempt to achieve the following objectives:

- Help control emotions and arrive at a situation which they feel comfortable.
- Provide emotional support and information..
- Enable them to understand the implications of proposed treatment for themselves, their family and for children born as a result.
- Balanced information on prevention and various treatment options on infertility should be provided as it will empower the couple to make appropriate decision for undergoing treatment and if not successful then going for assisted reproductive techniques (ART) or adoption.
- Clinics can have take-away information brochures in simple languages

Basic principles during assessment of infertile couple

- Assessment should be done by a dedicated team in a comfortable setting.
- Couple centered approach to be used.
- Process should be stress-free for the couple.
- Listen carefully, respect and encourage couples to express their concerns.
- Discuss with them the evaluation and treatment plan.
- Psychological and sexual counseling to be done.

Assessment approach towards an infertile couple

- Take complete medical, reproductive and sexual history.
- Both partners should be interviewed separately, as well as jointly, to elicit important facts that one partner might not wish to reveal to the other.
- Review thoroughly past medical records.

- Clinical/physical examination of the couple for systemic disease, genetic abnormalities or androgen dysfunction.
- Discuss issues like efficacy, cost, ease of use, and side effects of therapy.
- Remain realistic about prognosis.
- Sometimes patients can become abusive or cynical. It is important to note that these reactions are normal and should be received with empathy.
- An infertile partner, particularly the female, may feel guilty of letting the other partner down, e.g., couples who have had a termination of their first pregnancy and cannot conceive a second time
- Women are particularly vulnerable, become isolated, losing contact with reality, thus suffer from chronic depression with acute episodes. They develop poor self-image and feeling of unfulfillment.
- Ignorance about sexuality, timing of sexual intercourse and the compulsion to have sexual intercourse on demand may affect both partners.
- Insemination, whether by partner or donor sperm may result in loss of esteem and fear of losing wife or partner.
- Explain that infertility treatment does not produce immediate results. Emphasize that with patience, positive attitude and appropriate treatment, most infertile couples can eventually become parents

Content of counseling in infertility

- Emphasize to the couple that infertility is a shared concern. Hence evaluating both partners is mandatory. Problem could lie with either or both.
- Discuss about normal anatomy of male and female reproductive system, fertile period (how to track number of days in her menstrual cycle, monitor appearance and texture of cervical mucus, which becomes clear, watery and copious around ovulation), physiology of conception, sexuality; lifestyle factors affecting reproduction like body weight, effect of smoking, exposure to high temperature and role of STI or RTIs in causing infertility
- Give information on how often to have intercourse and its timing. The best period is around 11-17 days of a 28 days menstrual cycle. To avoid unnecessary stress, the couple can be advised to have intercourse two or three times a week.

- Clear common misconceptions and doubts like:
  1. Do not use lubricants during intercourse, as they decrease the chances of pregnancy
     - Birth spacing methods do not cause infertility.Some hormonal oral, injectable contraceptives and implants can delay fertility by a few months but fertility will eventually return.
     - Barrier methods protect against STIs, hence against tubal infertility.
     - IUCDs are also safe and effective method of birth spacing and do not cause any pelvic infections by themselves or contribute to infertility but may accelerate ascending infection in women that are at risk of STIs leading to tubal infertility. Such women should use barrier methods and receive adequate treatment for STIs and pelvic infections.
  8. Psychosexual counseling for problems such as erectile dysfunction, premature ejaculation and vaginismus.
  9. Therapeutic counseling to help couples understand investigation and treatment schedules.
  10. Genetic counseling should be offered when there is an increased risk of passing on an inherited disease to the offspring
- Counseling on pregnancy after infertility treatment as couples are anxious about risk of miscarriage, multiple pregnancies and fetal abnormalities.
- They need to be given hope, but at the same time should be explained about all available realistic options, including sensitization about adoption by giving a third party example. This gives them adequate time, knowledge and helps in final decision making.

Assessment of male factor infertility: Male Genital System (Fig 6)

The male partner usually feels uncomfortable and vulnerable when asked to undergo investigations or treatment. More awareness among the community about the male causes of infertility is hence needed.

It consists of the penis (1), the testicles (2), the epididymis (3), the deferent canals (4), the seminal vesicles (5) and the prostate. Semen (the ejaculate) is constituted of seminal fluid secreted by several glands - the prostate and seminal vesicles - and spermatozoa, mobile cells produced in the testicles. Normally, 1 ml semen contains 20-100 million sperms, among which at least 40% are mobile.

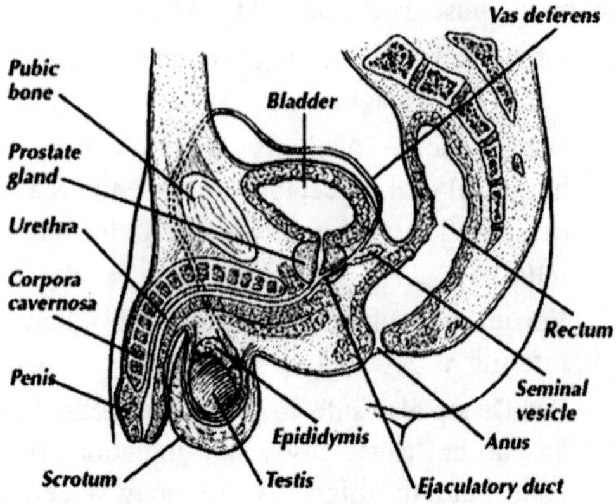

A side view of the male reproductive organs.

Fig 6: Male genital system

Varicocele: It is a dilatation of the pampiniform venous plexus and the internal spermatic vein. It is a well-recognized cause of decreased testicular function affecting 15-20% of all males (40% of infertile males). In fact, scrotal varicoceles are the most common cause of poor sperm production and decreased semen quality. Varicoceles are easy to identify and to correct surgically.

The testes are the paired male genital organs that contain sperm, cells that produce and nourish sperm (spermatogonia and Sertoli cells, respectively), and cells that produce testosterone (Leydig cells). The testes are located in a sac called the scrotum. The epididymis is a small tubular structure attached to the testes that serves as a storage reservoir wherein sperm mature.Sperm travel through the vas deferens, which connects the epididymis to the prostate gland. The vas deferens is in the scrotum and is part of a larger tissue bundle called the spermatic cord. It contains the vas deferens, blood vessels, nerves and lymphatic channels.

The pampiniform plexus is composed of the veins of the spermatic cord. These veins drain blood from the testes, epididymis, and vas deferens and eventually become the spermatic veins that drain into the main circulation of the kidneys. The pampiniform venous plexus may become tortuous and dilated, much like a varicose vein in the leg. In fact, a scrotal varicocele is simply a varicose enlargement of the pampiniform plexus above and around the testicle. Two other veins, the cremasteric and the deferential, also drain blood from the testicles; however, these are rarely involved in the varicocele process.

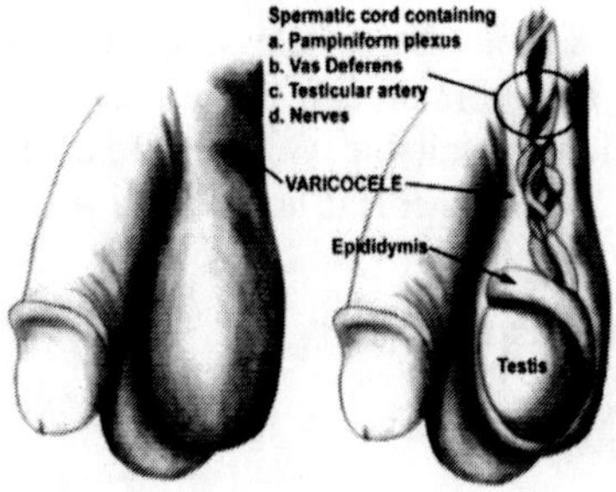

Fig. 7: Penis, the testicles & the epididymis

Causes of Male infertility: These include:

- Oligoasthenospermia- Proper sperms are not there, e.g., decreased sperm count & decreased motility.
- Spinal injuries.
- Congenital bilateral absence of Vas Deferens.
- Obstructive azoospermia-Absence of sperms due to blockage, which can be corrected with surgery.
- Untreated Recurring episodes of Sexually Transmitted Diseases like gonorrhea, chlamydia and tuberculosis may cause obstruction and difficulty in passage of sperms.
- Chronic alcoholism, smoking/drug abuse reduces sperm quantity & quality.
- Psychosexual disorders (erectile dysfunctions, decreased libido).
- Environmental toxins, including pesticides and lead.
- Health problems such as mumps, serious conditions like kidney disease, or hormone problems.
- Lack of ejaculation, premature or retrograde ejaculation, erectile dysfunctrion.
- Anatomical abnormalities like hypospadiasis, epispadiasis and phimosis or other local factors that prevent normal deposition of semen in the vagina.
- Systemic illness like diabetes and hypertension.
- Medicines, radiation treatment and chemotherapy for cancer, age, obesity, etc. are associated with low testosterone levels. In massively obese individuals, reduced spermatogenesis associated may favour infertility. Moreover, the frequency of erectile dysfunction increases with increasing body mass index.

Management of male factor infertility

History taking: A good history helps in coming to a diagnosis. It is very important to cover all the important factors during history taking, so that maximum information is available. General ill health can also affect sperm count; therefore a detailed medical history is a must in every couple. (see flowchart)

A. General information –

1. Age
2. Religion
3. Occupation
4. Previous marriages & their outcome

B. Occupational / Environmental exposure –

- Exposure to hot temperature & environmental toxins (furnaces, bakeries, solvent or chemical industries)
- Sauna
- Tight pants
- Dietary habits
- Smoking
- Alcohol
- Caffeine
- Drug consumption
- Testicular trauma

C. Family History –

- Infertility
- Birth defects
- Spontaneous abortions & still births
- Genetic diseases
- Mental retardation

D. Fertility History -

5. Primary or secondary infertility
6. Duration of infertility
7. Number of confirmed pregnancy losses
8. Knowledge of reproductive cycle
9. Previous evaluation & treatment

E. Past medical history -

- Tuberculosis
- Mumps
- Chronic infection
- High fever (in past 6 months)
- H/o increase in scrotal size with / without pain
- Allergies
- Diabetes, Hypertension
- Renal & liver diseases
- Neurological diseases
- Drugs – e.g. anti hypertensives, anti diabetics, ketoconazole, sulfasalazine, spironolactone, allopurinol, colchicine & antibiotics like nitrofurantoin, erythromycin, gentamicin
- H/o chemo or radiotherapy in the past

F. Surgical / Urologic History -

- Precocious or delayed puberty
- Orchitis due to Mumps etc
- Penile discharge / burning micturition/ ulcerative lesions over genitals
- Testicular trauma / torsion

1. Inguinal hernia operation
2. Varicocelectomy
3. Vasectomy
4. Prostatectomy

- Hydrocele, varicocele
- Cryptorchidism, orchiopexy

5. Bladder operations

G. Contraception - temporary as condom or permanent as vasectomy

H. Sexual History -

- Knowledge & use of fertile period
- Coital frequency & timing
- Use of lubricants
- Erection & ejaculation problems
- Nature & volume of ejaculate
- History of previous marriage or extra-marital sexual relations.

Table 4: General examination

Factors	*Significance*
Height	Genetic defects eg. Klinefelters syndrome, Noonan's syndrome
Weight	Endocrine disorders eg. Bardet-Biedl syndrome, Laurence-Moon syndrome
Vital parameters, BP	General health, Hypertension
Secondary sexual characteristics	Genetic / Endocrinological disorders
Gynaecomastia, nipple discharge or tenderness	Hyperprolactinemia
Thyroid enlargement, nodule or tenderness/ scars	Thyroid disorders
Respiratory system / Cardiovascular system / Abdominal examination	General health, Hernia

Genital examination

- Penis - size, structural abnormalities: hypospadias, chordee, plaques
- Scrotum – size, consistency, lesions
- Testis - size, location, consistency, masses
- Epididymis - complete/ partial, distended/ normal, nodularity
- Vas deferens - presence, nodularity
- Varicocele
- Inguinal examination – swelling, hernia
- Digital rectal examination for cysts, seminal vesicle abnormalities, prostate size, consistency and tenderness

Investigations

Semen analysis - Instructions to the male partner for collection of semen Husband / male partner should be given clear written and spoken instructions

1. Minimum of 2 days and a maximum of 7 days of sexual abstinence
2. For additional samples, number of days of sexual abstinence should be as constant as possible at each visit
3. Obtained by masturbation and ejaculated into a clean, wide-mouthed container made of glass or plastic, from a batch that has been confirmed to be non-toxic for spermatozoa
4. Semen sample needs to be complete and loss of any fraction of the sample should be reported.

Semen sample collection

5. Sample should be collected in a private room preferably near the laboratory, in order to limit exposure of semen to fluctuations in temperature and to control time between collection and analysis
6. Following information should be recorded on the report form - man's name, birth date and personal code number, period of abstinence, date and time of collection, completeness of sample, any difficulties in producing the sample, and the interval between collection and start of semen analysis
7. Specimen container should be kept at ambient temperature, between 20 °C to 37 °C and avoid large changes in temperature that may affect spermatozoa after they are ejaculated into it
8. Note in the report if sample is incomplete, especially if the first, sperm-rich fraction is missing. If the sample is incomplete, a second sample should be collected, again after an abstinence period of 2–7 days

If the result of the first semen analysis is abnormal, a repeat confirmatory test should be offered. It should ideally be undertaken 3-4 weeks after initial analysis. However, if gross spermatozoa deficiency (azoospermia / severe oligozoospermia) is detected, it should be undertaken as soon as possible. (GPP).

Other investigations include:

- Hormonal tests like FSH, testosterone to differentiate between central (e.g. hypothalamic) and end organ (e.g. testicular) cause
- Doppler USG of scrotum to rule out varicocoele
- Fine needle aspiration cytology (FNAC) or biopsy of testis, especially in cases of azoospermia, is indicated very infrequently

WHO reference values for semen analysis (2010)

Table 5: Reference limits for semen characteristics

Parameter	*Lower reference limit*	*Range*
Volume	1.5ml	(1.4-1.7 ml)
Sperm concentration	15 million spermatozoa/mL	12-16 million spermatozoa/mL
Total sperm number	39 million spermatozoa/ ejaculate	33-46 million spermatozoa / ejaculate
Total Motility	40%	38-42%
Progressive Motility	32%	31-34%
Normal Morphology	4%	3-4%
Vitality	58%	55-63%

Treatment – It depends on:

- Age, overall health and medical history
- Extent of the disease
- Tolerance for specific medications, procedures or therapies
- Expectations for the course of disease
- Patients opinion or preference

There is a range of treatment options currently available for male factor infertility; Drug therapy

Treatment – It depends on:

- Age, overall health and medical history
- Extent of the disease
- Tolerance for specific medications, procedures or therapies
- Expectations for the course of disease
- Patients opinion or preference

There is a range of treatment options currently available for male factor infertility; Drug therapy

- It may include gonadotrophin therapy, antibiotics (for any infection), or other medication deemed appropriate
- Men with hypogonadotropic hypogonadism should be offered gonadotrophin drugs . Discussion about the duration of treatment and cost involved, must be done with the couple, as the therapy may continue for 2-3 years and it may cost up to Rs. 2-3 lakhs.
- Men with idiopathic semen abnormalities should not be offered antioestrogens, gonadotrophins, androgens, bromocriptine, or kinin-enhancing drugs.
- Antioxidants like Co- Q, vitamin E and trace elements like zinc, selenium etc may be helpful in some cases
- Men with leukocytes in their semen should not be offered antibiotic treatment unless there is an identified infection (confirmed by doing culture studies), because there is no evidence that this improves pregnancy rates.

Erectile dysfunction –

- First-line treatment of consists of lifestyle interventions (weight loss, increased exercise, and smoking cessation), discontinuation or changing of medications that may cause erectile dysfunction
- Psychogenic factor may be an important contributory cause, especially in infertility management during peri-ovulatory period,

due to excessive stress of performance on specific days. In most cases this can be effectively managed by proper counseling, and only a few may additionally require phosphodiesterase type - 5 (PDE5) inhibitors

- Diagnostic workup include fasting serum glucose, lipid profile, thyroid-stimulating hormone test, and a morning total testosterone level
- Oral PDE - 5 inhibitors should be first-line treatment especially in patients with diabetes mellitus, spinal cord injury and sexual dysfunction associated with antidepressants
- Alternative therapeutic options include intra-urethral and intra-cavernosal injections of alprostadil, vacuum pump devices, surgically implanted penile prostheses and psychotherapy

1. Surgery
   - It is designed to overcome anatomical barriers that impede sperm production and maturation or ejaculation
   - Operative procedures include surgeries to remove varicocele, ejaculatory duct obstruction or hypospadias
2. Artificial insemination / Intra uterine insemination (IUI)
   - Placement of relatively large numbers of healthy sperm either at the entrance of the cervix or into partner's uterus, bypassing the cervix, to have direct access to the fallopian tubes
3. Assisted reproductive technologies (ART)
   - IVF – Retrieved oocytes are exposed to an optimal concentration of processed high quality, motile sperm outside the female's body and embryo is transferred back to the uterus.
   - Microsurgical fertilization / Intracytoplasmic sperm injection (ICSI) Facilitates sperm penetration, by injection of a single sperm into the oocyte, under microscope to fertilize it in cases with low sperm count & motility.

Donor insemination vs ART vs adoption

- Couples should be offered information about the relative merits of ART like *IVF* and ICSI versus less expensive options like donor insemination or adoption, in a context that allows equal access to both treatment options.
- Couples considering donor insemination should be offered counseling from someone, independent of the treatment unit, regarding all

physical and psychological implications for themselves and potential children.

(Details are given in details in the ICMR ART guidelines 2005).

Donor insemination

- One parent has a biological and genetic link with the child.
- Relatively simple and usually painless procedure requiring neither surgery nor a stay in hospital.

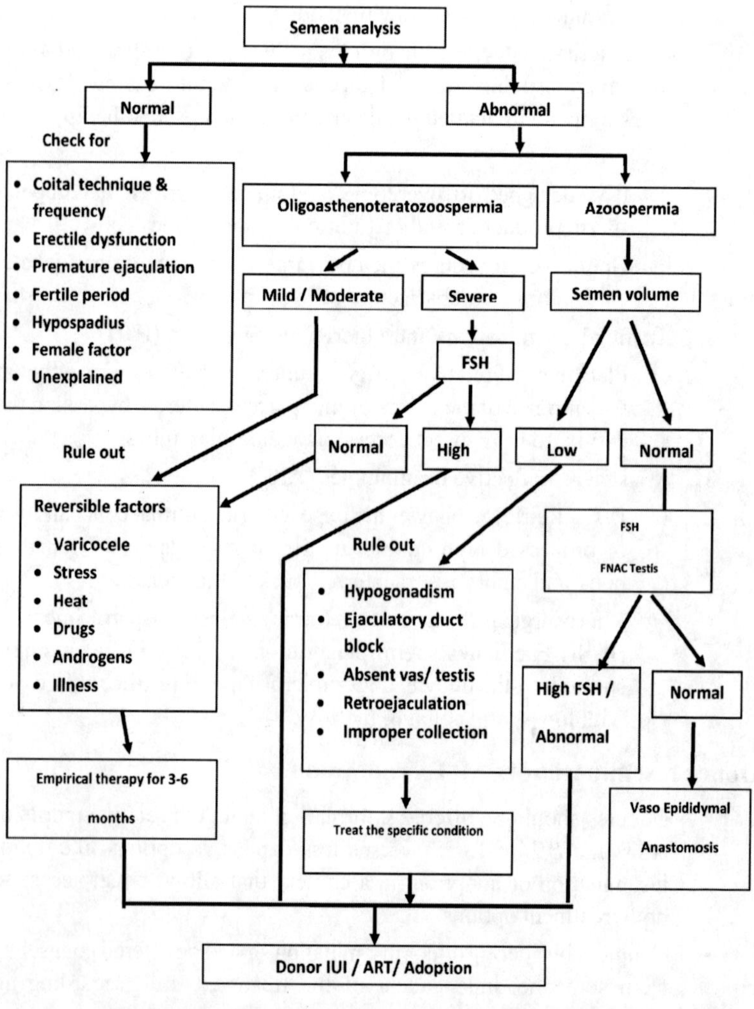

Fig 8: Algorithm for management of male factor infertility.

- Anonymity of donor ensures against any legal, material or emotional claim by him on the couple or child and vice versa.
- Mutual acceptance is of utmost importance.

Adoption

- This option must be given to couples, as some might prefer it, than complicated and expensive technologies which are not always successful.
- Also they may feel adopting a baby is a more human action.

Some general tips for the couple

- If couple is young and recently married, don't take unnecessary stress.
- Have a carefree attitude
- If female is 30 or above, plan early pregnancy
- Plan 1st child as soon as possible after marriage
- Don't abort if early pregnancy happens
- Don't go for abortion for your 1st pregnancy especially if you are < 25 years
- Avoid late marriage and try to conceive before age of 35 years
- Keep track of menstrual cycle
- Avoid cigarette smoking, air pollution and ionising radiation

Some tips for the husband-

- Think of job change if working in hot surroundings
- Avoid keeping the mobile phone on or near body. Use speaker/ headphones whenever possible. Avoid excessive use of laptop and gadgets.
- Exercise regularly
- Wear cotton underwear (Avoid synthetic inners)
- Avoid tight inner wear
- Eat healthy diet (Avoid obesity, junk and oily foods)
- Avoid cigarette smoke or tobacco use
- Limit proximity to ionizing radiations/heat
- Maintain good personal hygiene

Fertility specialists say that thousands of couples may be sabotaging their best efforts at conception with simple errors like this. Some doctors may unwittingly play a role in enhancing these mistakes, too. Luckily, many of these goofs are not only fixable but don't require a high-tech or pricey solution. Finding the right doctor can make a world of a difference to fertility treatment. This is why spending time researching the best fertility doctor in the best clinic is very important. Unfortunately, many patients go to doctors who lack any special expertise to treat their fertility issues. Most gynecologists can provide the basic infertility workup and testing. But they do not have the proper credentials to provide more advanced care that an infertile couple needs. Infertility can be a complex problem. To get the proper care without wasting precious time and valuable money it is vital to seek the help of infertility specialists.

Male involvement- Here it is worth mentioning that male involvement is very much necessary in treatment of infertility. It is not like that only female is responsible or to be blamed for infertility. Husband should escort his wife to the hospital. Treatment of infertility involves some investigations of husband too. It would not be wrong to emphasize that support of whole family is needed in such cases. Family members should support the couple emotionally. Also couple should ensure that they don't blame each other for failure to conceive.

They need to be told, "You have willfully married each other and you need to be together in this time of crisis. Try to move through this together. Be mentally strong and fight this battle together. There is some purpose for your coming into this world. Don't let this failure over power you. Be strong. Take life as it comes your way. Everything that happens to us is for some good. Doctors will try their best but your support and strength is constantly needed."

Lastly, for those couples who remain devoid of this happiness, they need to be told, "Understand that there is life even after infertility. Find ways to fulfill yourself –with or without children. Learn new ways of relating to each other as it will deepen your relationship in years to follow. And of course you always have adoption as a choice."

FEW MISTAKES THAT INFERTILE COUPLES MAKE

- Getting Fed-up and giving up: Infertility is likely to be one of the first major life shocks you will encounter, when you have to confront your biological frailty. Moreover, it's a problem that will not go away by throwing money at it, since the technology is still not perfect. How well you cope with this adversity will depend largely on your adversity quotient, and your need to develop coping skills. Joining a support group can be a very valuable source of emotional strength.
- Not Getting a Second Opinion: While it's an excellent idea to trust your doctor; this should not be left to blind faith. It's always

worthwhile to get a second opinion from an infertility specialist, to make sure you are on the right track. It's even better to get an opinion from a specialist who is not going to be treating you; this is much more likely to free of bias.

- Losing Control: Patients who have unrealistic expectations from their treatment go through highs and lows that they find difficult to cope with. You need to have a plan of action, in which you hope for the best, but prepare for the worst. Don't think of any treatment on a single cycle basis.
- Let's Try Something New This Time: Some patients want to try every new treatment every time they read a report in the newspaper. Remember that newspaper reports are deceptive and often give a one-sided view that emphasizes the successes. It's foolhardy to trust media hype. Don't act as a guinea pig - let the technology mature. If it's really good, it will be even better in another two years. Many fads come and go, and not all of them are truly helpful for patients (though they often help some doctors rake in quick bucks because it's the latest thing to be in vogue!).
- From having too much sex, to not having sex often enough**:** Some of the most common mistakes the patients make when first trying to conceive a baby are related to -

Timing: In a 28-day cycle, ovulation generally happens on day 14. But don't assume that time clock necessarily applies to you. So, in order to figure out the exact day you ovulated, you'd actually need to count back 14 days from the day you started your period. If your cycle's fairly regular, though, you can use this technique to estimate when ovulation happens each month.

Going to the specialist soon enough: If you're under 35, it's completely normal for you to take up to a year to be pregnant. It's also completely normal to feel frustrated after month 6 or 7 — but if you don't have any underlying health problems, you should probably wait it out. If you're over 35, go ahead and set up an appointment with a specialist after six months instead of a year.

Waiting too long to go to the specialist: There are definitely exceptions to the one-year-wait rule: If your cycle is shorter than 25 days or longer than 35 days, if you get very painful or heavy periods, or if you've had a significant pelvic infection in the past, it's a good idea to head to the doc sooner rather than later to get everything checked out.

Hanging on to unhealthy habits: Kick those obviously bad habits like smoking, drinking, and/or drug use once you get pregnant. But remember that other common lifestyle factors play a role in affecting your fertility, too. Patients avoid extremes in weight (either being too thin or overweight), along with keeping a balanced and relatively healthy diet (skip the fad diets). Other things to keep in mind: Ease up on the caffeine (studies show it affects your ability to absorb iron, a key pre-natal nutrient) and try to curb that artificial sweeteners habit.

Obsessing about positions: If you've taken to standing on your head, lifting your legs in the air, or bending into any other coital or post-coital position to up your baby-making odds, we've got some news for you: You may be wasting your time. The truth is, the majority of a man's sperm goes toward the woman's egg the moment he ejaculates. And as for that left-over liquid that comes out after? It won't actually have much sperm left in it anyway. So if you want to do it missionary-style or prop a pillow under your hips, go right ahead; but don't stress out about it.

Only having sex on the exact day (you think) you're ovulating: Even if you have a super-regular, 28-day cycle, there's a chance you might ovulate one or two days before or after the day you think you will. Plus, even if you do ovulate on day 14, sperm can live inside your body between 24-48 hours (and in some cases, up to a week!) after sex. If you're hoping to up your fertility odds, start to have sex 4 to 6 days before ovulation and then continue until 4 to 6 days after.

Having sex everyday: Believe it or not, too much sex can decrease man's sperm count which can then take a few days to rebound! Once you get the timing down, trying to have sex every other day (alternate day), instead of every day, in the week leading up to ovulation and during the week after.

Assuming "the problem" is with you: A lot of couples focus their fertility investigation on the woman — but in reality, 40% of the time fertility problems can actually be attributed to the man. So if you haven't conceived after a year of trying and are under 35, you should both head to the doctor. Your partner will probably need a semen analysis to rule out any problems on his end.

Waiting too long to try: We get it – you've probably got a lot left on that pre-baby to-do list (establishing a career, beefing up your savings, buying a bigger house, etc.). But, if you're in a stable relationship and want a child, don't wait just because you think it won't be a problem to get pregnant later in life.

Some common mistakes usually made by physicians when they have tried to treat infertile couples. This information should be used to ensure that that time and money are not wasted.

- Not getting a semen analysis right away. It is estimated that 20-30 percent of infertility cases are due to the male factor.
- Over-diagnosing anovulation, a condition in which the ovary does not release a ripened egg each month as part of a woman's normal

cycle. Many doctors will diagnose anovulation by using a blood test for a hormone called progesterone which is only elevated in women after they have ovulated. However, many doctors will mistakenly tell a woman she has not ovulated if her progesterone level is less than 10. "This is a very common mistake that results in women being misdiagnosed, having unnecessary tests performed, and being treated incorrectly,"

- Hormone levels in women change according to the time of the menstrual cycle. Every test needs to be timed precisely. Failure to recognize this fact results in hormonal testing being performed with un-interpretable results. This causes delays and incorrect treatment to be given.
- Some doctors may not be up to date with the latest IVF tests, procedures, technologies and medications. For example, the post coital test looks for sperm in a woman's cervix after a couple has had intercourse. In the past, it was believed that failure to find moving sperm could be a sign of a woman "killing off" her partners' sperm. However, several rigorously performed studies have shown that the test is worthless. Despite the fact that this has been well known for decades, some doctors still use the test today.
- Spending too much time on one IVF procedure. A commonly used fertility medication is Clomid. The vast majority of women who will conceive taking clomid will do so within the first four to five months of use. However, some doctors will keep patients on Clomid for many months and even years. Besides being a poor treatment option after the first few months, long-term treatment with this medication is potentially harmful. Even the manufacturers say that it should not be used for more than 6 cycles.
- Failure to be more aggressive with older patients (age 37 and above). As women age, their fertility decreases. It is important to be more aggressive in their treatment. Treatments should be considered sooner.

Waiting too long to see a specialist: Patients need to be referred to a fertility specialist, such as a reproductive endocrinologist, if they are unable to conceive within a year. This still makes sense for people under 35, but if there are hidden fertility issues (even obvious issues like previous surgery), waiting a full year can set you back unnecessarily, heightening your anxiety and squandering precious time. If you're over 35, see a specialist after six months of trying to conceive. And if you're over 40, "There's nothing wrong with checking in immediately,"

Women who have had a prior pregnancy are particularly likely to wait longer than they should. They assume if they were fertile in the past, they don't have fertility problems. But we see a lot of secondary infertility—the inability to conceive or bear a subsequent child. Remember, you're older now than when you had the first pregnancy—and your eggs are older, too.

Just because you have a period does not mean you are ovulating or that the eggs you release are of a high enough quality to ensure pregnancy. This myth is often held among women of older reproductive age. Women think they must be fertile if there cycles are normal. But women can go on having periods as much as a decade after they've stopped producing good, healthy eggs.

Women of any age can experience so-called "anovulatory" cycles, during which no egg is released, meaning pregnancy can't occur. Such cycles can produce some bleeding, which results from a buildup of the uterine lining.

Believing that good health habits will extend your pregnancy prospects Fertility declines with age: A healthy 25-year-old engaging in unprotected sex has about a 20 to 25 % change of conceiving in any given month; a 30-year-old's chances are 10 to 15 %; by age 40 it's down to 4 to 8 %; and over age 43 it's less than 2 %. Yet many women believe that their healthy ways will help them beat their declining odds regardless of age. Many patients in their late 30s or early 40s come in and say they've taken care of themselves, never smoked, and eat well. They've just gotten married and are shocked that they can't accomplish their goal of starting a family. Taking care of yourself is important for optimizing your fertility, but "it won't make your eggs younger or guarantee a pregnancy at age 42.

Psychological Aspects of Infertility

In the pre-marriage stage of their lives, both girl and boy are only concerned about their studies, job and life style. During this phase, they are least concerned about their reproductive health. In arranged marriages, the basis of establishing a good relation is often based on being physically comfortable because there is hardly any time to have the emotional connect with each other. The couples find themselves in a very awkward situation by having preconceived notions about sex which are mostly based on imagination or hearsay.

During the initial phase of their martial life, the couple goes through many changes, starting from adjustments, meeting the expectations from in-laws, friends, relative and society, etc. to creating an environment of compatibility among themselves. Even before the girl could establish her own identity in the new home, the so-called well-wishers', i.e., neighbors, relatives, etc. start teasing the couple about having baby and think about family planning with the most prominent *dialogue " Abb do se teen, jaldi ho jao"*. This mounts pressure on the newly-wed couple. Especially the expectations of mother in-law are very high. Mostly, the in-laws pressurize the girl to give them "*ghar ka chirag*" as if it's mandatory to conceive immediately after marriage. This comes as an external pressure for the couple, especially for the girl.

Fortunately, if the couple is not having any financial liability, stress, depression etc. they try to plan their family immediately after marriage. But in few cases where the couples are career oriented, or have financial liabilities, etc. family planning is never a priority. In these cases the couple is usually tagged as infertile irrespective of their conscious decision.

But in few unfortunate cases if the couple is actually infertile then the painful struggle starts which may further lead to stress, tension, depression, and guilt, lack of self-esteem, anger, and resentment, single or in combination. The pain is similar to the grief over losing your loved one, but it is more painful because it is a recurring pain.

Infertile people grieve the loss of the baby that they never had. They grieve the loss of that baby who would had mommy's nose and daddy's eyes. But, each month, there is the hope that maybe that baby will be conceived this month. No matter how hard they try to prepare themselves for bad news, they still hope that this month will be different and bring good news for them. Then, the bad news comes again, and the grief engulfs the infertile couple again. This process happens month after month, year after year. For infertile couple it is like having a deep cut that keeps getting opened right when it starts to heal. Infertility can be a real test of a couple's relationship. It may shake the foundation of marriage. Irrespective of whosoever is liable for infertility the society always blames the female partner primarily. Especially, in Indian society the family members make the female accountable irrespective of analyzing the facts. It is known that in 50% cases male partners are infertile but still our society tags the female as *Banjh*. And just for the sake of status and self-esteem of her husband the female hides the reality and takes all the blame on herself.

As the couple moves into infertility treatments, the pain increases while the bank account depletes. The tests are invasive and embarrassing for couple. They feel as if doctor has taken over their bedroom. This comes as a mental as well as physical stress for the couple. And for all of this discomfort, you pay a lot of money, which adds to financial stress as well.

Some couples will sooner or later resolve the infertility by eventually conceiving. Others stop the infertility treatments and choose to live without children, and few find an alternative way of parenting, such as by adopting a child. Reaching a resolution can take years, so infertile couples need your emotional support during this journey. Most people don't know what to say, so they end up saying the wrong thing, which only makes the journey so much harder for the infertile couples.

Comments such as "plan a family now; *Ab do se teen ho jao*" create even more stress for the infertile couple, particularly the woman. The woman feels like she is doing something wrong when, in fact, there is a good chance that there is a physical problem preventing her from becoming pregnant.

Failure to conceive a baby is a very painful journey. Infertile couples are surrounded by families with children. These couples watch their friends give birth to two or three children, and they watch those children grow while the couple goes home to the silence of an empty house. These couples see all of the joy that a child brings into someone's life, and they feel the emptiness of not being able to experience the same joy. Comments and pressure from family and friends do not offer comfort. Instead, these comments make infertile people feel like they are criminal and it's their fault that they are not able to conceive.

One of the cruelest things people say to a girl is, "Maybe God doesn't intend for you to be a mother." Who gave society the right that they can tag a girl as "*baanjh*" /"barren" Infertility is a medical condition, not a punishment from God .

Infertility treatments are very private and embarrassing, which is why many couples choose to undergo these treatments in secret. Men especially are very sensitive to letting people know about infertility testing, such as sperm counts. No couple can endure infertility treatments forever. At some point, they will stop. This is a painful decision to make, and it involves even more grief. Once the couple has made the decision to stop treatments, support their decision. Don't encourage them to try again, and don't discourage them from adopting, if that is their choice. Once the couple has reached resolution (whether to live without children, adopt a child) they can finally put that chapter of their lives behind them. Don't try to open that chapter again.

Having a baby is one of the most exciting times in a couple's life, but for couples coping with infertility and infertility treatments, the circumstances are different. The physical, emotional and financial stress of infertility can, hurt your relationship with your partner, if you're not careful and do not support each other. It would be easy to turn to one another and shout, "It's your fault!" But the reality is that no matter who plays the blame game, you both lose.

Does it really matter whose "fault" it is? After all, this is not something you have much control over. And it may be too late to change the few things you might have once controlled. The reality is what you're facing today.

So, stay away from turning down the blame lane and reassure your partner that you are both in it together. Remember how you feel about your partner, why you love him or her, why you want to have a child together. Most importantly talk about your frustration and anger openly. Studies show that couples who keep their feelings hidden are much more likely to have problems related to the stress of infertility. Face the infertility issue as a united front. That means going to appointments together, coping with side effects together, grieving together, and sharing the news together with friends and family.

There *are* ways to protect your relationship from the potentially damaging stress of infertility, e.g.:

Focus on yourselves- Remember that the two of you came first, before any thought of a baby. Even if you do have a child, the two of you still need to be a healthy couple before you can be good parents.

Schedule non-infertility dates. On these dates, neither of you is allowed to talk about children, infertility, medical treatments, adoption or anything to do with what you're going through. **Bring spontaneity back into sex.** Let the fresh air energize you romantically. The key is to make it so much fun.

Take a break. You and your partner might consider taking a month long break from trying to get pregnant. Reducing the stress and anxiety in your sexual relationship now will ensure that your sex life will remain a source of pleasure and relaxation for years to come.

Do physical workout together. Exercise is a fabulous stress buster. Take up tennis, dancing etc. Consider taking a yoga class together. It will not only strengthen your body but also teach you deep breathing, which is helpful in relaxing and focusing. Of course, there's nothing wrong with long walks either. Just remember to hold hands.

Respect your differences. Each of you will deal with the situation differently. Just because he doesn't cry or talk for hours about the infertility doesn't mean he isn't hurting. Men are more likely to distance themselves from the issue and become irritable. Understand that this may be *his* way of coping.

Talk-He cannot read your mind. If you need him to be more supportive, tell him, but be specific. What do you mean by supportive? If you need time to be alone because you're angry and upset and don't want to take it out on him, *tell him* so he doesn't think you're shutting him out. If you have a hard time verbalizing your feelings, try writing them down in an e-mail or letter to him.

Agree on how far you'll go in term of financial stress. You can easily exhaust your bank account, marriage and emotional reserves through infertility treatment. **From the Male Perspective**

Sometimes it may seem as if your wife or partner is the only one experiencing infertility. She's the one who gets the hugs and flowers; she's the one who is asked about her feelings, her health, her emotional state.But what about you? Chances are, you're suffering too. A recent study found that the male partners of infertile couples were quite likely to feel depressed and to have erectile dysfunction and other sexual relationship problems. Unfortunately, too often men try to distance themselves from infertility, keep their feelings to themselves and focus on plans to "solve" the infertility, all of which are less than ideal ways of coping that can harm your relationship. Discussing your feelings with your partner will allow you to bond over feelings of being out of control.

Yoga for Fertility

Yoga is supposed to be good for fertility issues. *Hatha yoga* is more beneficial if you're trying to conceive instead of vigorous forms like Power yoga. Couples suffering from fertility issues or just trying to conceive have a lot on their plate – doctor's appointments, monitoring ovulation cycles, timing intercourse. This is the time to take extra care of yourself and try to keep yourself calm and happy. Yoga is just the thing you need to keep yourself healthy and happy as you try to conceive.

Doctors generally recommend using yoga with other medical treatments to help women de-stress and enhance the chances of pregnancy. Certain studies have shown that women who tried yoga while trying to conceive were three times more likely to conceive than those who did not do yoga.

Benefits of yoga for those trying to conceive

- Stress can interfere with your ovulation and menstrual cycle, while stress can also affect your husband's sperm producing capability. Yoga will help both of you to de-stress.
- f a couple does yoga together, they can not only strengthen their relationship, but can help each other cope with the anxiety as they try for a baby.
- There are specific yoga poses that can prepare the woman's body for conception. Yoga *asanas* can remove stress from the region of the ovaries, uterus and fallopian tubes, and can soften the abdomen. Poses where you need to recline stretch the abdomen and increase the circulation of blood to the reproductive organs.
- Yoga poses can be used after intercourse to increase your chances of conception. *Viparita Kirani* (Legs up the wall posture), where you need to put your legs up the wall, is good for conception.

- Yoga can be good for you if you have certain hormonal problems that are restricting conception. Yoga *asanas* improve the function of the glands.
- While yoga may not be the only way to increase your chances of fertility, fertility focused yoga can help you conceive.

Here are a few yoga poses to cope with fertility issues -

Ardha Matsyendrasana (Half Lord of the Fish Pose)

This posture is good for back problems. It is not only good for conception; this asana improves appetite and digestion, relives menstrual discomfort, asthma and strengthens the back and spine. A good pose for energizing the entire body.

Supta Padangusthasana (Reclining Big Toe posture)

This posture is not only good for the spine and for conception, it also strengthens the knees, reduces menstrual problems, sciatica and blood pressure; and stimulates the prostrate glands.

Paschimottanasana (Seated Forward Bend)

This asana is also good for conception and fertility issues.

Adoption - An option to manage infertility

With proper diagnosis and treatment, the majority of couples managed for infertility will achieve pregnancy and for those who do not respond, Assisted Reproductive Techniques (ARTs) are available. However, ARTs have their own inherent problems, so adoption should be discussed as an available realistic option. Components of adoption should be discussed by the treating team with the couple from the initial visit itself. It helps to sensitize couple to this option, so that they have adequate time and knowledge when it comes to decision making.

'Adoption' has been defined by the Juvenile Justice Act as follows: 272

"A process through which the adopted child is permanently separated from his/her biological parents and becomes the legitimate child of his adoptive parents with all the rights, privileges and responsibilities that are attached to the relationship."

The eligibility criteria of a person competent to adopt and the list of documents required for the same are provided in annexure 10.

Important issues to be discussed with adoptive parents

1. Discussion about adoption should be held from the beginning itself for educating the adoptive parents about the requirements for adoption

2. Financial and legal aspects should be discussed with counselling regarding the health, upkeep and future of the adopted child
3. Couples should be referred to proper agency, either public or private for understanding the procedure systemically.

Adoption laws in India and legal system

The latest legislations for adoption or taking a child in custody in India come under:

Juvenile Justice (Care and Protection) of Children Act, 2000 (56 of 2000): Guidelines Governing the Adoption of Children, 2011

(i) The Juvenile justice Act -1986 was meant for the protection of the vulnerable children but its implementation revealed many gaps, hence it was re-enacted in 2000 and later amended in 2006 as Juvenile Justice (Care & Protection of Children) Act33,34.

(ii) Apart from improving the provision of children's home, food, education training and medical care and efforts to relocate them in their families if possible the new law also provides for secular adoption.

Criteria for the Child to be adopted (Sec.41 (5) of the Act)

- Abandoned child - If two members of the Committee declare the child legally free for placement.
- Surrendered child - If the period two months for reconsideration by the parents is lapsed.
- Child who can understand and express his consent - If his/her consent is obtained in this regard.

Agencies

Central Adoption Resource Authority (CARA) is under the Ministry of Woman & Child Development, Government of India. It functions as the nodal body for adoption of Indian children and is mandated to monitor and regulate in-country and inter-country adoptions. Others include:

- LAPA - Licenced Adoption Placement Agency
- RIPA - Recognised Indian Placement Agency
- AFAA - Authorised Foreign Adoption Agency
- SARA - State Adoption Resource Agency

Adoption expenses

The Prospective Adoptive Parents (PAPs) are required to bear following administration expenses in the process of adoption:

- Registration fee for PAPs for in-country adoption, of approximately Rs.1,000
- In addition, around Rs. 5000 for the Home Study Report and post adoption follow-up services
- PAPs shall be required to contribute towards the Child Care Corpus (CCC), maintained by the agency from where they are adopting the child. This amount shall also cover all expenses incurred to finalize the adoption. However, the agency may decide to waive off or reduce this amount in exceptional cases. The amount contributed by PAPs is as under-
    - Towards CCC in case of in-country adoptions: around Rs. 40,000/-
    - Towards CCC in case of inter-country adoption: US$ 5000/- (approx.)

Modalities for payment is mentioned in Schedule –xvi of the Guidelines

Adoption road map

The duration for completion of adoption process depends on problems, fitness, availability of the baby as per the couples need and legal system.

Adoption procedure in country

↓

Couple enrols and gets information guidelines form

↓

Parents submit application form 4 files of application to RIPA / LAPA

↓

Parents' registration [Fee]

↓

Home study by social worker

↓

Child matching by RIPA LAPA

↓

Pre-adoption foster care

↓

(Contd...)

Social worker revisits the family

↓

After petition gets filed, one copy goes to 'Indian Council of Social' Welfare (ICSW)

↓

After re-evaluation of all documents by District Registrar, Judge

↓

verifies petition file and issues Adoption order after hearing

↓

Adoption deed is prepared after lawyer, gets the order

↓

Birth registration, Change of names of Parents

Fig 9: Day from the date of admission to the child placement

- If you want to adopt a child you need to register with any one Specialized Adoption Agency, preferably nearest to your home or online at www.adoption india.nic.in
- You can check your eligibility on the website of CARA39
- To enable you to take an informed decision, the Agency provides pre-adoption counseling. You can clarify with them any apprehension that you might have
- You would need to complete certain documentation
- The Social Worker of the Agency will visit you in your home to assess your social and family background, and suitability for adoptive parenthood
- This home study is conducted within two months from the date of registration
- The Agency will locate a suitable child and you will receive a referral
- Once you see the child and decide to adopt, the child can be medically examined by any doctor of your choice
- The legal process then starts and you can take the child in pre-adoption foster care
- The Competent Court legally places the child in adoption by a Court decree
- For a period of two years, the Agency will keep in touch with you and provide post adoptive services

Eligibility criteria and list of documents required for adoption

Who can Adopt?

In accordance with the guidelines governing the adoption of children, (2011), provisions of sub-section (6) of section 41 {Juvenile Justice (Care & Protection of Children) Act}, the Court may allow a child to be given in adoption:

(a) to a person irrespective of marital status; or

(b) to parents to adopt a child of the same sex irrespective of the number of living biological sons or daughters, or

(c) to a childless couple

Additional Eligibility Criteria

(a) 2 years of stable relationship in case Prospective Adoptive Parents (PAPs) are married

(b) To adopt children in the age group of 0-3 years, the maximum composite age of the PAPs should be 90 years wherein the individual age of the PAPs should not be less than 25 years and more than 50 years.

(c) To adopt children above three years of age, the maximum composite age of the PAPs should be 105 years wherein the individual age of the PAPs should not be less than 25 years and more than 55 years.

(d) A single PAP desiring to adopt should not be less than 30 and more than 50. The maximum age shall be 40 years to adopt children in the age group of 0-3 years and 50 years for adopting children above 3 years.

(e) PAPs should have adequate financial resources to provide a good upbringing to the child;

(f) PAPs should have good health and should not be suffering from any contagious or terminal disease or any such mental or physical condition which may prevent them from taking care of the child;

(g) A second adoption is permissible only when the legal adoption of the first child has been finalized;

(h) Single male is not permitted to adopt a girl child

List of documents required for adoption

- Proof of identity (voter card/pan card/passport/driving license)
- Proof of address indicating residence in India exceeding 365 days

- Marriage Certificate
- Family Photograph
- Health certificate by a registered medical practitioner certifying that the Prospective Adoptive Parents (PAPs) are not suffering from any contagious or terminal disease or any such mental or physical condition which may prevent them from taking care of the child.
- Three recent postcard sized photographs of the adoptive family.
- Two letters of recommendation from persons who know the family well (not from immediate relatives of either spouse)
- If the PAPs are self-employed, IT statement for the last three years and if they are employed, Income Certificate from the employer also indicating the date of superannuation.
- Financial statement including copies of bank statement for the last six months, details of movable and immovable property owned by the family and details of loans taken by the PAPs.
- Written consent of the biological and/or adopted child/children and if they are above 7 years of age.
- Adoption decree, if the couple have adopted child/children earlier.
- Divorce/legal separation decree in case of single PAP if applicable.
- Letter from close relative of single PAP stating that in the event of any unforeseen circumstance, the relative would take care of the child.

(Infertility certificate is not required from the PAPs wishing to adopt a child)

Above documents are required to be produced in original along with two self-attested copies by the PAPs.

Chapter - 5

Training Package for Minor Disorders in Pregnancy

— Avinash Rana, Vanita Suri,
LK Dhaliwal, Amarjeet Singh

With the rapid pace of industrialization and urbanization in today's society, the joint family system has broken down. Earlier, elderly women in joint families used to guide/tell pregnant women about maternity/child care. In every family, there used to be many married women living together who shared their experiences and helped each other regarding various aspects of motherhood/ maternity. With the breakdown of joint family system, there is usually no one in the family to guide the women on these issues.

Such problems are particularly faced by the women who become pregnant for the first time .It has been reported that primigravida women often lack knowledge on various aspects of pregnancy, labor, postpartum care and neonatal care e.g. diet, rest, precautions, appropriate postures while working during pregnancy, recognition of true labor pains, diet and hydration during labor etc. Now, all this has been medicalized. The traditional birth attendants who used to take care of maternity related issues in families are also vanishing. The role of the family members & TBA has been taken over by the hospital set up. Nurses and doctors are now expected to tell primigravida women about maternity care which was considered earlier an internal family matter. However, most of the time of nurses/obstetricians is spent in clinical care. Consequently, they have little time to attend to routine day to day advisory needs of pregnant women. The situation is particularly more critical in India where because of its population size hospital is overcrowded. Moreover, in government health care set up in India, female doctors are scarce and are overworked; they are not able to devote adequate time to individual pregnant women. Consequently, in this set up, preparedness of most primigravida for safe motherhood leaves much to be desired.

Health education during pregnancy seeks to enable the pregnant women to actively participate in their own antenatal care with or without the help of nurse or obstetrician. In fact, for primigravida her pregnancy is fraught with many uncertainties. For her the course of pregnancy is an unknown path .There are so many physiological changes during pregnancy and so many likely complications that may occur during antenatal period. However, do's & don'ts during labor are not known to many women, particularly the first timers. Many women are not aware of the guidelines pertaining to these issues. This makes them apprehensive about the course and outcome of the pregnancy. Their anxiety level is also high. Proper knowledge about these things will prepare the women adequately for labor. There are many things women may be taught so that it improves the outcome. e.g. what to eat, what to wear, how to prepare for labor, how to recognize the onset of, labor, what to do when one has cramps, what test to get done etc.

In this context, a study was conducted by Dr Avinash Rana, to ascertain the effect of self-care interventions on preparedness safe motherhood among primigravida mothers. An RCT was done. The study was conducted by the investigator, a trained (M.Sc Psychiatric Nursing) in five visits during 2005 – 2007 in the, Antenatal Clinic OPD. Clean Labor Room, Maternity & Gynae Wards, Nehru Hospital PGIMER, Chandigarh.

In, the initial visit (13 – 20 weeks of gestation) (232) primigravida mothers were recruited. They were randomized into two groups (A only SIM; B SIM + Counseling). Baseline data was collected. The respondents were administered the training packages at various stages i.e. package at 13-20 weeks, the topics of training package 2 at 30-32 week, and training package 3 on the first day after delivery. PI also ascertained their practices during labor. On the spot observation was also done.

The respondents (mother and baby) were examined / interviewed in postnatal follow-up clinic / home visit at six weeks after delivery. PI ascertained their postpartum self-care activities / practices. The information on outcome variables was collected during visits 2-5. These pertained to the items on which the training was given to the respondents during earlier visits e.g. change in knowledge of the respondents regarding recognition of minor disorders like backache, cramps, varicose veins, fainting spells, heartburn, constipation, piles, swelling on face / hands / feet, insomnia, craving, skin changes, warning signals. The investigator also sought to document any impact of the acquired knowledge on the related practices of the respondents e.g. measures taken by them for the remedy of minor disorders, ability to undertake self-care activities for hygiene, bathing, dental care, wearing loose cotton clothes, diet, hydration, correct posture, rest, sleep were also assessed.

Majority (60%) of women had 6 or more symptoms whereas six percent reported only one symptom and 3 mothers did not experience any symptoms. It shows that training improved the correct activities to overcome the symptoms of minor problems which mothers faced in pregnancy. It also shows improvement in their self-care activities.

Overall results indicate pregnant women faced a variety of minor symptoms ranging from weakness, swelling in the face, hands, legs and feet. Naturally, they are very much troubled by these & often seek medical advice for the same. This is particularly more worrying for primigravida. Most of these symptoms can be managed by women themselves without any medicine if they are aware how to deal with them. The present study demonstrated successfully that the pregnant women can easily be trained to manage these symptoms themselves.Training provided in their study improved the percentage of women who took correct actions to overcome the symptoms of minor problems which mothers faced in pregnancy. Primigravida women and their families appreciated the one to one, phone call based and home visit based training by the PI. They also liked the information signed throughout the manual (copy enclosed hereunder).

TRAINING PACKAGE – 1; Visit – I

Minor Disorders in Pregnancy

1. **Backache**

   - As your baby grows your posture changes.
     This puts extra stress on your back and thighs.
   - Hormones of pregnancy relax your joints.
   - As breasts gain in size and weight, the result is a stooped posture.

   Above 3 changes are the possible causes of backache.

WHAT YOU CAN	DO DON'T
Wear low-heeled shoes/slippers with equal level of sole.	Lift heavy weight e.g. bucket full of water
Do abdominal wall exercises (blow out exhale and pull in your abdominal wall for the count of 5).	Do heavy exercises
Practice pelvic tilt exercises	
Do shoulder circles forwards and backwards.	
Stand with your back against a wall. Place a hand in the small of your back then drop your hand.	
Bend your knees when lifting, (basket/bucket)	Lift weight without bending knee

Hold objects as close to your body as possible when you want to lift it.	Hold objects away from your body while lifting
When standing for long periods rest one foot on a stool	Stand for long periods
Regularly rotate your feet in small circles	Rotate your feet too fast
Use the strength of your legs when getting up.	

Correct postures

Most of the problem of backache are due to wrong posture. It can be prevented if correct posture is maintained.

A. STANDING

DO'S	DON'TS
Stand comfortably	Stand on slippery floor
Keep your feet straight on the floor	Bend your shoulders forward and backward
Keep your arms straight by the side of the body	Bend your arms
Keep your neck and head straight	Bend your neck and head forward

B. SITTING: Sit comfortably on the floor, chair/sofa, bed, *peedhi/chownki*

Floor

DO'S	DON'TS
Sit on clean floor	Sit on slippery floor
Keep your buttocks touching the floor level	Keep your buttocks above the floor
Keep your legs straight flexed on the floor	
Sit in a butterfly position (Pix. 1)	

Chair/sofa

DO'S (Pix. 2)

Sit comfortable on the Chair /sofa
Support the back against the back of the chair/sofa
Keep feet on the floor or on the *peedhi / chownki*

DON'TS (Pix. 3)

Sit on too small a chair
Sit on broken chair/sofa
Let feet hang in the air
Leave a gap between your back and the back of chair/sofa

Chownki / peedhi

DO'S	DON'TS
Sit on *peedhi / chownki* as you like	Sit on very small *peedhi / chownki*
Keep your buttocks on it	
Keep your feet touching the floor	Use broken *peedhi / chownki*

LYING DOWN (Pix. 4)

DO'S	DON'TS
Rest in hard bed with firm mattress	Lie down in too loose bed *navar / cane* bed
Lie down in lateral (either position)	Lie down in straight posture 9 2
Keep one / two pillows under head\knee	Keep too many pillows under the head / knee

GETTING UP FROM BED (Pix. 5)

DO'S	DON'TS
Get up slowly	Get up very fast
Change positions slowly	Change positions too fast
Roll over to your side. Use your arms to bring your body to a sitting position.	Do a "sit up"
Bring your legs down/feet should touch the floor	
Sit for 2-3 minutes on the bed and then get up from the bed	Start walking immediately when you get down from bed

2. Cramps in legs

Cause:

- Increased pressure on the nerves in your abdomen by the growing baby.
- Extra strain on your legs due to standing for long duration

Symptoms:

- Sudden pain in the calf muscles (lower leg)
- Difficulty in walking

DO'S	DON'T
Take rest in between where long standing required	Stand for long time
Take three glasses of milk in a day	Forget to take milk.

HOW TO RELIEVE CRAMPS

(a) With the help of another person (Pix. 6)

During cramps another person forces the foot upwards towards the abdomen with one hand on the sole of the feet below the toes, while the woman keeps legs straight by putting pressure on the hand of that person

(b) By self (Pix. 7)

Gently push your feet against a firm surface
Gently stretch your leg against wall/chair
Keep your hands on the wall /chair
Put pressure against the wall
Stretch your legs
Keep your feet on the floor
Put your feet up several times during the day

3. Varicose veins

- The flow of blood from the peripheral parts of the body to heart is slowed because of pressure exerted by your growing baby on the veins.
- The increased fluid in your blood stream and slowed blood flow cause swollen veins.

Symptoms

Pain and tiredness in the lower extremities

- Feeling of heaviness in varicosities in the vulva and perineum
- Redness heat and tenderness at the site.

DO'S	DON'TS
Regular walk	cross your legs/feet while sitting
Put your feet up several times a day on a stool/*peedhi*	Stand / sit in one position for long period
Elevate your legs with hips when you sit	
During long sitting / standing periods (unavoidable reason) walk frequently to promote venous return to the heart	
Do foot exercises (As given in self-care) **(Pix. 13)**	Do foot exercises if ankle is injured

Steps (foot exercises)

DO'S	DON'TS
(A) Dorsiflex the feet (pull upwards) Hold above position for 3 seconds then release Repeat above exercise for 8-10 times each day	Do dorsiflex the foot too forcefully

(B) Lie down with your legs elevated Keep too many pillows while on pillows and place one pillow lying down under one hip elevated (to avoid compression of the veins)

4. Varicosities of vulva and anus

- Aches and sense of heaviness on the vulva and perineum

DO'S	DON'TS
Take lots of water	Forget to take fluids
Apply perineal pad for support	Leave the varicosities of vulva and anus without support
Lie down in Sim's position i.e. keep one pillow under the head. Lying down in left side straighten the left leg and place the left arm at the back side slightly in flexed position. Flex and place your right arm and leg on the one pillow under each.	Lie down in straight position

5. Fainting spells

- Feeling of dizziness for few seconds.

DO'S	DON'TS
Lie on your left side	Lie down supine or straight on your back
Sit down immediately and lower your head between the legs, when you feel uneasy / dizzy.	Start walking immediately
Take sweet/sugar immediately	Be in hurry

DO'S	DON'TS
Take glucose water	Take extra sweet/sugar if you have diabetes
Get blood pressure checked up	

Prevention

- Arise slowly from resting position
- Change positions slowly
- Avoid prolonged standing in warm/stuffy environment
- Make sure you are eating and drinking enough at regular times
- Always keep some toffees in your pocket/purse
- Wear loose clothes

6. Heart burn

Burning and irritation in the food pipe which goes upwards leaving bad taste in the mouth.

Cause

- Due to displacements of the stomach by enlarging uterus.

DO'S	DON'TS
Eat small and frequent meals	Take those food that make you feel uncomfortable.
Walk for 10-15 minutes in the room after each meal	Lie down 2 hours after a meal
Sleep with your head raised on a pillow	Take medicine unless suggested by doctor
Take last meals at least 2 hours before bed time	Take fried / fatty food

Remedy

- Drink adequate amount of fluids each day.
- Take frequent sips of milk / water
- Take 10ml chilled milk without sugar
- Take one table spoon antacid (Gel) before meal.

7. Constipation

- Difficult to pass hard stool.

Causes:

- As your baby grows, it puts more pressure on your bowel obstructing it.

DO'S	DON'TS
Drink 6-8 glasses of fluids every day.	Forget to take water / fluids
Take a glass of warm water in the morning before tea/breakfast	Take any medicine unless advised by doctor
Add more fruits and vegetables (spinach, cabbage, *sag* etc) in your meal	Take *maida* made stuff such as pizza, bread etc.
Exercise regularly 3 to 4 times a week	
Go for morning and evening walk	

8. Piles

Pressure on blood vessels in your rectum can cause a slowing of the blood flow and swelling of the veins.It cause burning, itching and sometimes bleeding

DO'S	DON'TS
Lie on your side while resting	Sit / stand too long
Do pelvic floor exercises.	Do fomentation
Reduce the swelling by raising your hips and legs several times a day advice	Take any medicine without doctor
Apply ice / cold packs and hemorrhoid cream	
Take advice if you have severe pain	
Go to doctor if piles persists	
Avoid constipation	

9. Swelling (feet, hands, ankles)

Some swelling on your feet below the ankle is normal but if it is increasing; involves your hands and face, consult a doctor.

Cause

- Extra fluid in your body
- Pressure on blood vessels in your pelvis by your growing baby

DO'S	DON'TS
Get blood pressure checked frequently	Stand/walk for long periods
Put your feet up as often as possible	Stay in one position for long periods
Go to doctor if finger ring is tight	Add extra salt in diet and avoid potato-chips, soft drinks preserved meats and pickles
Rest and sleep on your left side	Reduce your fluids
Use normal amount of salt	Wear tight clothes rings / shoes
Exercise regularly.	
Wear support stockings. Put them on before you get out of bed in the morning	

(Sudden excessive swelling may be a sign of HIGH BLOOD PRESSURE, see your doctor immediately)

10. Sleeplessness or insomnia

DO'S	DON'TS
Daily walk in the evening	Do exhaustive walk in the evening
Take a glass of warm milk at bed time	Take rest less than 2 hours
Read story book	Read books till late night
Wear loose clothes at night	Wear tight clothes
Take frequent rest in between before you become overtired	

DO'S	DON'TS
Use extra pillow for comfort when lie on your side. Place one or two pillows	Use more than two pillows on your head side
under your head and another small pillow between your knees and one behind your back	Forget to do regular exercise
During the day take short breaks with your feet up.	
Exercise regularly	
Reduce caffeine intake	Take too much caffeine.

11. Cravings (pica)

When you crave for certain foods or unnatural substances such as clay (*mitti*), coal, *rajasthani mitti, pickles* etc

Causes: Due to changes in the body

DO'S	DON'TS
Eat well balanced diet	Eat unnatural substances too much
Take advice from doctor / nurse if you consume too much unnatural substances If you are crave for unnatural substances	Feel shy to ask the doctor/ nurse.

12. Skin changes

- Dark discoloration on face, breasts abdomen and thighs.

Causes

- Due to stretching of the skin during pregnancy

DO'S	DONT'S
Wear loose clothes	Scratch on the abdomen
Apply cold cream	Neglect if itching present along with yellow discoloration of the skin (it may be due to jaundice or more at night time may be scabies).

13. Frequent passing of urine

- As your baby is pressing on your bladder

DO'S	DONT'S
Drink 6-8 glasses of fluid in a day	Reduce the amount of fluids that you drink
Do pelvic floor exercises (pull up and tighten the pelvic floor muscles as if you are stopping the flow of urine)	Take too much caffeine
Repeat this exercise 5 to 10 times, several time a day	Practice the exercise while passing urine
Wash your perineal area with soap water and dry it after voiding.	Forget to wash your perineal area
Wear clean under wear.	

Consult doctor, if pain, burning or hematuria occur	Delay to consult doctor, if pain burning or hematuria occurs.

14. Dyspnea

- "Shortness of breath during pregnancy".

Cause

Decrease in thoracic space due to the upward displacement of diaphragm due to enlarging uterus.

DO'S	DON'TS
Use good posture	
Do tailor reach exercise	Overexert while doing domestic / official activities
*Sleep in semi-flower position with extra pillows under the head and shoulder	
Lie down on left lateral position	
Eat small meals at frequent intervals	
Consult the doctor if dyspnea is continuous	

* All position explained in self care during pregnancy.

Fatigue and drowsiness

- Feeling of weakness

DO'S	DON'TS
Take rest, before you become overtired	Become overtired
Take short break during the day time with your feet up	
Eat well balanced diet (including Take extra coffee fruits, vegetables, milk, juices etc.)	
Do exercise regularly	
Use extra pillows for comfort during sleeping	
Lie on left lateral side	

DANGER SIGNALS IN PREGNANCY & THEIR MANAGEMENT

(Things to be kept in mind when you are shifting to hospital because of emergency)

- Do not panic.
- Keep clean perineal pad (in case of bleeding / leakage per vagina).
- Always lie down on left lateral position during transportation.
- Keep some help ready (Extra hand / money).

Danger Signals in Pregnancy

- Every delivery is a risk situation
- Risk can lead to death or disease of the MOTHER & BABY

- This can be avoided or minimized by early detection of such risks and relevant remedial measures.

1. Vaginal bleeding before the birth of the baby

Any type of bleeding per vagina before the birth of the baby can be dangerous for the mother / baby. It may be with / without pains. **If you have such bleeding, rush to the hospital immediately** (or consult a doctor).

What to do (till you reach hospital)

- Keep clean perineal pad
- Lie down in left lateral position
- Save all the perineal pads and show to the doctor when you reach hospital (to estimate loss of blood)
    - Tell the doctor whether bleeding p/v started before or after onset of labour pains
- Move to the hospital as early as possible
- Do not eat or drink anything except water
- Avoid internal examination by *dai* or others

2. Premature rupture/break of bag of water

- In the womb baby floats in a bag of water. This bag can rupture any time anywhere during pregnancy with / without labour pains. Warm liquid may also dribble out or gush profusely with / without labour pain.

What to do

AT HOME	IN HOSPITAL
Note the time when leakage started	Show the perineal pad to the doctor
Keep a clean pad as you keep during menstruation	Tell the doctor what time the leakage started
See the color of leakage whether it is like clear water, green / yellow in colour	Lie down on left lateral side
If it is clear / green / yellow / blood stained in colour without delay come to the hospital immediately	Do not take any anything by mouth (there may be the need of operation)
Lie in left lateral position during transportation	

3. Greenish fluid comes out of vagina before the birth of the baby

- Normally baby do not pass stool inside the womb. But under stress the unborn baby passes stools in the womb. It indicate that there is some problem inside the womb. If transportation to the hospital is delayed the unborn baby may aspirate this greenish fluid. This can kill the baby. Immediate action has to be taken.

What to do

IN HOME	IN HOSPITAL
Keep clean perineal pad	Show the perineal pad to the doctor
Lie down in left lateral position	Lie down in left lateral position
Do not take any thing by mouth (There may be need of operation)	Do not panic if operation is advised

4. Any change in fetal movements

- Any change in fetal movements indicate fetus is at stress. Always keep record of your baby's movements.

How to count fetal movements

Sit comfortably on the chair or bed one hour after each meal(breakfast, lunch, dinner) OR

- Lie down on left lateral side.
- Keep pen/pencil and a diary or paper
- Keep your hand on upper abdomen
- Feel whenever baby moves and record with pencil on the paper
- Record the fetal movements for 3 hours (till one hour after every meal – breakfast, lunch and dinner) if the count is less than 10-12 movements in three flows/less than 3 movements per hour approach the doctor.

What to do

IN HOME	IN HOSPITAL
Keep a record of fetal movements with date and time. (6th month onwards)	
Lie down on lateral side to feel fetal movement for 1 hour.	Show the fetal movements chart to the doctor.
Count for another hour if no movements then immediately come to the hospital	

5. Persistent headache, blurring vision, sudden and severe vomiting

- If you have these together, these are the signs of high blood pressure.

What to do

AT HOME	IN HOSPITAL
Immediately lie down on left lateral side	Don't be anxious
Immediately come to hospital with one/two family members if you have headache	Lie down in lateral side

6. Premature labour pains

When labor pains start before 9th months it is known as premature labor. The lady may have -

- cramps (may feel like menstrual cramps/gas pain)
- low back pain and uterus becomes hard
- fluid gush or leakage of fluid from birth canal
- change/increase in vaginal discharge
- full/heavy feeling in the birth passage (vagina)

What to do at home

AT HOME	IN HOSPITAL
Immediately rush to the hospital	
Don't panic	Lie down in lateral position.
Keep clean perineal pad in underwear if there is leakage or blood discharge p/v.	
Lie down in lateral side	
Be prepared. Baby may be too small. It will need special care/incubator care.	

7. Prolonged labour (More than 12 hours)

- When labour pains are very strong and contractions are painful but ineffective to open the mouth of the uterus and last more than 12 hours without result.

What to do

AT HOME	IN HOSPITAL
Take deep breath during labour pains through nose and exhale through the lips	Give complete history (since how long continuously labour pains are there)
Lie down on lateral side	Lie down on lateral side
Move to the hospital without any delay	Do not take anything by mouth

8. Pain in abdomen

- Never ignore pain in lower abdomen in pregnancy. It can be dangerous for your baby.

What to do

AT HOME	AT HOSPITAL
Note the characteristic of pain – Does it start from back & comes forward.	Give complete history of abdominal pain whether it was accompanied with bleeding per vaginally
Note if there is any bleeding per vaginally. Keep pad in the undergarments	Lie down on lateral position
Lie down on left lateral side	
Don't take any medicine to relieve the pain.	

SELF CARE IN PREGNANCY

1. Hygiene

- Daily hygiene is important during pregnancy because of the increase in perspiration and vaginal discharge caused by hormonal changes.

2. Bathing

- Take daily bath with soap & water.
- Sit on the stool/*chownki* while taking bath.
- Keep your feet very carefully against slipping in the bathroom.
- Always wear rough surface sole *chappal* (avoid slippery soles).
- Regular scrubbing of the bathroom floor should be done.

3. Breast care

- Keep your breasts clean.
- Wash them daily with soap & water while taking bath.
- Wear well fitted/supportive bra.
- Examine for any abnormality.
- Do nipples exercises if nipples are inverted (nipples are facing inward).

Nipple Rolling (Fig. 1)

- Gently pull them between thumb and index finger.
- Hold them in this position for 1-2 minutes.
- Repeat this for 5-6 times during bath.

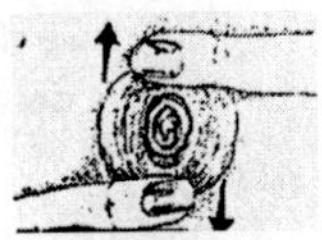

Nipple-Stretching (Fig. 2)
Place thumb/index fingers opposite each other near the edge of the dark part (Areola) of the breast.

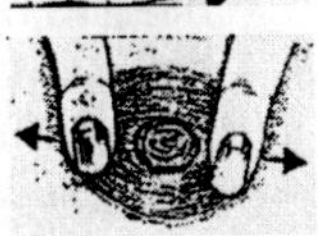

- Press the breast and stretch outward.
- Hold then in this position for 1-2 minutes.
- Repeat this for 5-6 times during bath.

4. Care of perineum

- Wash the perineal area with soap and water (from front to back).
- Change undergarments everyday.
- Wear cotton undergarments.
- Remove pubic hairs throughout the pregnancy.

5. Dental care

- Brush your teeth everyday in the morning.
- Brush your teeth after dinner also.
- Use soft toothbrush.
- Avoid tooth extraction during pregnancy.

6. Clothing

- Wear loose and light cotton clothes [*kameez* and *salwar*].
- Wear loose undergarments.
- Tie the salwar/petticot below the umbilicus.

7. Shoes

- Wear comfortable flat/low heel shoes/*chappals* with rough sole surface.

8. Travel

- Avoid long traveling in the 7th, 8th and 9th months of pregnancy.
- Travel in the train is more comfortable than bus. Do not travel in auto rickshaw
- If you are traveling in the train walk in the train at regular interval while holding the railings.
- *If there is bleeding p/v the traveling should be avoided.*
- If travel in car, after every few hours take a break and walk for sometime.
- Apply seat belt one part above the umbilicus and other below the umbilicus (Pix. 8).

9. Rest

- Rest for two hours in day time and 10 hours in night time.
- Rest in lateral (right/left side; preferably left side).
- Keep one pillow under the head. Turn your body either left/right side.
- Keep another pillow in between the knees.

10. Sleep

- Sleep in well ventilated room.
- Lie down on hard mattress / *gadda*.
- Wear loose clothes during night.
- Sleep in right/left lateral position (preferably left side).

11. Diet

- Do not skip any food.
- Take meals in small quantity but at frequent intervals.
- Take any fruit such as apple, orange, banana 3-4 times a days.
- Take a glass of juice.

- Take at least 2 glasses of milk.
- Do include lots of green leafy vegetable e.g. spinach, *methi* for iron, fresh fruits for vitamins, jaggery for energy. Gram (*chana*)

12. Supplements

- Take the diet as advised by doctor.
- Take tablets of iron and folic acid and calcium per day.
- Iron tablets cause constipation and black stools.
- Take lot of fluids regularly.

13. Household activities (Pix. 9)

A. Avoid lifting heavy objects.

B. Lift objects from the floor in following manner

- Bring the object near the body.
- Keep your back straight
- Bend your knees.

C. Cleaning the floor

- Clean the floor in sitting position.

D. Cooking

- Do not cook for long time in standing position.
- Do cooking in sitting position.

14. Injection tetanus toxoid (TT)

- Have two doses of Injection T-T with a gap of 4-6 weeks between the two doses. First dose should be as early as possible.

15. Coitus

- Sexual intercourse is not prohibited in pregnancy.
- However, avoid sexual intercourse in last one and half months of pregnancy.

16. Drugs

- Do not take any medicine without advice by doctor.

17. Smoking

- Do not smoke during pregnancy.
- Ask the husband and the family members not to smoke in that room where you sit/sleep.

18. Correct postures

Standing

- Put equal weight on both legs.
- Keep your feet apart.
- Both abdomen and buttocks tucked in.
- Keep your shoulders relaxed at the side and down.
- Choose comfortable chair; Sit close to your desk / table to avoid bending forward.
- Support your back against the back of the chair.
- Thighs should rest on the chair.
- Keep the knees slightly higher than hips.
- Keep your feet on the floor or *peeddi*.
- On easy chair, support your head with pillow and raise your legs on the stool.

19. Lying down

Side – Lying Position (Pix. 4,5)

- Keep one pillow under the head and another under the arm.
- Straighten the lower leg.
- Flex upper leg.
- Keep one pillow under the upper leg.

Half Back Lying Position (Pix.. 10)

- Keep 2-3 pillows under the head.
- Keep one pillow under the back and another under the knees.
- Straighten the legs.

Getting Up From Lying Position (Pix. 5)

- Bend your knees
- Roll on to one side.
- Put the pressure on one elbow joint to prevent strain on back and abdomen.
- Hand of another arm should touch the bed.
- Sit for 2-3 minutes, then walk if you want.

20. Antenatal exercises

Guidelines for Exercises

- Do regular exercises (at least 3 times a week)
- Stop exercise when you feel tired.
- Exercise in safe and in cool surroundings.
- Drink extra fluid before and after exercising.
- Avoid exercises with jerking, bouncing and jumping.
- Avoid any type of exercises that cause a loss of balance, falling or mild abdominal injury.
- Avoid exercises that require you to lie on your back after 3rd - 4th month of pregnancy.
- Empty your bladder before exercises.

Pelvic Tilting or Rocking Exercises

- Lie down in half lying position.
- Bend knees with feet flat on the bed / floor.
- Place one hand under the small of your back.
- Place another hand on the top of your abdomen.
- Tighten the abdomen and buttocks.
- Lift the buttocks about 3-4" from the surface.
- Press the small of the back down on to the underneath hand.
- Breathe normally, hold for up to 10 seconds than relax.
- Repeat up to 10 times.

Pelvic Floor Exercise

- Sit, stand or half lying down with legs apart. Do these exercises after urination
- Close and draw up around the back passage as though preventing a bowel action.
- Repeat around the front two passages as preventing the flow of urine.
- Hold up to 10 seconds, breathing normally and relax.
- Repeat up to 10 times.

Abdominal Tightening

- Lie down in half lying position.
- Breathe in and out.
- Pull in the lower part of the abdomen below the umbilicus while breathing normally and then breathed out.
- Hold breath for 10 seconds and then relax.
- Repeat up to 10 times.

Breathing Awareness Exercises

- Sit comfortably with eyes closed
- Take deep breath in from the nose and breathe out from mouth.
- Listen to your breathing especially outward breath.
- Recognizing short pause before inward breathing naturally follows.

Foot and Leg Exercises (Pix. 11)

Sit or half lie with back supported.

Bend and stretch the ankles at 10-12 times.

Circle both feet at the ankle at least
10 times in each.

Inner thigh Stretches (Pix. 12, 13)

- Sit in a butterfly position with heels together.
- Pull the knee close to your body.
- Gently press both knees towards the floor.
- Relax.
- Repeat this for 10 times.

Tailor Reach Exercise (Pix. 14)

- Sit with legs crossed at ankles.
- Stretch arms over head.
- Reach up with right arm, then with left arm.

FOLLOWING PICTURES ILLUSTRATE THE THINGS TO BE DONE BY WOMEN FOR MINOR DISORDERS IN PREGNANCY

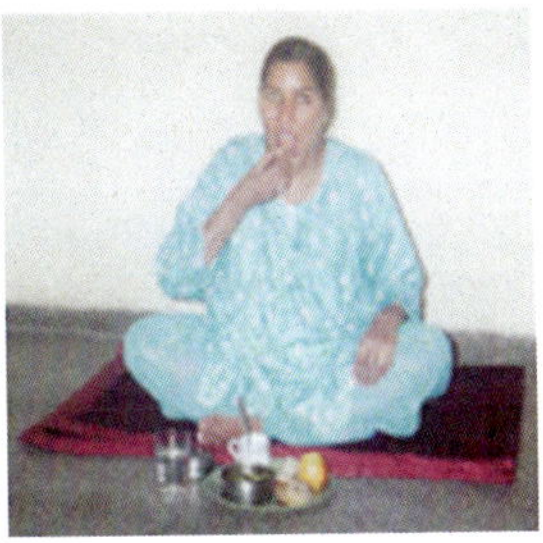

Pix. 1: Sit comfortably on the floor.

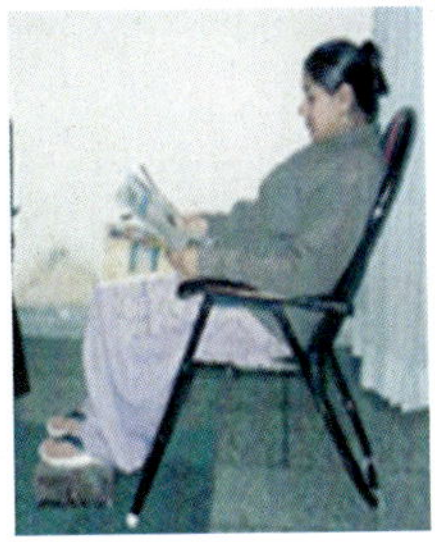

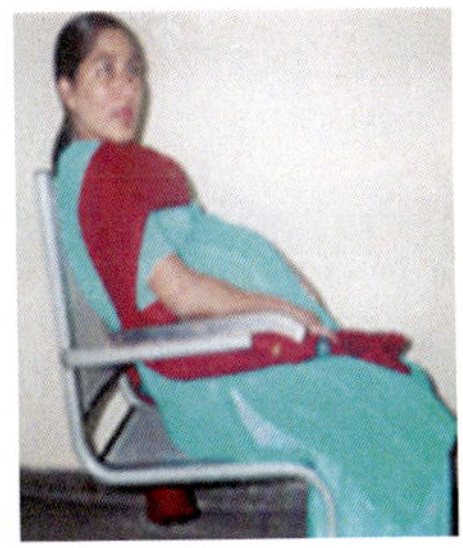

Pix. 2-3: Sit comfortably on the Chair

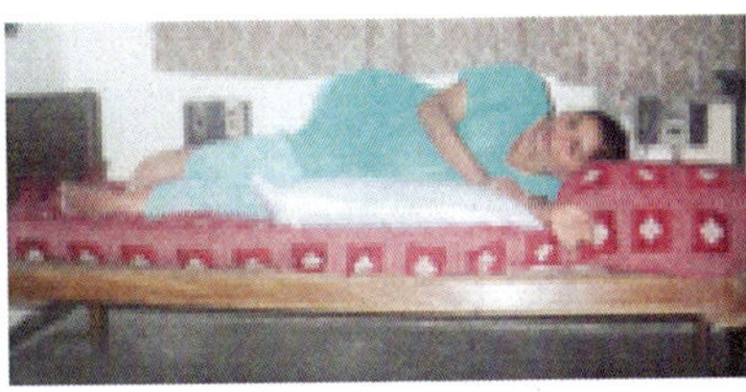

Pix. 4: Lying Down.

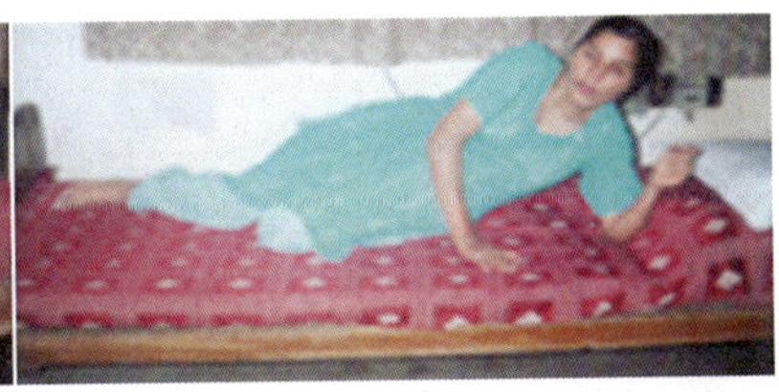

Pix. 5: Getting Up From Bed.

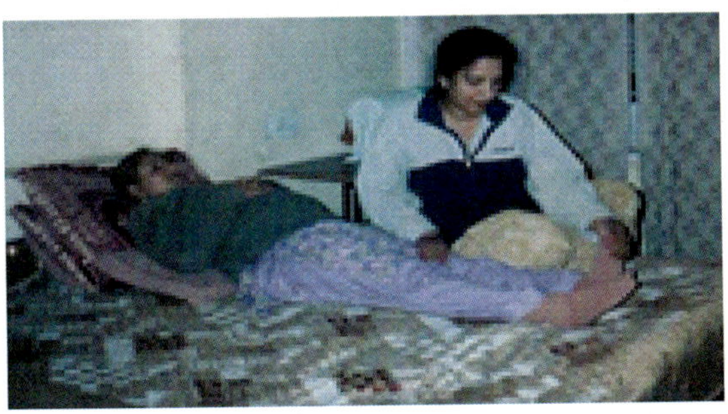

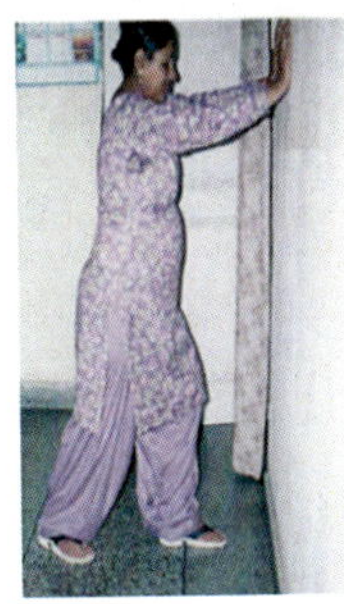

Relieving Cramps — (a) Pix. 6-With the help of another person (b) Pix. 7 -Alone.

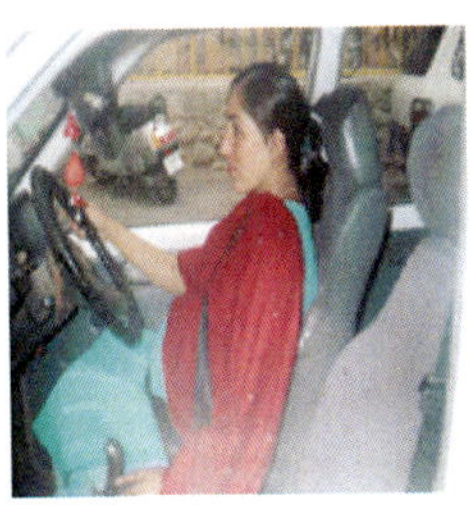

Pix. 8: Driving posture.

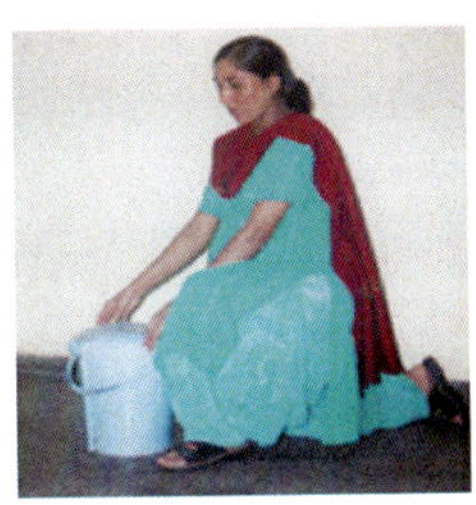

Pix. 9: lifting heavy objectsfrom the floor.

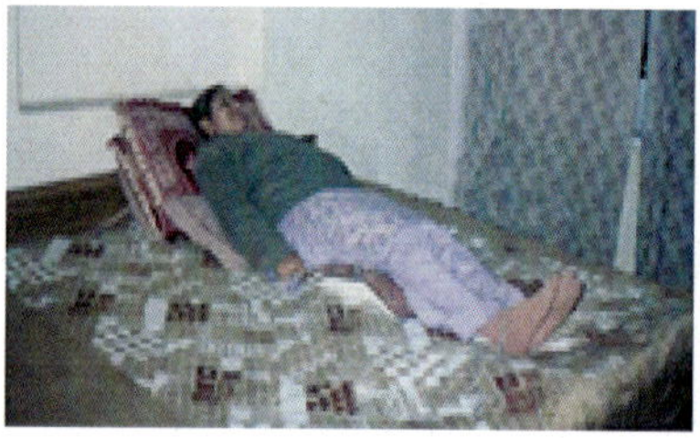

Pix. 10: Half Back Lying Position.

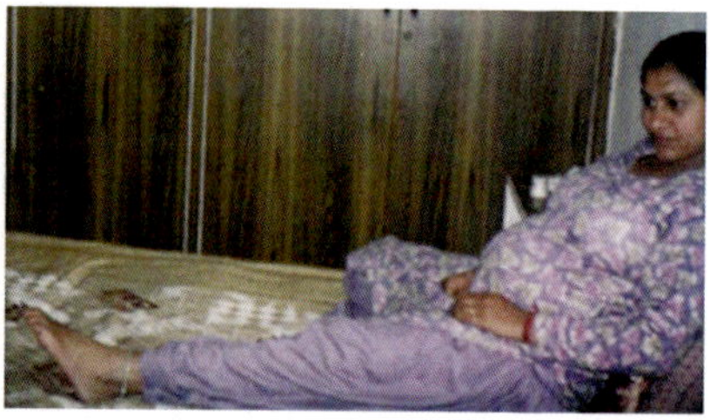

Pix. 11: Foot and Leg Exercises.

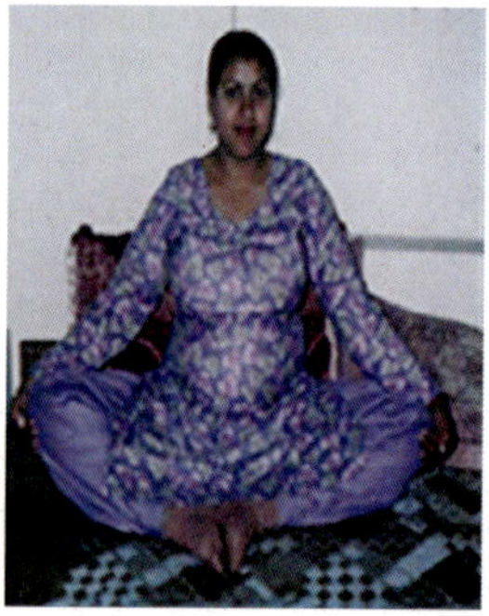

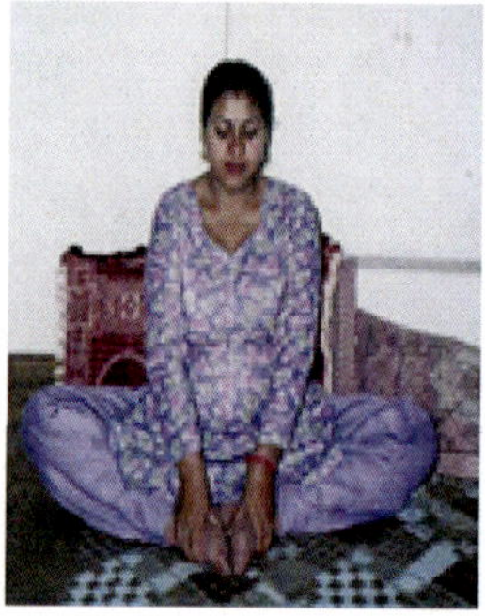

Pix. 12-13: Inner thigh Stretches(butterfly position)

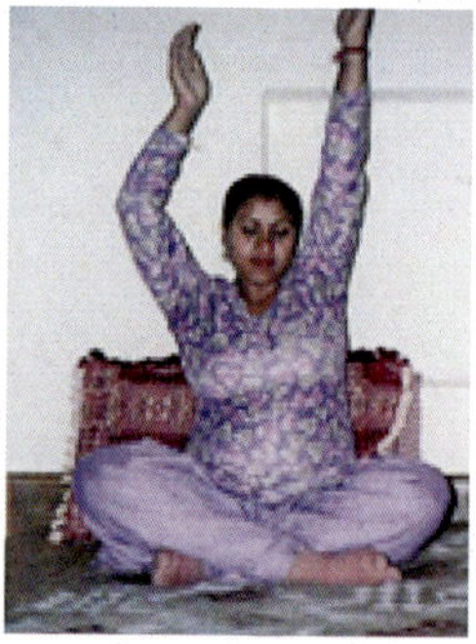

Pix. 14: Tailor Reach Exercise.

Chapter - 6

Intervention package for the Health and Fitness of Ante - And Post-Natal Women

— *Pradeep Sarkar, MS Dhillon, Paramveer Singh, Vanita Suri, Amarjeet Singh*

Introduction

Pregnancy brings about many changes in mothers' body which continues even after baby is born. After a vaginal delivery, taking good care of mother is an essential part of postpartum care and to maintain overall fitness. This is the time of restoration of muscle tone and connective tissue to the pre-pregnant state. Although change is subtle during this phase, a woman's body is not fully restored to pre-pregnant physiology until about 6 months post-delivery. But full restoration of fitness is not always possible; women usually loose shape of her body permanently. In modern era almost every woman wishes to bring back and maintain her shape as it was pre-pregnant state. Even the women from well to do family do not receive any fitness advice because in India we do not have basic infrastructure to deliver fitness packages.

Birth preparedness is advance planning and preparation for delivery which helps ensure that women can reach professional delivery care when labor begins.

This will also help reduce the delays that occur when women experience obstetric complications. Here comes the role of health care providers which almost untouched in Indian scenario. So we need to develop a management package which is scientific and evidence based, so that at pre-natal and post-natal stage, mothers suffer less complications and recover from the health complications as early as possible. This will help the mother to maintain and improve their fitness level as normal as possible and also stay fit in future. An attempt has been made by the authors to bring together all training related interventions to see their impact.

In the first few weeks after delivery, gentle lower belly and pelvic exercises are all it takes to help the mother's body to recover. It has following beneficial effects:-

1. Boost mothers' mood by increasing the levels of feel-good chemicals (endorphins)
2. Help to lose weight and regain pre-baby figure.
3. Protection from aches and pains.
4. Improve strength and stamina, which helps looking after newborn easier.
5. Helps to control the bladder and bowel in antenatal and postnatal stage.

The most important exercises in the first few days after birth are pelvic floor exercises. Start doing them as soon as she can. Strengthening pelvic floor will help to protect against having accidental urine leaks. Pelvic floor exercises will also help perineum and vagina to heal more quickly. That's because the exercises improve circulation to the area, helping to reduce swelling pain and bruising. If mother have stitches, gentle pelvic floor muscle exercise won't put any strain on them.

In this regard, there is plenty of scope and potential in the discipline of physiotherapy to maintain and bring back the fitness of pre & post-natal women. Another important aspect is whatever the books, journal and information regarding maintenance of fitness are available that are mostly generic in nature prepared for all women. There are no special applicable guidelines for sports women or working mother. Ideally the fitness program should be need based. This is the era of customized or individualized fitness programs which are required for the modern women.

Following pregnancy related problems can be rectified by physiotherapeutic intervention, as described here under-

Prenatal stage

- Women with pregnancy related abdominal weakness/overstretching of the rectus abdominus muscles
- Women with pregnancy related carpel tunnel syndrome
- Women with pregnancy related bladder problems (urinary incontinence)
- Low and mid back pain
- Leg cramp
- Sacro-Iliac Joint (SIJ)pain (+/- sciatica), Pubic Symphysis pain

- Piriformis muscle spasm
- Shifting of center of gravity anteriorly/Postural changes
- Respiratory distress

Intranatally

Ease of delivery in stage II

Postnatally

- Back, shoulder and neck pain
- SIJ, pubic symphysis or piriformis pain
- Rectus Diastasis
- Abdominal bulging during movement
- Post caesarean pain (after healing)
- Perineal pain and discomfort
- Bladder/bowel control difficulties and constipation/straining (stress/urge urinary incontinence)
- Obesity
- Pelvic organ prolapse (prolapsed uterus)
- Thoracic pain
- Rib pain
- Varicose vein

Earlier the focus of the health care planners was on maternal mortality which did not address individual problems of women. As the society progresses, quality of life of the women becomes an important factor which needs attention of the health care providers. Often some problems precipitated during pregnancy or puerperium continue throughout life. Their health is always at risk after pregnancy. Some of them are forced to leave or change their profession just because of lack of fitness. There is a need to develop a package of intervention to help women regain their fitness level after delivery.

To deliver this fitness program in scientific way help of an expert hand is important. It is also important to develop the program according to the need of the subjects. As we know, the sportswomen need to develop the fitness in respect of their sports field, a teacher need to develop the fitness so that she can stand in the class room for longer duration, an actress needs to remain fit for various role she may play, a house wife also needs to develop in a way so that she can easily carry out the household work and so on for each and every woman. Hence, customized development of fitness program is important.

Self Instruction Manual (SIM)/Intervention package

Before starting the exercise program following components has to be taken care:

Do's

- All The exercises should be done on a hard bed or a flat surface
- Take rest as often as she can with feet up slightly higher than the level of the hips.
- To get out of bed, draw tummy in, keep knees together, roll on the side and get up by taking the weight on the arms.
- Stand tall with buttocks and tummy tucked in and knees relaxed.
- Always sit with the back fully supported with a cushion or pillow.
- Maintain a gap of at least one hour between meal and exercise.
- Always do the exercises after breastfeeding the baby (for lactating women).
- Do the exercises 2 times a day.

Don'ts

- High impact exercises like jumping, running, fast lateral movements.
- Sudden changes in direction of movements.
- Extremes of joint bending and straightening.
- All activities that cause discomfort and increase in low back pain.
- All activities that cause vaginal bleeding.
- Do not stand or sit for long periods.
- Always take frequent rest while doing work and exercise.
- Do not stoop. When lifting, she should bend knees, keep the back straight.
- Keep her back straight and pull up pelvic floor as she takes the weight of the object.
- Do not lift or carry heavy weights.

EXERCISES DURING PREGNANCY

1. Breathing exercises

Deep breathing exercises during pregnancy help women to relax. This exercise should be done throughout the prenatal and post natal stage. This will help to avoid any breathing trouble. It will also help to control pain.

This ensures a steady intake of oxygen into our body system. This also prepares the woman to maintain uniform and rhythmic breathing during labor.

Exercise steps

- Breathing exercise is done in sitting position with back supported with legs straightened out on a horizontal surface.
- Keep hands on the mid chest with palms facing the bone (on the sternum), elbows show be in straight line horizontally.
- Breathe in slowly through nose for longer duration and breathe out through mouth.
- Do the exercise for 10-15 repetitions.
- Do it twice daily.

2. Active Foot and Ankle exercise

These exercises reduce swelling, improve blood circulation, decrease patient discomfort and fatigue. These increase circulation in the legs and reduce edema of the feet.

Exercise steps

- Active foot and ankle exercise can be done in
  - (a) sitting position with back supported and legs hanging down as sitting on chair...OR
  - (b) sitting position with legs straightened out sitting on a bed with back supported...OR
  - (c) lying position with back supported and legs straightened out.
- The effects of this exercise on circulation can be enhanced if the legs are supported and raised higher than the hips. This way gravity assists in return of blood flow to heart.
- Movements of ankles and foot should be done in 3 steps:
  - (1) Flexion (upwards towards the leg)
  - (2) Extension(opposite or downwards away from leg)
  - (3) Rotation in wide circles, first in one direction (clockwise) and then the other (anticlockwise).
- Repeat it 10 to 12 times slowly.
- Do it twice daily.

3. Stretching exercises

(a) Leg and Abdominal Stretching Exercises

Leg and abdominal stretching exercises will improve flexibility as well as strengthen the stomach region.

Exercise steps

- Do this exercise in lying position.

- Lie down on back with arms at sides and legs extended (straightened).
- Then lift right leg up as high as possible. Be comfortable.
- Hold this position for a count of five.
- Bring leg back down and repeat with left leg.
- Repeat it 10 times on both the legs.
- Do it twice daily.

(b) Tailor press- Adductor stretching (butterfly exercise):

This increases mobility of the hip joints and stretches the adductor muscles as well as the perineal muscles. This ultimately helps in easier vaginal delivery.

Exercise steps

- Do this exercise in sitting position on bed or floor.
- Sit with knees bent pointing outwards on the sides and the soles of feet should be kept together at the centre in front of you.
- Grasp ankles by hands, pull feet gently toward the body.
- Then put your hands on the knees and gently grasp them.
- Keep spine straight and gently flap knees down and up, resembling the movement of a butterfly as it flaps its wings.
- Repeat this exercise 10 times.
- Do it twice daily.

4. Strengthening exercise

Pelvic tilt in supine position The pelvic tilt movement in supine position strengthens and tones the abdominal muscles. It also stretches the lower back muscles. It is most helpful for decreasing the lumbar lordosis, realigning posture, and reducing low back pain.

Exercise steps

(a) Isometric abdominal exercise

- The exercise should be done in lying position
- Knees bent at around 90 degrees pointing upwards and feet flat on the surface.
- Place a folded towel horizontally under your lower back.
- Then press the lower part of back against the folded towel
- Notice the upward tilting movement of pelvis and tightening in the abdominal part.
- Hold this position of pressing the towel for a count of five .Then slowly release.

- Repeat this exercise 10 times.
- Do it twice daily.

(b) Pelvic bridging exercises :

- This is to be done in lying position.
- Bend knees pointing upwards and place feet flat on the floor or bed.
- Contract abdominal muscles and hip muscles.
- Slowly lift the pelvis(hip) up of the bed surface till comfortably done.
- At the top i.e. with pelvis up, hold for a count of five.
- Then release.
- Relax down with back (lying) on the surface.
- Repeat the exercise up to 10 times.
- Do it twice daily.

EXERCISES AFTER DELIVERY

1. **Breathing exercises**

   Same as explained in the exercises during pregnancy

2. **Active Foot and Ankle exercise:**

   Same as explained in the exercises during pregnancy

3. **Stretching exercise**

   Cat and camel exercise in quadruped position:

The cat and camel exercise is to increase thoracic spine i.e. middle and upper back mobility, reduce stiffness and increase flexibility in trunk. It improves posture and helps to decrease and prevent back pain.

Exercise steps

- Get down on hands and knees on the floor or bed (as a cat does) Relax the head, and allow it to droop in between your shoulders.
- Inhale, tighten the abdomen.
- Then curve (round) the back up toward the ceiling as resembling a hump until a little stretch is felt in upper, middle, and lower back.
- Hold this stretch for a count of five and repeat it 10 times.
- Return to the starting position with a flat back while on all fours i.e. knees and hands.
- Then lower (curve down) the abdomen toward the floor
- Head extended with looking up at the ceiling.

- Hold this position for a count of five
- Repeat it 10 times.
- Do it twice daily.

(a) Strengthening exercise: 4 point kneeling - arm lift and leg extension

It activates transverse abdominis muscle and reduce the laxity of abdominal muscles.

Exercise steps — For arms:

- Kneel down on hands and knees resting on a flat surface at 90 degrees on bed or flat surface.
- Lift one arm out in front to horizontal plane.
- Hold it for count of five.
- Keep the back straight.
- Do not reach the arm above horizontal.
- Lower the arm slowly on the bed.
- Repeat it on other arm.
- Repeat it 10 times on both arms.
- Do it twice daily.

For legs

- Kneel down on hands and knees resting on a flat surface at 90 degrees on bed or a flat surface.
- Lift one leg from the bed at back and straighten it as far as comfortable.
- Do not make it too horizontal.
- Hold it for a count of five.
- Lower the leg slowly back to original position with knee on the bed.
- Do same on another leg.
- Repeat it 10 times on both legs.
- Do it twice daily.

(b) Leg lifts/side leg raisers

This exercise is to strengthen the weak hip stabilizing muscle i.e gluteus medius.

Exercise steps

- Do this in lying position on a bed or flat surface.

- Lie on the right side with shoulders, hips lined up straight and with bent knee backwards.
- Support the body by holding the head with folded right arm put below it.
- Place the left arm on the floor or on the bed in front.
- Slowly lift the left leg as high as comfortable (with knee straight).
- Hold it for a count of five and then relax.
- Repeat this exercise on the other side also.
- Do this exercise for 10 times and twice daily.

4. Isometric exercises of neck

These enhance stabilization. It boosts strength of neck and shoulder muscles. It also helps to alleviate neck pain. It includes

(a) Static flexion

(b) Static extension

(c) Isometric lateral flexion

Exercise steps

(a) Static Flexion –

- Join both hands together, clasp your finger, and put them with palms facing on forehead.
- Gently push forehead against the hands.
- Tighten the neck muscles.
- Do not to let the head move forward i.e. press back head with hands.
- Hold this position for a count of five. Rest the neck.
- Repeat it 10 times.Do it twice daily.

(b) Static Extension –

- Join both hands together, clasp your finger, and put them with palms facing on lower back of head.
- Apply slight forward pressure with hands and push head back against the hands.
- Be conscious that head does not fall backward.
- Hold the position for a count of five.
- Repeat it 10 times.
- Do it twice daily

Isometric Lateral Flexion –

- Place left hand on the left side of face or head, just near the left ear.
- Tighten the neck muscles.
- Try to move the head sideways.
- Resist the pressure by hand.
- Hold the position for a count of five.
- Rest the neck.
- Then repeat.
- Do the same procedure to the right side.

FOLLOWING PICTURES SHOW THE EXERCISES / POSTURE TO BE USED FOR FITNESS OF ANTE - / POST-NATAL WOMEN

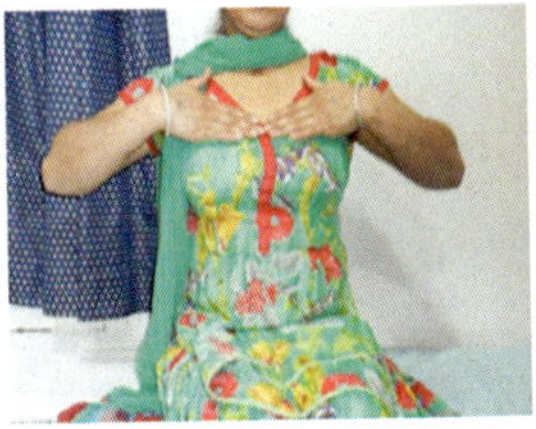

Pix. 1:
Breathing exercise.

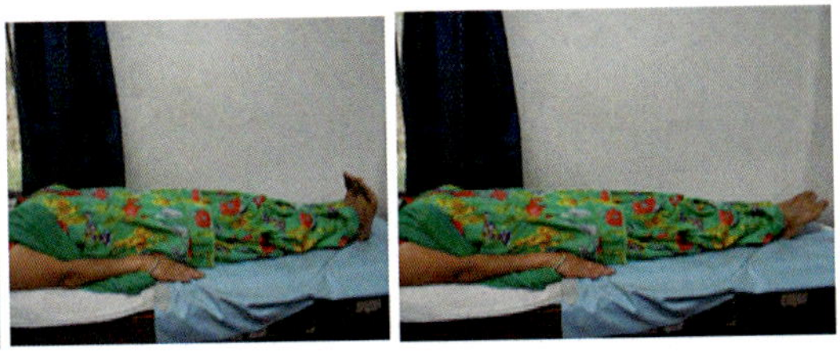

Pix. 2-3:
Active foot/ankle exercise (Flexion/Extension).

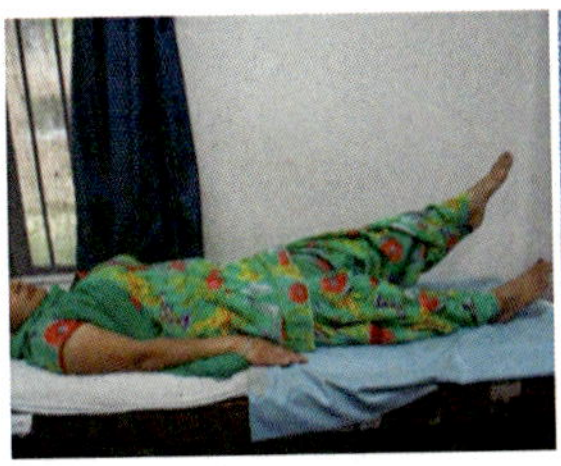

Pix. 4:
Leg / abdominal stretches.

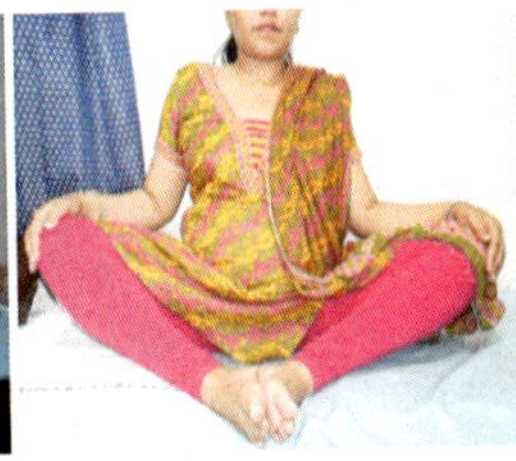

Pix. 5:
Adductor stretching.

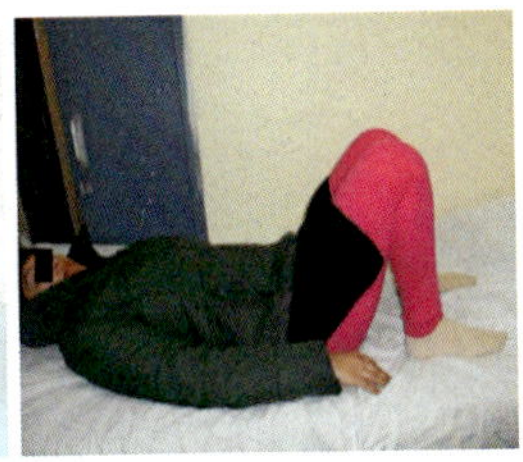

Pix. 6:
Isometric abdominal ex.

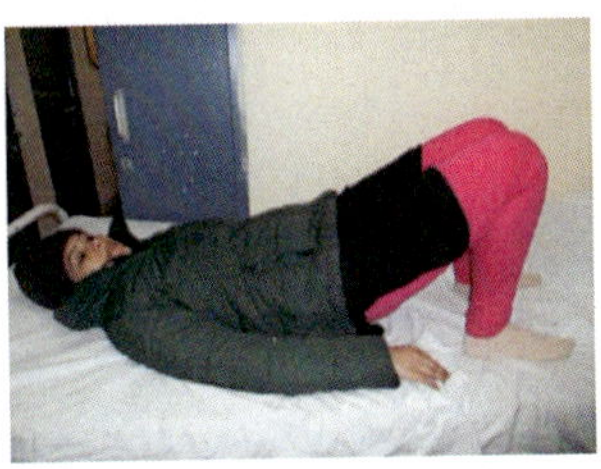

Pix. 7:
Pelvic bridging exercise.

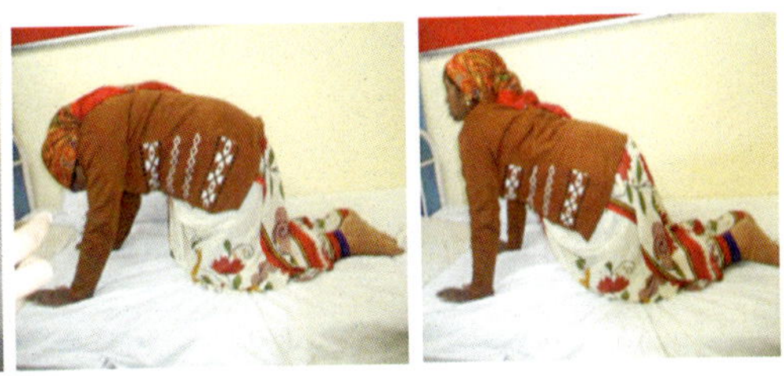

Pix. 8-9:
Cat and camel exercise

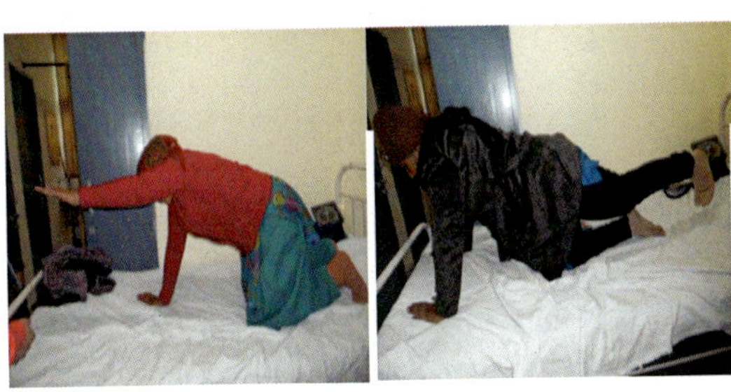

Pix. 10 -11:
4 point kneeling arm / leg lift exercises

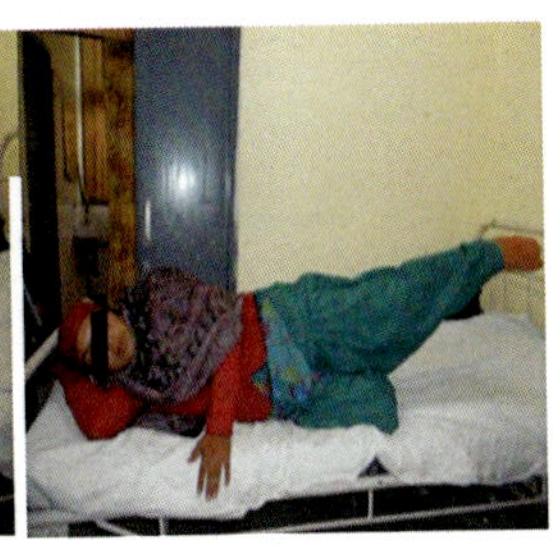

Pix. 12:
Side leg raise exercise.

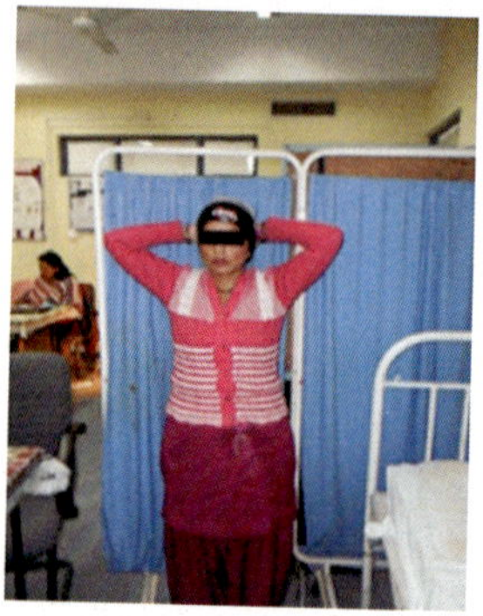

Pix. 13:
Static extension of neck.

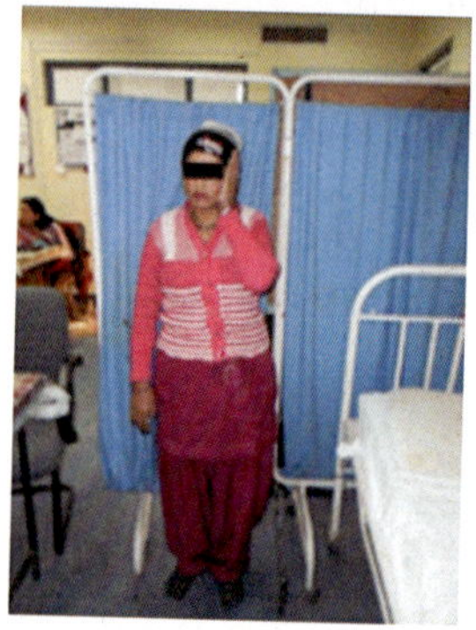

Pix. 14: Isometric lateral flexion of neck.

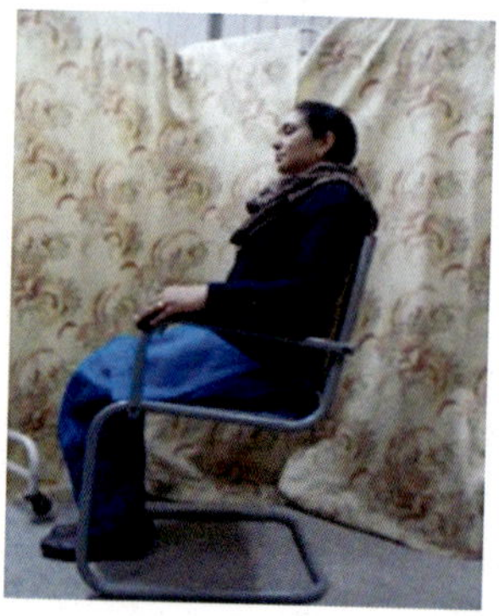

Pix. 15:
Correct sitting posture.

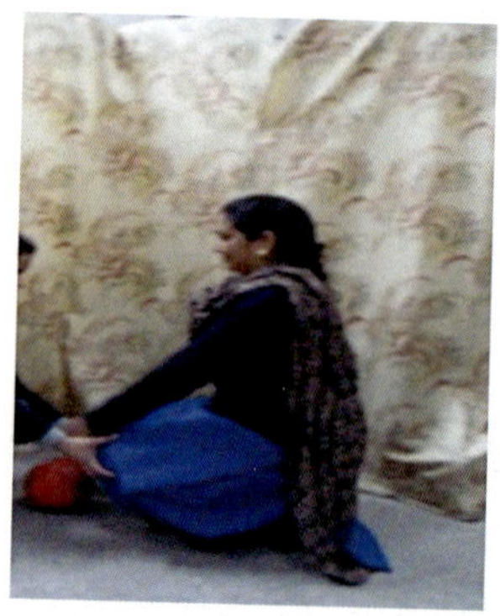

Pix. 16: Correct posture for picking up an object.

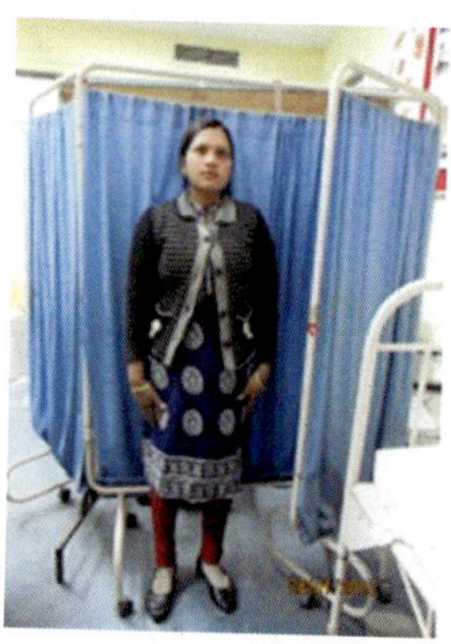

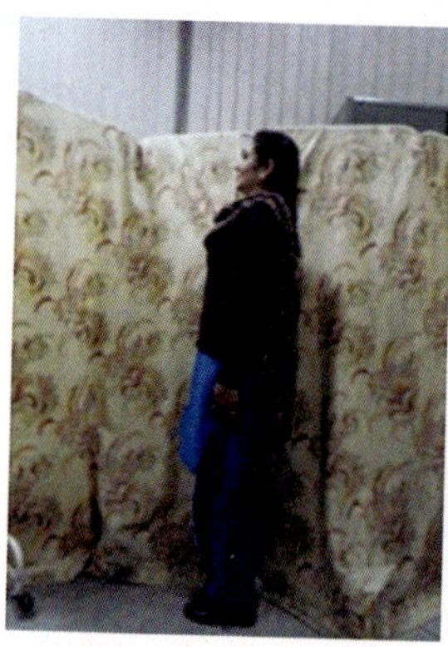

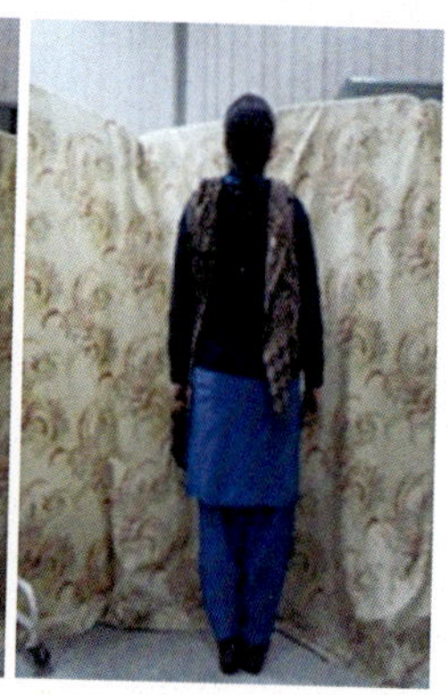

Pix. 17: Correct standing posture.

Chapter - 7

Behavior Therapy for Urine Leakage (Urinary Incontinence)

— S Kumari, V Jain, AK Mandal, AJ Singh

Urinary incontinence (U.I.) is one of the most common health problem affecting millions of women worldwide. The involuntary loss of urine can vary from the occasional nuisance of losing a few drops of urine to a more serious problem of losing larger amount of urine several times a day. Urinary incontinence is often severe enough to have significant social and/or hygienic consequences for women. It is a major clinical problem in most obstetric/ gynecology departments. It affects all age groups and is particularly common among elderly. Approximately 15-30% of older women suffer from urinary incontinence. In two studies conducted in North India urinary incontinence was reported in 40% and 54% of uterine prolapse cases, with a population prevalence of 3.1% and 5.2% for stress incontinence among women 18 years and above. In a study from Chandigarh prevalence of 11.6% was detected. Prevalence studies show that urinary incontinence is endemic among women of every age group. Overall, irrespective of definition, the reported prevalence was at least 30% i.e. almost 1/3rd of women suffer from urinary incontinence.

Incontinent individuals are often reluctant to seek help because they view it as a normal part of the aging process. Many do not report the problem until they have had the symptoms for a long time. Unfortunately, those who do seek help frequently do not receive the attention they deserve. Incontinence remains largely a neglected problem despite the fact that it is treatable and often curable. Urinary incontinence is a chronic health problem which severely reduces the quality of life of women. It is an embarrassing symptom which is grossly under-reported by women.

Types of incontinence

Stress incontinence: This is an involuntary loss of urine on exertion, e.g. coughing, sneezing, and running, laughing and jumping. Leakage occurs when there is increase in intra-abdominal pressure caused by physical activities. It is most common in younger women and the second most common in elderly women and is also known as outlet incompetence. It is usually due to pelvic muscle or ligament laxity. Small volume of urine is usually lost.

Urge incontinence: This term is used to define the symptoms that result from involuntary contractions of the bladder muscle which may occur spontaneously. A patient with urge incontinence usually reports the loss of large volume of urine with each episode of incontinence. If a person does not reach toilet in time, urine leak occurs.

Mixed incontinence: In this type of incontinence the symptoms of both stress incontinence and urge incontinence are present.

Risk factors for urinary incontinence:

(a) Predisposing Factors:

Gender: Women are at least thrice as likely to suffer from incontinence as compared to males. A female to male ratio of approximately 4:1 exists at ages below 60 years and a ratio of 2:1 occurs at age 60 years and older.

Age: Prevalence of urinary incontinence increases with age. Prevalence of incontinence increases with age. After the age of 40 yrs incontinencc is 2-4 times more common. In a study, the UI prevalence of 3.4% in age group 20-24 yrs. increased to 23.7% in people aged 65 years and above. Age more than 75 years has 70% increased risk for urinary incontinence.

Race: A very low prevalence of UI was reported (4.5%) from Singapore, suggesting the ethnic advantage of studied group. The racial difference in the investigation revealed an incontinence rate of 1.1% for Malay Singaporeans, 1.6% for Indian and 5.2% for Chinese Singaporians. Indian females are more prone to develop stress urinary incontinence as compared to Black women. It was reported that Pakistani females using commode type of toilet had a higher incontinence (28.5%) than those voiding in squatting position (12.3%).

(b) Inciting Factors:

Radical pelvic surgery and radiation are identifiable as inciting factors for pelvic floor dysfunction, but are applicable to only a small subset of women. Clearly, vaginal delivery is the major inciting factor for the development of pelvic floor dysfunction in the majority of women.

Parity: Most studies show significantly increased risks for urinary incontinence related to parity. Parity 3 or above has twice the risk.

Vaginal Childbirth: Urinary incontinence and stress urinary incontinence is strongly associated with vaginal childbirth. Forceps delivery or instrumental delivery has been reported as risk factor for urinary incontinence, when compared with those women who had normal delivery. Heavy weight of children delivered by vaginal delivery and a wider circumference of fetal head also has been reported to predispose to prolapsed uterus.

Several studies have shown that prevalence of stress urinary incontinence increased during pregnancy and declined after delivery. In a study from UK stress urinary incontinence during pregnancy was 43.7% and postnatal prevalence was 14.8%. In another study from Denmark stress urinary incontinence during pregnancy was 32% and it was 3% one year after delivery. Among women who reported stress incontinence (SUI) during pregnancy, less than 5% remained incontinent one year after delivery. In contrast, among women who reported onset of SUI after delivery 24% remained symptomatic after one year. This indicates that the increased pressure from the growing uterus on the bladder may cause temporary leakage during pregnancy. The women who have onset of symptoms after delivery are at increased risk for urinary incontinence in later life.

(c) Promoting Factors:

Promoting factors are the ones which aggravate the already existing urinary incontinence.

Constipation: There is a growing body of evidence linking chronic constipation with urinary incontinence, fecal incontinence and pelvic organ prolapsed (2-13 times higher risk).

Occupational and Recreational Stresses: Most reports have reported a higher prevalence of Incontinence in athletes.

Obesity: Obesity is a commonly cited risk factor related to the development and recurrence of urinary incontinence in women(2-3 times higher risk).

Surgery: Hysterectomy has twice the risk of UI.

Chronic Lung Disease and Smoking: The relationship between cigarette smoking and chronic respiratory problem is irrefutable. Smokers are likely to develop persistent cough and stress urinary incontinence. Those who suffer from chronic lung disease are more likely to develop stress urinary incontinence. More violent coughing promotes the earlier development of the anatomic and pressure transmission defect leading to stress urinary incontinence. Due to cough, there is increase in intra-abdominal pressure which is transmitted to bladder and urethra which is unable to sustain adequate pressure under exertional circumstances.

Infection: Evidence suggests that acute urinary tract infection is associated with acute urinary incontinence of both stress and urge variety in about 1/4th of the infected women. Successful treatment of infection has been shown to relieve urge and stress incontinence. A history of previous urinary tract infection has been significantly associated with urge urinary incontinence.

Menopause: Menopause and estrogen depletion leads to atrophy of mucosal tissue that lines both urethra and vagina. It results in weak urethra and reduces urethral pressure. In a study it was revealed that women with stress urinary incontinence have an altered tissue metabolism causing decreased collagen production, which may result in insufficient support of urogenital tract. Urinary incontinence has been reported to be more prevalent among menopausal women. Postmenopausal hormonal replacement appears to increase the risk of developing urinary incontinence.

(C) Decompensating Factors

A variety of factors extrinsic to the pelvic floor and independent of changes in pelvic floor structure or function cause the compensated, although less than perfect, patient to decompensate and become symptomatic.

Some medicines like non-steroidal anti-inflammatory drugs, calcium containing antacids, or iron can cause constipation and predispose the patients to urinary incontinence. Some drugs can cause severe nonproductive cough. Diuretics can cause more production of urine and it becomes difficult for older patients to reach toilet in time. Decreased mobility may prevent an otherwise compensated individual for going to toilet in time leading to urinary incontinence. Co—morbid conditions such as diabetes, vascular insufficiency or congestive heart failure may overwhelm fragile continence reserve with a sudden increase in urine output. Diabetes as a risk factor has been reported by some studies. Hypertension as risk factor for urinary incontinence has also been reported. Arthritis has been reported to be associated with urinary incontinence. Arthritis patients are 70% more prone to urinary incontinence.

Diet: An association between high caffeine intake and detrusor instability has been found.

Family history of urinary incontinence is also reported by some studies as a risk factor. The relatives of incontinent women displayed a higher prevalence of SUI (71.4%) among mothers and (24.6%) among sisters of operated women for SUI as compared to 40.3% among mothers and 11.6% among sisters of continent women. It suggests that heredity may play a significant role.

Impact of Incontinence on Quality of Woman's Life

Urinary incontinence substantially compromises the overall quality of life of women. There is a great amount of fear and stress among the incontinent women for coping with embarrassment and restriction of daily activities induced by incontinence.

Physical Impact: In immobilized patients and those recovering from illness urinary incontinence leads to disturbed sleep. More than 50% incontinent women are bothered by night time voiding leading to disturbed sleep. More frequent urge incontinence episodes may increase the risk of falls among elderly in the bathrooms leading to nursing home admissions.

Psychological Impact: The psychological impact of urinary incontinence may not be directly proportionate to the severity of incontinence. It involves more than hygiene. Patients, whose activities are limited, find it difficult to speak about their condition. Many patients suffer silently with symptoms for years, believing treatment to be ineffective. It poses a threat to self-esteem. Fear of odor of urine is most common because of which incontinent women feel embarrassed and ashamed.

Social Impact: Women with urge or mixed incontinence often limit their social activities. The performance of daily activities that most people take for granted necessitates elaborate planning or simply becomes impossible because of incontinence. Traveling by public transport becomes very difficult, limiting options for shopping or visiting friends and family. Finding accessible public toilet (toilet mapping) can be a prime source of anxiety. Most of women avoid going to public places with unknown restrooms. It also affects their hobbies, vacation and attending church or temple. It is most bothersome during journey.

Incontinence also has an impact on family life. In one study, 324 sexually active women were surveyed and 24% reported incontinence during sexual activity. Thus, sexual relations are also affected. Usually urge incontinence is more bothersome than stress incontinence.

Patients with urge incontinence finds urinary leaks to be of greater problem than do those with stress incontinence because urge incontinence is less predictable and large volume of urine leak occurs. Urge incontinence often occurs at night, resulting in loss of sleep and the need to change clothes and bedding. This indicates that there is reduced quality of life and increased coping behavior among women with urge and mixed incontinence.

Financial Impact: Urinary incontinence is a costly condition because of the use of absorbent products, laundry cost, urinary tract and skin infections and drugs needed to manage incontinence. Supplementary costs which are more difficult to quantify include caregivers' time and women's isolation due to negative social stigma and hygienic problem associated with it. The financial burden is further compounded by the poor mobility, coordination and vision problem common among elderly persons who are at risk for falls and other accidents as a result of urge incontinence.

Diagnosis of Urinary Incontinence

Urinary incontinence is a complex condition that can result from multiple interacting causes, including physiological, behavioral, emotional, social and environmental factors. Its successful management is dependent on a thorough evaluation that accurately characterizes the type of incontinence, and if possible, identifies the underlying etiology. The assessment process includes history and physical examination, measurement of post void residual, voiding diary, laboratory and perineal pad test and if indicated a urodynamic evaluation.

History

Diagnosis of UI can be made according to symptoms alone, without referring to a specialist or invasive processes. Symptom analysis can detect 81% cases of genuine stress urinary incontinence accurately.

Voiding Diary

A three day voiding diary is a simple and practical method of obtaining information on UI. Approaching diagnosis through the evaluation of symptoms obviates the invasive and expensive procedures requiring specialist referral.

Home pad testing

Pads can be used to evaluate objectively the amount of urine lost. This can be combined with history to evaluate incontinence.

Barrier to treatment seeking for women in India

In India, women in their natural role as mothers, sisters, wives and daughters have been accepted as the principal providers of good health to their families and indirectly to the community. Yet when it comes to their own health, women in India receive low priority. Women consider most of their reproductive morbidities as 'normal' and a part of their destiny. They may not seek treatment or may not report their symptoms. Even If they perceive it to be abnormal, they may conceal it out of guilt or shame as they take it as a punishment to their past deeds (theory of *karma*).

There is often a low consultation rate for any morbidity related to private parts. Women usually feel shy to discuss their health problems with male health team members. Like other Indians, women here also have a fatalistic attitude and that of "ignorance is bliss" Other reason for non-consultation is poverty, lack of financial independence, and "culture of silence" In general; there is a scarcity of female doctors and urologists in India. And even they are often too busy to patiently listen and understand the problems of women and provide the treatment.

In India, surgery of any kind is usually a dreaded proposition and people tend to avoid it as far as possible, probably because of which women continue to suffer and tolerate the symptoms of any sort before resorting to operation, if at all when the situation becomes unbearable. Women give low priority to their health. They tend to suffer silently without seeking health care until it reaches severity, because of their shyness, poverty and dependence on their husband. In many instances lack of education and information may limit women's understanding of the benefit of health services. Thus, education is an important determinant in the utilization of health services.

Thus, there is poor utilization of health services not only because services are inaccessible to poor women but also because they are culturally inappropriate to women's needs and expectations Moreover, as indicated above, various handicaps and compulsions in women's lives force them to develop a tolerant attitude and a "culture of silence" towards their reproductive health problems..

Treatment of urinary incontinence

Treatment goals for incontinence management are the elimination of symptoms and improvement of the quality of life. For urge and mixed incontinence, two approaches are used: pharmacological and non-pharmacological. But the effectiveness of either treatment may take as long as four weeks to become apparent. For stress urinary incontinence, surgical, pharmacological and non-pharmacological therapies are used. Treatment ranges from minor life style changes to surgery.

Non pharmacological management

Life style modification: It is targeted towards reducing or eliminating risk factors like reduction of intake of caffeine or other dietary irritants (such as acidic fruit juices, colas, coffee and tea), smoking cessation, weight reduction. . Constipation and straining during bowel movement increases pressure on the bladder. Regulation of bowel movements helps to prevent urinary incontinence.

Behavioral Therapy

Behavioral intervention should be considered the first line of treatment for urinary incontinence for patients who are motivated enough to devote time and effort for behavioral therapy in order to avoid invasive procedures.

Behavioral therapy describes a group of treatments that are based on the idea that incontinent patient can be educated about the condition. Strategies are developed to conservatively minimize or eliminate the incontinence. It is sometimes erroneously equated with and reduced to the combination of fluid restriction and timed voiding. But actually it is a far richer therapy. In fact, one of the main problems with the term "behavior therapy" is that it has been used so differently by practitioners that its meaning has become dilute and vague. There is no standard protocol or best methodology for behavior therapy of urinary incontinence. Behavioral therapy must start with instruction about normal urinary tract anatomy and function. Patient needs to understand the role of the bladder and pelvic floor muscles. A voiding diary is used to teach patient about his or her bladder function. This diary becomes a basis for evaluation and goal setting for desired voiding interval. Repeated evaluations are made in which patient's performance is compensated with goals and new goals are set, providing positive reinforcement. Patients are taught urge inhibition. Kegels exercises are a part of such therapy.

Bladder training: It is strongly recommended for the management of urge and mixed incontinence and also recommended for stress incontinence.

Pelvic floor muscle exercises: These are strongly recommended for women with stress urinary incontinence.

As the table 1 illustrates the utility of behavioral therapy can be realized when we compare it with the surgical and drug therapy for incontinence. Women with pure stress incontinence respond well to surgical therapy with cure rate of 35-95%. Women with urge incontinence benefit from drug intervention, with cure or improvement of 50-60%. However both drugs and surgery have side effects and risks are involved hence, behavior therapy should be considered as initial step for management of incontinence before considering surgical or medical intervention.

Table 1 Comparison of different modes of treatment for Urinary incontinence

Variables	*Modes of Treatment*		
	Medicine	***Surgery***	***Behavior Therapy***
Consultation & need of Follow-up(no.)	Multiple contacts needed	Multiple contact needed	Only one contact needed
Specialist consultation required	Yes	Yes	No
Invasive investigations required	Yes	Yes	No
Side effects & Complications	Headache, dry mouth, nausea, vomiting, blurred vision, constipation	Injury to bladder, hematoma, infection, urine retention, fistula, recurrent stress incontinence, urge incontinence	None

(Contd...)

Fear of surgery	No	Yes	No
Easy & Acceptable	No	No (fear of surgery)	Yes
Cost	Yes	Yes (Rs. 20,000 -30,000)	No
Success rate	50-60%	30-90%	50-90%
Relapse	Yes	25-50%	10-15%
Duration of treatment	Long	One time surgery	8-12 weeks daily exercise and then a habit is formed

Impact of Behavior Therapy

A study conducted by the authors at PGIMER Chandigarh concluded that behavior therapy intervention led to a rapid and highly significant improvement in the severity of urinary incontinence in the study group. Out of total mild cases, 77% were fully cured and rest had no leak episode since training. 71% of moderate cases were completely cured and 16% changed into mild. Out of total severe urinary incontinence cases 34% became continent and 1/3rd became mild. At the end of follow-up, overall 52.5% women were continent and 24.4% became mild. So, 77% cases were benefited by intervention. Out of these cases 73% respondents reported complete relief from incontinence immediately after the 8 weeks intervention phase (weekly session one contact) was over.

Involuntary loss/leakage of urine is called **Urinary Incontinence**. It is a significant social and hygienic health problem among women. It can vary from occasional botheration/problem of leaking a few drops of urine to a more serious problem of leaking ample amount of urine several times a day. It has severe economic and psychosocial impact on women's lives. It is a heavy emotional burden for women in terms of embarrassment, social isolation and diminished self-prestige. Such women are often not willing to seek help. Some view it as a routine part of their lives. Many do not report it as health problem to doctors because in Indian society it is not considered good to discuss women's illness with strangers.

Why leakage occurs: Leakage of urine occurs as **pelvic floor muscles** become weak with age and repeated childbirths. Moreover, hormonal changes associated with menopause also cause weakness of muscles leading to incontinence.

Affected women often feel embarrassed and ashamed. They go on suffering without telling anyone. If it is left untreated for long, it gets worse and operation may be needed.

But one should know that it is very simple to control and correct this defect without operation. This can be achieved through special exercises which all women can do easily. These exercise helps in strengthening **pelvic floor muscles**. This manual describes how women themselves can get rid of this problem by self-care.

Three types of urinary incontinence are there:

1. **Stress urinary incontinence:** It is sudden leakage of a small amount of urine. It usually occurs with coughing, sneezing, laughing, lifting weight, bending and standing from sitting position.
2. **Urge incontinence:** It is characterized by a strong desire to pass urine that occurs immediately prior to leakage of urine. Such individuals tell that they cannot reach the toilet on time and leakage occurs. Some may report frequent need to go for urination. Some even report passing urine in the bed during sleep.
3. **Mixed incontinence:** It refers to a combination of stress incontinence and urge incontinence symptoms.

HOW THE BLADDER WORKS

You must have observed small children passing urine in bed and even in clothes. They do so because in children, the bladder gradually fills with urine, the bladder expands and signals spinal cord that it is getting increasingly full. Bladder filling continues as it reaches a critical point, when spinal cord signals bladder to empty itself. This is called as voiding reflex. Our brain has no control over it. At this stage urine control is without any connection to brain as it occurs in babies.

When a child is 2-3 yrs old we teach him where and when to pass urine. Slowly, over time, children learn to control urine and pass urine when they reach toilet.

To control when the bladder empties, person must learn to control voiding reflex. This learning takes place in early childhood. Through their parents/caretakers children learn to void when they reach toilet. Even if voiding reflex is there, it is the brain which controls continence and muscles help by keeping in them closed until you reach toilet. Continence is, therefore, a learned behaviour and habit.

But you must know, this training will help you to control your urine leakage problem. But it will not give instant result. As you will continue exercise you will notice improvement in 2-3 weeks. Be patient and continue with your exercises.

STRUCTURE OF URINARY SYSTEM

To understand the exercise therapy for cure of incontinence, it is important to understand the structure & functioning of urinary system especially the lower urinary tract in women.

The urinary system in human performs the task of collecting waste and removing them from body in the form of urine. It consists of two kidneys, two ureters, a urinary bladder and a urethra (Fig. 1). Pelvic floor consists of muscles and connective tissue that stretches from tail bone to pubic bone like a sheet. These muscles and the connective tissue support the lower urinary tract organs (urinary bladder & urethra) as well as the uterus and rectum (Fig. 2, 3).

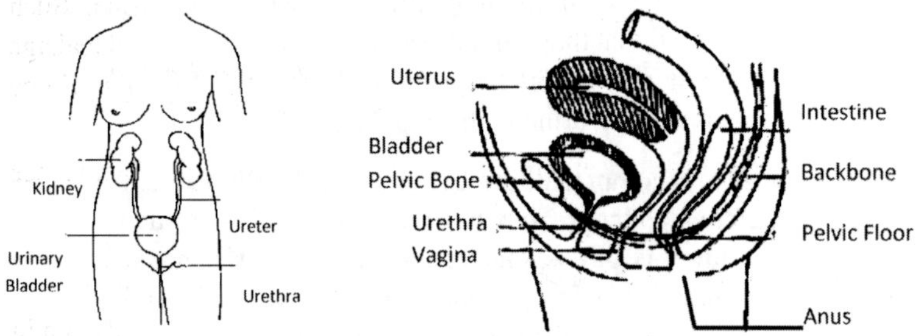

Fig. 2 & 3: Views of the Pelvic Floor.

The urinary bladder is a hollow bag like organ. It has muscles in its lining. When the bladder is full the urine is expelled through urethra by contraction of the bladder muscles (Fig. 4).

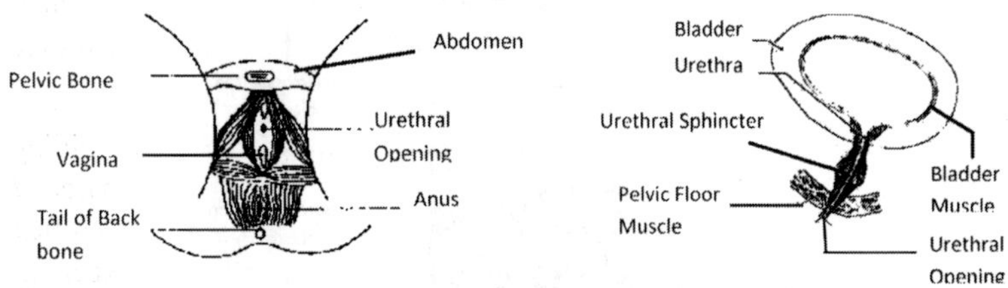

Fig. 4: Urinary System.

Female urethra is a short tube about 3 to 4 cm (1 to 1.5 inch) in length consisting of layer muscles. It is encircled at middle part by the external **urethral sphincter**, a voluntarily controllable muscle (a kind of valve/lid/ plug) which controls leakage of urine.

THERE ARE TWO PHASES IN URINATION

1. Storage Phase: (1) During this phase bladder fills gradually with urine which is formed in kidneys. (2) Bladder muscle remains inactive, although it

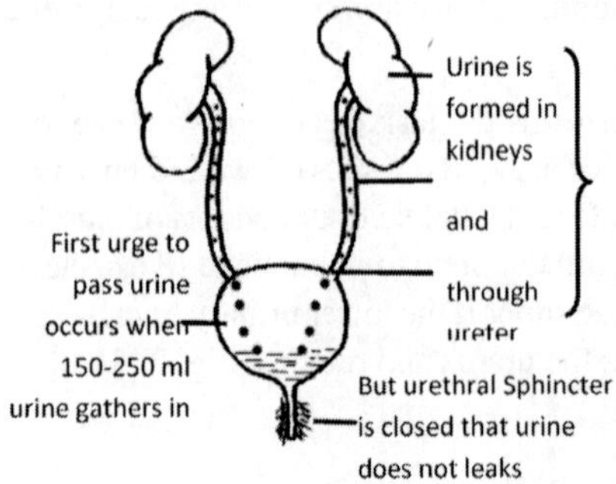

Fig 5: Collection of urine in Bladder.

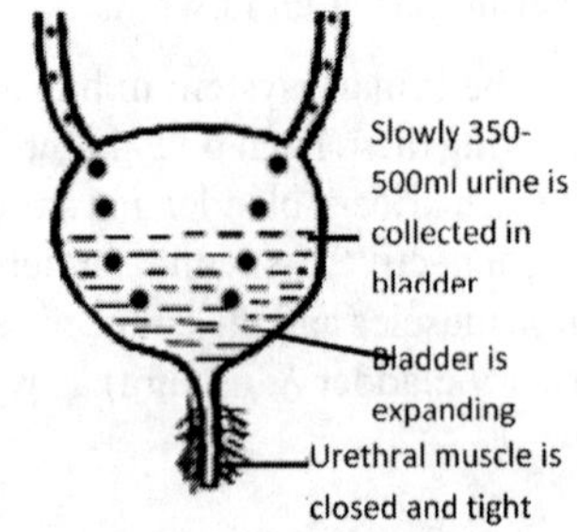

Fig. 6: Bladder is full with urine but urethral sphincter is closed.

expands passively to accommodate urine (Fig. 5, 6). Usually 150-250 ml urine can be stored before bladder pressure begins to rise and first desire to urinate is perceived. During this time sphincter increases its resistance and signal from brain allows bladder to fill up to maximum capacity (350-500 ml)

2. Expulsion Phase : When the bladder is full to its capacity signal goes to brain and getting OK from it, bladder muscle contracts pushing urine out of bladder and the bladder neck sphincter relaxes, allowing urine to pass through urethra (Fig. 7). It means passing urine is controlled by brain.

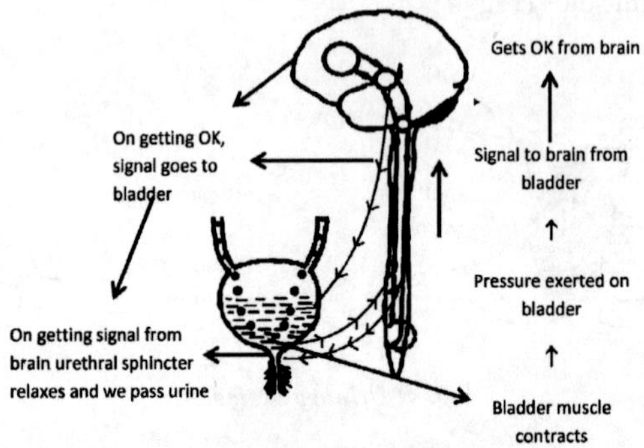

Fig. 7: Process, controlling the urinary system by Brain.

Normally, a person passes urine 5 to 7 times per 24 hours. Thus, there is a 3 to 4 hours interval between passing urine when we are awake. During night a person may go for urination before going to bed and then after getting up in the morning. Urination may be more frequent during winter and rainy season than in summer. Urination frequency also depends on liquid intake.

BLADDER TRAINING TO CHANGE URINATION HABIT

Normally a person passes urine every 3-4 hours. Bladder training involves finding an interval during which there is no leakage and gradually increasing this interval to a normal urination pattern of every 3-4 hours. Women who leak urine knowingly or unknowingly may go for urination more frequently than necessary. They believe that having less urine in the bladder decreases the chances of leakage. However, on the contrary, more frequent urination leads to development of a habit where brain sends a signal to go for urination even when less urine is there in bladder.

Usually, the first desire to urinate occurs when bladder is half full (150-250 ml). So when you get the first feeling to go for urination take deep breath and divert your attention from going to toilet. But if the urge is very strong you may go to toilet. Slowly, increase the interval between urination. Your target is to achieve an interval of 3-4 hours between urination within 6 weeks.

It is the **brain that controls your urination signal. Bladder muscles work according to the signal**. So it is important to correct your habit of frequently going to toilet by increasing the interval so that your bladder gets trained to hold normal amount of urine and your voiding interval of three to four hours is achieved. This can be facilitated by keeping a urination diary.

MYTH – More frequent urination prevents leakage.

REALITY – Rather, this leads to leakage of urine. Frequent urination sends wrong signals to brain.

WHAT TO DO – Do not pass urine frequently. Train your bladder to hold.

Actually rushing is the worst thing you can do.

- Rushing jiggles your bladder, increasing your awareness of how full it feels and making the urgency worse.
- Movement can stimulate the bladder to contract and empty.
- Rushing put extra-abdominal pressure on bladder and tends to push urine out.
- Rushing interferes with concentration that you need to control bladder.

Six simple steps to do when desire to urinate is felt.

1. Stop what you are doing, sit down when possible or stand quietly.
2. Contract your pelvic floor muscles quickly several times. Do not relax fully in between.
3. Take a few deep breaths.
4. Concentrate on suppressing the desire to urinate.

5. Wait until desire to urinate subsides.
6. Walk to bathroom at normal pace. Do not rush, continue contracting you pelvic floor muscles while you reach toilet.

Bladder training is like forming a habit, just like teaching a child to control his urination. So you have to learn to pass urine at regular interval. But be patient as results are not instant, Results will be noticeable offer 2-3 weeks. So be patient and continue your training.

HOW TO PREVENT URINE LEAKAGE

(a) Lifestyle changes & dietary modifications for prevention of urine leakage

Leakage of urine can be prevented by changing our life style/activities. Often a person with incontinence restricts the liquid intake thinking that it will prevent leakage. This practice is harmful. This not only reduces bladder capacity but also increases the risk of constipation and bladder irritation leading to leakage.

1. Increase fluid intake to 8-10 glasses per day i.e. 1.5 – 2 liter. This helps not only to dilute bladder irritants but also to increase bladder capacity. (Do not take too much liquid at one time but take it at equal and regular intervals). Sufficient water/liquids should be taken to satisfy your thirst.

   DO NOT RESTRICT FLUID INTAKE

2. Take fiber rich diet e.g. whole grains, fruits and vegetables and salads to relieve constipation. Constipation itself can precipitate incontinence. Constipation is a risk factor for leakage of urine.

   AVOID CONSTIPATION – AVOID LEAKAGE

3. Do not smoke as it can produce cough and exaggerate incontinence.

   SAY NO TO SMOKING AND STAY DRY

4. Always lift heavy objects with care or get help for lifting, if needed. Lifting weight increases intra-abdominal pressure leading to incontinence.

   BE CAREFUL WHILE LIFTING – AVOID LEAKAGE

5. If you are overweight, try to reduce your weight to normal.

   OBESITY IS A RISK FACTOR FOR LEAKAGE

6. Avoid irritable fluids such as tea, coffee and cold drinks. These fluids cause bladder irritation leading to leakage.

   TEA, COFFEE, COLD DRINKS LEAD TO – LEAKAGE

7. Avoid infection. Keep genital area/private part clean. Change and wash your undergarments daily. Wear cotton underwear. Maintain menstrual hygiene.

   INFECTION CAN LEAD TO URINE LEAKAGE

8. Avoid mental stress.

URINATION DIARY

To know your success with training, you are required to maintain urination diary.

Instructions

Please record each time you drink fluid, each time you pass urine in toilet or leak accidentally. Do this for three consecutive days.

- Whenever you drink water please P in column 1.
- Whenever you drink tea,coffee, cold drink, milk, *lassi* put P in column 2.
- If normal urine is passed in toilet put P in column 3.
- In the column of "urine leak" tick under column (o) for a drop or two, (O) for enough requiring you to change clothes or smell (in column 4).
- If you had sudden urge to void and you could not reach toilet in time. Tick P in column 5.
- In "activity" column 6 tick if leak occurred during (e.g. coughing, sneezing, laughing, lifting heavy objects, rising from chair, washing hands, hearing running water).

Day 1 – Count from the time you got up from bed.

Table 2: Urination Diary

Time	***Fluid Intake***		***Normal***	***Urine Leak***			
	Water	***Cold drink Tea/Coffee***	***Urination in Toilet***	***Could not reach toilet***	***Urine Leak***		***Activity when leak***
	1	2	3	4	5		6
6 AM		200ml			o	O	Cough
7 AM							
8 AM							
9 AM							
10 AM							

PELVIC FLOOR MUSCLE EXERCISE (KEGEL'S EXERCISE)

These simple exercises can help in preventing leakage.

Basic information

- Pelvic floor muscle exercises can strengthen the muscle around vagina & increase your ability to contract & relax these muscles completely.
- Pelvic floor muscles are special in women because they support the organs in the pelvis (uterus, bowel & bladder). Keeping these muscles strong can help prevent urine leakage and even a uterine prolapse.
- With age, weakness develops in pelvic floor muscles due to normal wear & tear and child birth. The bladder, uterus & rectum begin to slip down and get squeezed into lower region of pelvis. Women can develop stress incontinence, urge incontinence or both. Performing exercises can help to prevent and relieve these symptoms.

TIPS FOR PRACTICING PELVIC FLOOR MUSCLE EXERCISE

How to identify correct muscle which needs to be exercised?

- To get the feel of the muscle alternatively start and stop urinating while using the toilet by tightening the muscle. If you can slow the stream of urine, even slightly, you are using the right muscle.

OR

- When you have urge to pass flatus in a gathering but you hold back the flatus by squeezing muscles around your anus; so that is the muscle we are talking about.

OR

- To find the muscle, place your finger inside your vagina or rectum and try to press your finger by contracting internal muscles. This is the muscle you have to exercise. This muscle is the same one you use to hold back gas or bowel movement.

Practicing the exercise

- Squeeze the muscle you have identified earlier for counts of ten (or ten seconds) then relax for ten seconds. Remember that, it is just as important to relax as it is to contract the muscle. Initially, you may not be able to hold this muscle for ten seconds. However, slowly over a period of two weeks you will be able to hold for ten seconds.

Start with 3 seconds and over a period of 2-3 weeks increase it up to 10 seconds.

- Practice the tightening and relaxation while sitting, standing, walking and watching T.V. and even lying down. While lying down on your back with knees bent and feet 12 inch apart, arms resting on your side you can perform the exercise. Start with five times each and gradually work up to ten and then up to twenty times each time.
- Give a gap of 2 minutes after 5-6 contractions.
- Do fifteen exercise in the morning, fifteen in the afternoon and twenty at night or do the exercise for ten minutes 3 times a day or you can try to work up to twenty five exercises twice a day.
- In time, you will learn to practice effortlessly. Eventually, you will be able to work these exercises in as part of your lifestyle like brushing your teeth or eating a meal.
- If you leak urine when you cough or sneeze or laugh you should squeeze the muscle before coughing or sneezing or laughing. Once the muscle become strong and has some endurance you will have lesser amount/episodes of leakage. Do the pelvic muscle contractions whenever you anticipate extra pressure on your pelvis.
- **Remember:-** Never use your stomach, leg or buttock muscles for exercise. The most common mistake is to use too many muscles. To find out if you are also contracting your stomach muscles, place your hand on your abdomen while you squeeze your pelvic floor muscle. If you feel your abdomen move, then you are wrongly using these muscles. If so, you must change your technique.
- This exercise can be practiced any time, in any place. Since this muscle is internal, no one can notice you exercising this muscle.
- Build strength slowly. Do not expect results right away. You can notice a little bit of change after two weeks and by six weeks, benefits will be visible.

Do not hold breath while doing exercise, take normal breath.

Can these exercises harm me?

No, these exercises cannot harm you in any way. Most patients find them relaxing and easy. If you have stomach pain or back pain after you exercise, then you are probably trying too hard or using stomach and back muscles. If so, again try to find the correct muscles. Remember, exercise should feel mild and easy. Do not exercise under tension. Remember to focus on relaxation as well as squeezing the muscle. When you will learn to practice effortlessly the exercises can be a part of your lifestyle like brushing teeth or eating a meal. This will help you to remain OK for a lifetime and there will never be a urine leakage problem.

You may be tempted to stop exercising your pelvic floor muscles. But remember! You have worked hard to strengthen these muscles. If you stop exercising, now, they will weaken again. So only way to maintain strength of your muscles is to keep exercising them regularly. This was you will remain coninent and leaking will not occur.

How to maintain record of your exercise: You are provided with a form where you will

- Tick mark three times if you are exercising three times daily.
- Tick mark two times if you are exercising two times daily.
- Tick mark one times if you are exercising once daily.
- Put cross mark if you are not exercising.

Table 3: Follow up chart

Day	*Date*	*Exercise*		
		Sitting	*Lying Down*	*Standing*
1				
2				
3				
4				
5				
6				
7				
8				
9				

Limitation of behavior therapy is that it is most effective in mild and moderate cases of incontinence. Those who do not have improvement after 4-6 weeks should consult the doctor. But behavior therapy is safe and it could be continued along with medication and after surgery to prevent recurrence of problem.

Conclusion: Incontinence causes a lot of distress, embarrassment and inconvenience among the affected women. It remains one of the most common social and hygiene problems of women. Incontinent women need not suffer silently. They must be encouraged to seek help and to discuss their problems openly with their health care providers. In fact, most of the mild and moderate cases can be managed conservatively at the primary care level.

References

1. Rowe J.W., Besdine R.W., Ford A.B., Gartley C.B., Consensus Conference, Urinary Incontinence in Adults. JAMA 1989; 261: 2685-90.
2. Sampselle C.M. Behavioral intervention in young and middle age women; American Journal of Nursing. (Supplement).2003; 103: 9-19.
3. Mittal.N, Hota.D, Urinary Incontinence, Drugs Bulletin. 2008; 31: 1-16.
4. Morkved S., Urinary incontinence during pregnancy and after delivery, effect of pelvic floor muscle training in prevention and treatment PhD Thesis, Norwegian University of Science and Technology 2003.
5. Thakar R., Stanon S., Management of urinary incontinence in women. British Medical Journal, 2000; 321: 1326-30.
6. Resnick NM, Yalla SV. Management of urinary incontinence in the elderly. The New England Journal of Medicine, 1985; 113: 800-805.
7. Newman D.K., Giovannini. D. The overactive bladder: A nursing perspective". Am J of Nursing, 2002; 102: 36-45.
8. Bump R.C., Norton P.A. Epidemiology and natural history of pelvic floor dysfunction. Obstetrics and Gynecology Clinics of North America 1998; 25: 723-740.
9. Brown J.S. Epidemiology and changing demographies of overactive bladder: a focus on the postmenopausal women. Geriatrics 2003 Supplement 1; 57: 6-12.
10. Haillot P.O., Bruyere F., Boutin I.M., Bertrang P., Lanson Y. Prevalence and risk factors of urinary incontinence in young and middle-aged women. British Journal Urology International 2002; 89: 61-66.
11. Skoner M., Thompson W.D., Caron V.A. Factors associated with risk of stress urinary incontinence in women. Nursing Research 1994; 43: 301-6.
12. Kumari.S, Impact of a behavioral training package on occurrence and severity of urinary incontinence, Ph.D thesis, P.G.I.M.E.R. Chandigarh(2007)
13. Samuelsson E., Victor A., Svardsudd K. Determinants of urinary incontinence in a population of young and middle-aged women". Acta Obstet Gynecol Scand, 2000; 79: 1208-15.
14. Hampel C., Wienhol D., Banken N., Eggersmann, C., Thuroff J.W. Prevalence and natural history of female incontinence. Eur. Urol. 1997; 32 (Suppl. 2): 3-12.
15. Henriette.J.Brummen.V. ummen.V. Bruinse.H.W, Pol.G.V.D, Peter.A.,Heintz.M, Huub.S, Vaart. V, Bothersome lower urinary tract symptoms 1 year after first delivery. Prevalence and the effect of child birth. British Journal of Urology International 2006; 98: 89-95.
16. Buchsbaum G.M., Chin M., Glantz C., Guzick D. Prevalence of urinary incontinence and associated risk factors in a cohart of nuns. Obstet Gynecol 2002; 100: 226-229.
17. Maclennan A.H., Taylor A.W., Wilson D.H., Wilson D. The prevalence of pelvic floor disorders and their relationship to gender, age, parity and made of delivery. British Journal of Obstetric and Gynecology 2000; 107: 1460-70.
18. Lukaaz E.S., Lawrence J.M., Cantreras R., Nager C.W., Luber K.M. Parity, mode of delivery and pelvic floor disorders. Obstet Gynecol 2006; 107: 1253-66.

19. Sharma S., Walia I., Singh A. A case control study on uterine prolapse in a Chandigarh Slum. Bulletin PGIMER, 2003; 37: 143-48.
20. Smith A.R.B., Hosker G.L., Warrell D.W. The role of partial denervation of the pelvic floor in the aetiology of genitourinary prolapse and stress urinary incontinence of urine. A neurophysiological study. British Journal of Obstetric and Gynecology, 1989; 96: 24-28.
21. Viktrup L., Lose G. The risk of stress incontinence 5 years after first delivery. Am J Obstet Gynecol 2001; 185: 82-87.
22. Brown J.S., Grady D., Ouslander J.G., Herzog A.R., Varner R.E., Posner S.F. Prevalence of urinary incontinence and associated risk factors in postmenopausal women. Obstet Gynecol 1999; 94: 66-70.
23. Snooks S.J., Setchell M., Swash M., Henry M.M. Injury to innervation of pelvic floor sphincter musculature in child birth. The Lancet 1984; 334; 546-50.
24. Hvidman L., Fddsprung A., Mommsen S., Nelsen J.B. Postpartum urinary incontinence. Acta Obstet Gynecol Scand 2001; 82: 556-63.
25. MacArthur C., Glazener C,, Don Wilson P., Lancashire R.J., Herbison G.P., Grant A.M. Persistent urinary incontinence and delivery mode, history: a six year longitudinal study. Br J Obst Gynecology 2006; 113:l218-224.
26. Viktrup L., Lose G. The risk of stress incontinence 5 years after first delivery. Am J Obstet Gynecol 2001; 185: 82-87.
27. Fischer J.R., Berg P.H. Urinary incontinence in United States air force female aircrew. Obstet Gynecol 1999; 94: 532-36.
28. Chaliha C., Kalia V., Stanton S.L., Monga A., Sultan A.H. Antenatal prediction of postpartum urinary & fecal incontinence. Obstet. Gynecol 1999; 94: 689-94.
29. Viktrup L., Lose G., Rolff M., Barfoed K. Symptoms of stress incontinence caused by pregnancy or delivery in primiparas. Obstet. Gynecol. 1992; 79: 945-49.
30. Bo K., Stien R., Hansen S.K., Kristofferson M. Clinical and urodynamic assessment of nulliparous young women with and without stress incontinence symptoms: A case control study. Obstet. Gynecol. 1994; 84: 1028-32.
31. Nygaard I.E., Thompson F.L., Sarah A.T.C., Svengalis L., Albright J.P. Urinary incontinence in Elite Nulliparous Athletes. Obstet Gynecol 1994; 84: 183-7.
32. Hannestad Y.S., Rortvert G., Dattveit A.K., Hunskaar S. Are smoking and other life style factors associated with female urinary incontinence? The Norwegian Epincont Study. British Journal of Obstet Gynecology, 2003; 110: 247-54.
33. Bump R.C., McClish D.M. Cigarette smoking and pure genuine stress incontinence of urine: A comparison of risk factors and determinants between smokers and non-smokers. Obstet Gynecol 1994; 170: 579-82.
34. Hannestad Y.S., Rortveit G., Sandvik H., Hunskaar S. A community-based epidemiological survey of female urinary incontinence: The Norwegian Epincont Study. Journal of Clinical Epidemiology 2000; 53: 1150-57.
35. Grodstein F., Lifford K., Resnick N.M., Curhan G.C. Post menopausal Haemon therapy and risk of developing urinary incontinence. Obstet Gynecol 2004; 103: 254-60.
36. Arya L.A., Myers D., Jackson N. Dietary caffeine intake and the risk for detrusor instability: A case control study. Obstet Gynecol 2000; 96: 85-87.

37. Ertunc D, Tok EC, Pata O, Dilek U, Ozdemir G, Dilek S. Is stress urinary incontinence a familial condition? Acta Obstet. Gynecol Scand 2004; 83: 912-16.
38. Singh A, Arora A.K. Effect of uterine prolapse on the lives of rural north Indian women. Singapore Journal of Obstetric and Gynecology.2003; 34:52-58.
39. Kumari. S, Walia I.J. and Singh A.J. Self reported uterine prolapse in a resettlement colony of North India. Journal of Midwifery and Women's Health.2000; 45: 343-350.
40. Wyman J.F., Harkins Stephen W., Choi S.C., Taylor J.R., Fantl JA. Psychosocial impact of urinary incontinence in women. Obstet Gynecol 1987; 70: 378-81.
41. Dubeau C.E. The continuum of urinary incontinence in an aging population. Geriatrics, 2003 (Supplement) 1; 57: 12-17.
42. Hilton P., Urinary incontinence during sexual intercourse: A common, but rarely volunteered symptom. British Journal of Obstetrics & Gynecology 1988; 95: 377-381.
43. Wilson L., Brown J.S., Shin G.P., Luc K., Subak L. Annual direct cost of urinary incontinence. Obstet Gynecol, 2001; 98: 398-406.
44. Versi E., Cardozo L., Anand D., Cooper D. Symptoms analysis for the diagnosis of genuine stress incontinence. Br J of Obstetric and Gynecology, 1991; 98: 815-19.
45. Fink. D, Perucchin. D, Schaer. G.N, Haller. V, The role of the frequency volume chart in the differential diagnosis of female urinary incontinence. Acta Obstet-Gynecol Scand, 1999; 78: 254-57.
46. Hawkins J., Gordone B. Shaw's Textbook of Gynecology, Padubidri. V.G., Daftary, S.N., (Editors) New Delhi. Elsevier India Pvt. Ltd., 13th edition: 187-193.
47. Davila G.W, Gurette N. Current treatment options for female urinary incontinence – A review. Int J Fertility 2004; 49: 102-12.
48. Fant J.A., Wyman J.F., Anderson R., Matt D., Bump R.C. Postmenopausal urinary incontinence: Comparison between non-estrogen supplemented and estrogen supplemented women. Obstet Gynecol, 1988; 71: 823-28.
49. Dmochowski R., Miklus J.R., Norton P., Zinner N., Yalein I., Bump R.C., Duloxetine versus placebo for the treatment of North American women with stress urinary incontinence. J Urology, 2003; 170: 1259-63.
50. Peattie A.B., Plevnik S., Stanon S.L. Vaginal cones: a conservative method of treating stress continence. Br Journal of Obstetric and Gynecology, 1988; 95: 1049-53.
51. Payne C.K. Behavioral therapy for overactive bladder. Urology 2000; 55 (Supple 5A): 3-6.
52. Burgio K.L., Pearce K.L., Lucco A.J., Staying Dry. A Practical Guide to Bladder Control. 1989 Baltimore, John Hopkins University Press: 1-120.
53. Fantl J.A., Wyman J.F., Mcclish D.K., Harkins S.W., Elswick R.K., Taylor J.R., Hadley E.C. Efficacy of bladder training in order women with urinary incontinence. JAMA 1991, 265: 609-13.

Chapter - 8

Promoting Health of Women – Conservative Management of Pelvic Organ Prolapse

— R Kashyap, AJ Singh and V Jain

Pelvic organ prolapse is one of the most common, but hidden, gynaecological morbidities. It is caused by weakening of the pelvic floor muscles. It is in fact, herniation of the pelvic organ or organs through the vagina below normal anatomical position. Some degree of descent occurs in most women who have experienced vaginal childbirth. It is a major public health problem for the nation. It seriously compromises the quality of life of the affected women, as the access to the treatment is restricted due to various social problems. Globally, 50% of all women who have delivered a child are affected by this malady. Symptomatic pelvic organ prolapse has important effect on general health-related quality of life and interferes as a disability with physical mobility, pain, emotional reaction, social isolation, energy, and sleep.

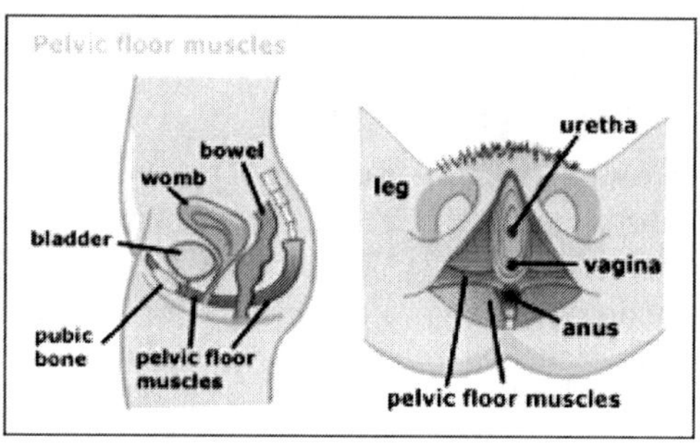

Fig 1 : Pelvic floor muscles

In this context a study was conducted by Dr R Kashyap between August 2010 and October 2011 to compare the effect of two packages of PFMT (One to one training and self instruction manual versus self instruction manual only) on clinical course of stage 1 to 3 POP, in the women attending gynecology OPD, PGIMER,Chandigarh, India (CTRI/2010/091/001190). The mean age of 140 participants was 47 years (SD 12).Maximum number of patients (39;27.8%) belonged to the age group of 41-50 yrs. Sixty (43%) patients were postmenopausal. Maximum number of patients (40;54.1%) had stage 1 pelvic organ prolapse in group A and 49(74.2%) in group B.

The most common type of pelvic organ prolapse was uterovaginal prolapse (48;34%),followed by cystocele (35;25%).Other types of pelvic organ prolapse were rectocele (10;7%) and cervical descent (4;3%).The most common combination of prolapse was cystocele and rectocele (25;18%) followed by cystocele and uterovaginal prolapse (9;6%) and cystocele,rectocele and uterovaginal prolapse in 7(5%) patients.

The most common symptom in both the groups at baseline was the feeling of something coming out of vagina which was present in 54(73.0%) patients in group A as compared to 50(76.0%) patients in group B. At the end of intervention, this symptom was present in 43% patients in group A and 64.1% patients in group B. There was relief in other symptoms also at the end of intervention in both groups.

There was a significant change in the mean POP-ss from baseline during follow up visits in both the groups exept follow up visit at 1 week in group A. The difference between groups regarding change in mean POP-ss score from baseline to follow up visits at 6 weeks,18 weeks and at 24 weeks follow up was significant. The comparison of mean PFIQ-7 score between the groups showed significant difference at 6th week follow up visit.

There was significant difference in the mean VAS score at follow up visits in group A except the follow up visit at 1 week. There was significant change in the mean VAS score at follow up visits at 6, 18 and 24 weeks in group B. There was no significant difference in the mean VAS score between group A & B compared at baseline and follow up visit at 6 weeks. However, the difference was significant at 18 and 24 weeks.

In group A, there was an increase in number of patients with mild symptoms from 30(40.5%) at baseline to 35(47.2%) at the end of intervention. The shift in category from moderate to mild symptoms was seen in 10(55.5%) patients and from severe to mild symptoms was seen in 5(83.3%) patients. The patients with severe symptoms decreased from 6(8.1%) at baseline to 3(4%) at the end of intervention.In group B, there was an increase in number of patients with mild symptoms from 24(36.4%) at baseline to 31(47%) at the end of intervention. The shift in category from moderate to mild symptoms was seen in 4(22.2%) patients and from severe to mild symptoms was seen in 3(50%) patients.

In group A downstaging was observed in five patients. One patient improved from stage 1 to stage 0 uterovaginal prolapse,2 patients with cystocele had improvement from stage 2 to stage 1 and 2 patients had improvement in stage 3 rectocele to stage 2. In group B, only one patient had improvement from stage 3 cysto-rectocele to stage 3.

So, the results of this study illustrates that POP can be demedicalised to quite an extent by involving paramedical personnel in treating the affected women. It is, in fact, an example of the success of low cost, low technology intervention. Its replicability is also likely to be high along with its potential use in the healthcare delivery system. It will save doctors' time in the hospital setting for other reproductive needs of the patients. With this simple therapy women will be able to get relief from a problem which has significant impact on the quality of life.

Causes of pelvic organ prolapse

Normally, the pelvic organs are held in place by the pelvic floor muscles and supporting ligaments, but when the pelvic floor becomes stretched or weakened, they may become too slack to hold the organs in place. A number of different factors contributing to the weakening of pelvic muscles over time are:

1. **Pregnancy and childbirth:** Pregnancy is believed to be the main cause of pelvic organ prolapse, whether the prolapse occurs immediately after pregnancy or 30 years later. The weight of the baby and the physical trauma of labour and birth are the causative factors.
2. **Obesity, large fibroids or tumors:** Women who are severely overweight, or have large fibroids or pelvic tumors, are at an increased risk of prolapse due to the extra pressure this creates in their abdominal area.
3. **Chronic cough and constipation:** Chronic (long-term) coughing, from smoking, asthma or bronchitis or the straining associated with constipation, increases a woman's risk of prolapse. If the stress and strain is ongoing, it may eventually weaken the pelvic support structures.
4. **Heavy lifting**: Heavy lifting can also strain and damage pelvic muscles and women in careers that involve regular manual labour or lifting, have an increased risk of prolapse.

5. **Genetic conditions:** Women with a genetic collagen deficiency (Marfan or Ehlers-Danlos syndrome) have an increased risk of prolapse even if they don't have any of the other risk factors. Collagen is a natural protein that helps keep tissues plump and elastic. Without it, the pelvic floor muscles become weak.
6. **Previous pelvic surgery:** Pelvic surgery, including hysterectomy or bladder repair procedures, may damage nerves and tissues in the pelvic area increasing a woman's risk of prolapse.
7. **Spinal cord conditions and injury:** Spinal cord injury and conditions such as muscular dystrophy and multiple sclerosis dramatically increase a woman's risk of prolapse. If the pelvic muscles are paralyzed or movement is restricted, the muscles waste away and cannot support the pelvic organs.
8. **Toileting habit**. In general, women in urban areas use the **'sit'** method while the rural women use **'squat'** toilets. Basically, squatting causes the angle of the pelvis to relax much better and give better pressure. When you are sitting, you do not have the right relaxation of the muscles and the angle of the pelvis. **'Squat' toilets are an excellent way** for women to exercise their perineum and pelvic floor muscles. **Sitting toilets increase the risk of Pelvic organ prolapse** because users are forced to strain for waste evacuation.

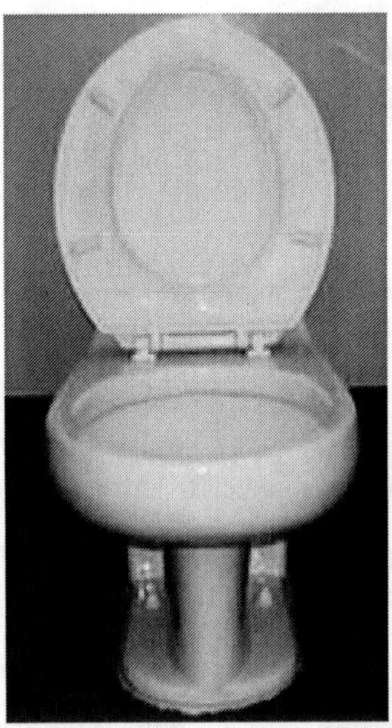
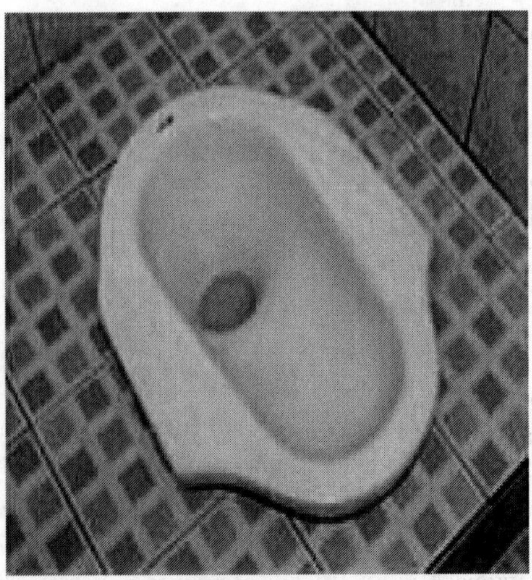

Pix 1 & 2 "Sit method" Squat method.

TYPES OF PELVIC ORGAN PROLAPSE

There are a number of different types of prolapse that can occur in pelvic area.

1. **Cystocele (bladder prolapse):**

   When the bladder prolapses, it falls towards the vagina and creates a large bulge in the front vaginal wall and is the most common type of prolapse in women.

2. **Uterine Prolapse:**

   Uterine prolapse is when the womb drops down into the vagina. It is the second most common type of prolapse.

Uterine prolapse is classified into three grades:

Grade 1: The uterus drops slightly. At this stage many women may not be aware they have a prolapse. It may not cause any symptoms and is usually diagnosed as a result of an examination for a separate problem.

Grade 2: The uterus drops further into the vagina and the cervix and the neck or tip of the womb can be seen outside the vaginal opening.

Grade 3: Most of the uterus has fallen through the vaginal opening. This is the most severe form of uterine prolapse and is also called procidentia.

3. Rectocele (prolapse of the rectum or large bowel)

This occurs when the end of the large bowel (rectum) loses support and bulges into the back wall of the vagina.

4. Urethrocele (prolapse of the urethra)

When the urethra (the tube that carries urine from the bladder) slips out of place, it also pushes against the front of the vaginal wall, but lower down, near the opening of the vagina. This usually happens together with a cystocele.

5. Enterocele (prolapse of the small bowel)

Part of the small intestine that lies just behind the uterus may slip down between the rectum and the back wall of the vagina. This often occurs at the same time as a rectocele or uterine prolapse.

6. Vaginal vault prolapse

The vaginal vault is the top of the vagina. It can only fall in on itself after a woman's womb has been removed. Vault prolapse occurs in about 15% of women who have had a hysterectomy for uterine prolapse.

Symptoms of pelvic organ prolapse

The terminologies mostly used by women to express their symptoms of prolapse are "*Neeche bojh padta hei*" (pelvic heaviness'), "*Shareer bahar aa raha hei* (uterine prolapse)," *Bachchadani bahar aa rahi hei*" (uterine prolapse),"*Bachadani khisak gayi hei* "(slipped uterus), "*Neeche se kuch bahar ata hei* (something coming out from below)," *Peshab ke raste hava bahar ati hei*"(wind comes out through urethra).

The women continue to tolerate prolapse for years together before seeking treatment. Thus, the quality of life of the affected women is seriously compromised. This is reflected by the following narration of women with prolapse:

1. "When I carry something heavy,"*shareer*" (uterus) comes down more. I can hardly walk then." "Squatting down to wash clothes and vessels is becoming agonizing"
2. "The body (uterus) touches the thighs while walking. After working for a while, I feel a desire to rest for some time. I can work only when I sit down and keep a cloth piece (pad) down below. I do not feel like doing hard work. Often I feel it is better to die."
3. "I am unable to do any work, and feel very depressed. Very often I get acute pain and burning sensation during urination. There is also profuse and smelly white discharge on many days"
4. "This year I could not go to the fields to work due to this problem (prolapse). My husband beats me daily as I am neither able to go to work nor willing to sleep with him. He refuses to believe that I am in pain. He says, what's wrong with you, you look healthy"
5. "After the delivery of my first child,. I had no rest even for a week, as no help was available. One day, I had to carry a huge basket of cow dung. As I bent down and lifted it up from the floor to put it on my head, I felt something give way"
6. "I went to the nearby hospital many times for my problem. They said I would get better with drugs and no surgery was required. I did not get any better. So I stopped taking the drugs also and problem aggravated."

Various interventions are available for preventing and treating pelvic organ prolapse, including medical devices and surgery. However, pelvic floor muscle exercises(**Kegel exercises**), which involves exercising the pelvic floor muscle, are the easiest to implement, since these exercises need no special equipment, additional health care infrastructure or other costly resources. It isn't just women who've given birth vaginally need to exercise pelvic floor muscles, but all the women. Slack pelvic floor muscles are the main cause of prolapse womb in women, and there is evidence that doing regular **Kegel exercises** avoid the need for hysterectomies, an operation which is becoming increasingly common these days. Hence, the precious time of the patients, concerned health staff is saved. Also, the impoverishment associated with the brunt of expenses for pelvic organ prolapse surgery can be avoided. Depending on the surgery, hospital stay usually lasts three to seven days, which adversely affects the child care. Most patients require at least some prescription for relieving pain for about one to two weeks after surgery. After surgery also, patients are asked to "take it easy" usually for 12 weeks to allow proper healing. This means no lifting more than 5 pounds, no intercourse, nothing in the vagina and no exercise other than walking. Since, the entire responsibility for caring of children, household activities is often with women and lack of concern shown by husbands; it is negatively associated with compliance to advices given by doctors.

If these exercises are done routinely, that grim future can be prevented and any current problems can be alleviated and improved. Doing these exercises regularly, prevents, limits progression and alleviates symptoms of pelvic organ prolapse.

Being non-invasive, easy-to-learn and an exercise that can be done practically anywhere anytime, Kegel exercise is an appropriate exercise for strengthening the pelvic floor muscles. Doing these exercises regularly, will enable women to have control over and improve their pelvic health.

Some degree of descent occurs in most women who have experienced vaginal childbirth. However, majority of these women have no symptoms. Early symptoms include feelings of heaviness or pelvic pressure, dragging sensation in the back and straining while passing urine.

Pelvic organ prolapse is curable. However, in countries like India, patients continue to suffer because of social stigma and "culture of silence" and "shame" associated with gynaecological problems. Even the most outspoken Indian female tends to close her lips when it comes to vocalizing her symptoms related to reproductive health. Most of the gynaecological problems are frustrating and embarrassing for the women. These problems seriously affect quality of life of women. Still the women do not seek any treatment. This is because of shyness, illiteracy, unawareness, lack of motivation among women in India, low socioeconomic status of the family and lack of easily accessible medical care in rural and semi-urban parts of India.

Women's lack of autonomy in decision making is also an important constraint on women's health seeking. Women are, by and large, taught self-modesty from an early age and are hence unlikely to acknowledge a health problem, and particularly a gynaecological problem. Lack of decision making, freedom of movement and time can restrict visits to the health centres, even where a health problem has been recognized. Moreover, pelvic examinations are strongly resisted by women. And even if a problem has been diagnosed, treatment is frequently not followed through because it is seen as an unnecessary expense or too demanding. Lack of concern is often shown by husbands regarding attending the clinic. They feel that the examination would cause pain, bleeding, and discomfort for the women and would make sexual intercourse painful. They also express their unwillingness to look after the children at home, if the woman goes to hospital for treatment. As a result, some women become frustrated and mentally depressed and do not show an interest in seeking health care. Religious belief, faith in spiritual healers, and remedies are also responsible for the low rate of consultation. Hence, the symptoms deteriorate.

In such a scenario, an effective conservative regimen (Kegel exercise) is a welcome option. This is a real health promotion measure for millions of women, which needs to be suitably utilised. Such an approach of conservative behavioural therapy of urinary incontinence in women has been found to be successful in Indian settings also (Kumari et al 2008).

It is required that similar approach of using Kegel exercise is tried for early stage of pelvic organ prolapse. Successful demonstration of use of such conservative regimen in hospital settings will go a long way in mitigating plight of women.

Operation (Surgery) is a dreadful pronouncement by the gynaecologist for the hopeless women who have who have pelvic organ prolapse. In general everyone fears surgery of any kind. For women (especially from rural area), it is a difficult situation. Because of her low social status in society and family, household commitments are often given more importance by her. Usually she postpones surgery on one pretext or the other and continues to suffer the symptoms.

Treatment modalities for pelvic organ prolapse

There are surgical and non-surgical options for treating uterine prolapse. The treatment chosen depends upon the severity of the condition, as well as the women's general health, age and desire to have children. Uterine prolapse may be treated surgically by removing the uterus (hysterectomy) when the women already has desired number of children and do not want any further pregnancy. Other procedures like Fothergill repair, anterior and posterior colporrhaphy involve putting uterus back into its normal position. These are done in women in whom family is not yet complete.

For mild cases of uterine prolapse (grade I & II), non-surgical conservative management is possible. Kegel exercises are recommended to strengthen the pelvic muscles in such cases. These exercises are easy to do. These can be done anywhere, at any time. Pessaries have also been used for management of milder pelvic organ prolapse. In menopausal women, taking oestrogens may help to limit further weakness of the muscles and other connective tissues that support the uterus.

However, despite all these modalities being available in India, most women do not seek treatment for pelvic organ prolapse, until their problem becomes severe. Even though reproduction and childbirth is considered a normal phenomenon in life of a woman, why are the health problems related to reproductive organs dealt with shyness? Women should talk and discuss with doctor or health care provider about problem at an early stage. Why to wait for a stage that .the life becomes miserable? Women should not have to" learn to live with it"

Advice from doctor should be sought, when following symptoms are noticed:

- Feeling of something coming out of vagina.
- Uncomfortable feeling or pain in vagina which is worse when standing.
- Heaviness or dragging feeling in lower abdomen.
- Heaviness or dragging feeling in lower back.
- Need to strain (push) to empty bladder.
- Feeling that bladder has not emptied completely.
- Feeling that bowel has not emptied completely.

How to prevent progression of prolapse when the problem is in early stage?

There are a number of ways to prevent a mild prolapse form getting worse:

- One of the most effective ways is to exercise pelvic floor muscles. Doing regular pelvic floor exercises (also called Kegel exercises), helps keep the muscles toned and strong.
- If overweight, try to lose weight. This will remove some of the pressure from your pelvic area.
- If you smoke, try to cut down or stop, as this will help reduce strain from coughing.
- Do not lift heavy objects. This can damage pelvic muscles.
- Eat a high fiber diet (fresh fruits, vegetables, bran) to help prevent constipation and reduce straining.

Prolapse doesn't necessarily worsen over time, so there's no need to seek aggressive treatments, unless symptoms are really bothersome. But if symptoms are mild or surgery is to be delayed or avoided, less invasive treatments can help. Women with prolapse but mild symptoms can practice Kegel exercises to reduce the chances of progression. The regular and correct performance of Kegel exercises has been proven to help in the prevention and progression of pelvic organ prolapse in women, as well as improving problems with bladder and faecal incontinence and poor sexual response.

What are Pelvic Floor Exercises (Kegel Exercises)?

Pelvic floor exercises (Kegel Exercises) help prevent prolapse by strengthening the muscles that support the pelvic organs. Kegel exercises reduce the chances of progression of prolapse. Since performing Kegel strengthening exercises is not visible to the naked eye, these can be performed while sitting, standing, or lying down. They can be done anywhere at any time.

But still, these exercises are not done by the women. Reasons given by the women are "I don't have the time out of my busy schedule throughout the day" "I've never heard of pelvic floor muscle exercises." "I've done pelvic muscle exercises in the past but they didn't make any difference, so, I stopped doing" "I tried but I can't do pelvic muscle exercises." "I don't know how to exercise my pelvic muscles. "I do so much of household activity everyday isn't it enough exercise for me? The answer to all the above excuses is just one...that is the lack of self-care attitude towards one's own health by the women. As doing exercises regularly, helps in building stamina, the same is true for these exercises for the pelvic floor. Doing these exercises regularly should be made as a part of routine activity. These exercises not only help keeping pelvic structures in place, but also help to control urine leakage, as well as improve sensation in the lower region for more sexual sensation. These exercise if done on daily basis helps to prevent pelvic floor complications later in life.

How to do Pelvic Floor Exercises (Kegel Exercises)?

The exercises are easy and quick to do, but it's important to do them correctly. Many patients make mistake while doing pelvic exercises. They start exercising the wrong muscle. Familiarizing with the muscles of each orifice gives a better chance of performing the exercises correctly.

Start by **locating the muscles you need to exercise**. There are a few different ways to do this:

- Place one or two fingers in your vagina and squeeze your muscles until you can feel your vagina tighten around your fingers. These are your pelvic muscles.

- Imagine you're trying to stop the flow of urine mid-stream. The muscles you tighten are your pelvic floor muscles.
- The other way to identify the correct muscles is to imagine you are trying to stop yourself from passing gas. The muscles you squeeze to do this are your pelvic muscles.

You should be able to feel your vagina tighten and your pelvic floor move upward. Then relax your muscles and feel your pelvic floor move down to the starting position. As your muscles become stronger and you become more experienced with the exercises, this movement will be more pronounced.

But don't make a habit of starting and stopping your urine stream, as a regular practice. Doing Kegel exercises with a full bladder or while emptying your bladder can actually weaken the muscles. It can also lead to incomplete emptying of the bladder, which increases your risk of a urinary tract infection.

If you're having trouble finding the right muscles, don't be embarrassed to ask for help from doctor to identify and exercise the correct muscles.

Once you've identified the correct muscles you're ready to begin. The exercises can be done while lying down, sitting or standing, with your knees together or slightly apart.

Remember to squeeze pelvic floor muscles whenever you sneeze or cough.

Step 1 —Slowly tighten your pelvic floor muscles and count to four, then let the muscles relax for a count of four. As your muscles get stronger gradually increase the count to 10 and relaxation for a count of 10.

Check that you're not tightening the muscles in your legs, abdomen or buttocks, as it's important to use only your pelvic muscles. Remember to keep breathing during the exercise.

Step 2 — Now, tighten and relax your pelvic muscles as quickly as you can, i.e., 10 times and relaxation for a count of 10 in between each contraction.

Try to do the exercises three to four times a day, but don't overdo it. Excessive exercising of the pelvic muscles can cause muscle fatigue and make the exercises less effective.

You can feel the changes in your symptoms like feeling of something coming down per vagina, dragging pain in the pelvis, heaviness or dragging sensation in the pelvis need to strain (push) to empty bladder, feeling that the bladder has not emptied completely, heaviness or dragging pain in the lower back and feeling that the bowel has not emptied completely, with time. **A minimum of 6 to 8 weeks** of therapy is necessary before improvement can be realized. Pelvic muscle exercises are like other muscles of the body that can be trained.

Preventive measures to reduce risk of prolapse:

- **Doing Kegel exercises during pregnancy**: Pregnant women should do Kegels because strong pelvic floor muscles help make childbirth, specifically pushing, easier and lowers chances of tears happening during labor. During the postpartum period, doing Kegels helps in healing from an episiotomy as well as prevent postpartum leakage and gives tone to outstretched vaginal muscles, thereby making sex better. However, these exercises should be done during pregnancy only after consultation with your gynecologist.
- **Doing Kegel exercises during menopause:** Kegel exercises, if done regularly and correctly, prevent the onset or progression of prolapse by strengthening the pelvic floor musculature. Doing these exercises should be made a part of routine activity.
- **Loose excess body fat with dietary modifications and regular exercise:** If you are significantly overweight, try to lose weight. This you can do by dietary modifications like decreasing your fat intake, increasing the intake of vegetables, fruits and salad. Regular exercise should be done so as to maintain appropriate weight. Maintaining the normal weight will remove some of the pressure from your pelvic area. Hence, prevent onset and progression of prolapse.
- **Eat a high fiber diet** (fresh fruits, vegetables, bran) to help **prevent constipation** and reduce straining .Drink plenty of fluid, eat lots of fruit, vegetables and fiber, and relax your tummy muscles to avoid straining when using your bowels.
- **Try to cut down or stop smoking:** If you smoke, try to cut down or stop, as this will help reduce strain from coughing.
- **Don't lift heavy objects**. When you lift heavy objects, this puts pressure on the pelvic muscles and weaken them and hence cause sagging of the pelvic floor organs. So, lifting of heavy objects should be avoided.
- **Treatment for underlying disorders:** Treatment should be taken for underlying disorders, especially those which produce raised intra-abdominal pressure like cough(due to asthma, chronic bronchitis or chronic constipation) in consultation with doctor.

Hence, it isn't just women who've given birth vaginally who need to exercise pelvic floor muscles, but all the women. Slack pelvic floor muscles are the main cause of prolapsed womb in women, and there is evidence that **regular pelvic floor exercises avoid** the need for unnecessary hysterectomies, an operation which is becoming increasingly common in these days .If you start to exercise your pelvic floor muscles routinely, that grim future can be prevented and any current problems can be alleviated and improved.

References

1. Cardozo L. Prolapse. In: Dewhurst editor. Textbook of Obstetrics and Gynecology for postgraduates. 5th ed. Oxford: Blackwell Science, ***1995; 642-52.***
2. WHO. Measuring reproductive morbidity. Report of technical working group WHO/MCH/90.4. Division of Family Planning, Geneva. Aug 30 – Sept 1, 1989; 1–39.
3. Dawn C.S. Practical highlights of genital prolapse. *J Obstet Gynecol India* 1998; 213 –15.
4. World Bank. India's Family Welfare Program: towards a reproductive and child health approach. Population and Human Resources Operations Division. South Asia Country Department II. 1995; Report no. 14644-IN.
5. Swift SE. The distribution of pelvic organ support in a population of female subjects seen for routine gynaecologic health care. Am J Obstet Gynecol 2000; 183:277–85.
6. Kumari S, Walia I, Singh A. Self reported uterine prolapse in a resettlement colony of north india.J Midwifery women's health 2000; 45:343-50.
7. Kegel A. A Progressive resistance exercise in the functional restoration of the perineal muscles. Am J Obstet Gynecol 1948; 56:238-46.
8. Hendrix SL, Clark A, Nygaard I, Aragaki A, Barnabei V, McTiernan A. Pelvic organ prolapse in the Women's Health Initiative: gravity and gravidity. Am J Obstet Gynecol 2002; 186:1160–6. 8 6
9. Suzanne H, Diane S, Cathryn G, Lesley S, Ian R. A randomized controlled trial of pelvic floor muscle training for stages 1 and 2 pelvic organ prolapse, Int Urogynecol 2009; 20:45–51.
10. Ghroubi S, Kharrat O, Chaari M, Ben AB, Guermazi M, Elleuch MH. Effect of conservative treatment in the management of low urogenital prolapse. Ann Readapt Med Phys 2008; 51:96–102.
11. Piya-Anant M, Therasakvichya S, Leelaphatanadit C, Techatrisak K. Integrated health research program for the Thai elderly: Prevalence of genital prolapse and effectiveness of pelvic floor exercise to prevent worsening of genital prolapse in elderly women. J Med Assos Thail 2003; 86:509–15.
12. John OL. The hidden epidemic of pelvic floor dysfunction: Achievable goals for improved prevention and treatment. American Journal of Obstetrics and Gynecology 2005; 192: 488-95.
13. Demedicalizing Women's Health. AJ Singh (Editor), (Mrs.) Indrajit Walia, LK Dhaliwal (Co- editors), New Delhi, Gyan Publishing House, 2010.

Chapter - 9

Empowering Women to Deal with Menopause Related Problems

— *Dr. Purnima Kaushal, Dr. Ruchi Sharma, Dr. Neelam Aggarwal, Dr. Seema Chopra, Dr. Amarjeet Singh*

1. Introduction

Menopause is defined as "the final menstruation." It is the final stoppage of menses in a middle aged woman. In reality, it is not a single event. This is a part of the ageing process. With age ovulation ceases. Thereafter menstruation also stops (meno = month; pauses = pause). Menopause is not a disease. Rather, it is a new but temporary phase in a woman's life. This natural process in women's life starts many years before menopausal symptoms actually begin to occur. Menopause happens to every woman. Menopause is something about which we have no choice. Every woman has to deal with this phase. Manifestation of various symptoms and problems at menopause is not uniform. Tolerance of different women for these symptoms also varies. That is why it is important to understand as much about it as possible.

Normally, with age, the ovaries start to slow the production of hormones like estrogen, progesterone and testosterone. Menopause occurs due to decline in female hormone levels. These levels fluctuate for several years before eventually becoming so low that the lining of uterus becomes thin and the bleeding stops. The average age of the natural menopause is between 47.8 years in India and 51.4 years in the Western Countries.

2. Terminology And Definitions Related To Menopause

The transition from regular menstrual cycle to cessation of menstrual period is rarely a sudden phenomenon. Most women can tell if they are approaching menopause when their menstrual periods start changing. For a year or two, periods may be regular. But scanty or less menses may occur at larger intervals or heavy menstruation with or without clots may be reported before menopause is reached.

Natural menopause is defined as the permanent cessation of menstruation resulting from decline in the function of ovaries. Natural menopause is recognized to have occurred after 12 consecutive months of amenorrhea, for which there is no other obvious pathological and physiological causes. Hence, we can say that a woman has attained menopause only in retrospect a year after the final menstrual period.

Induced menopause is the cessation of menstruation through either surgical removal of both ovaries with or without hysterectomy or by using medicines to stop ovary function e.g., by chemotherapy or radiation.

Early or premature menopause Menopause occurring before the age of 40.

Perimenopause (peri=around) is the period immediately prior to the menopause and the first year after menopause. This phase is characterized by irregular and unpredictable menstrual periods followed by stoppage of menses. Thereafter, the turbulent period of menopausal symptoms starts (caused by decline in hormone levels).

Postmenopause (post=after) is the period following the last menstruation.

3. Symptoms of Menopause and their Remedies

Experiences of women during menopause are often unique to them. Some women are able to undergo the menopausal transition without any problem. Some experience a variety of menopausal symptoms. The duration varies; for some women, the symptoms cease shortly after the occurrence of menopause, yet other women will continue experiencing them for many years. These menopausal symptoms may be unpleasant for some but not very bothersome for others. Though there are some common signs or symptoms at menopause, women may have different experiences about this phase of life. Degree and severity may vary. These symptoms are as follows:

1. Change in pattern of menstrual period

This might be what women may notice first. Periods may no longer be regular. They cycles may be shorter or longer than normal. Bleeding may be less or more than usual. These are all normal changes at menopause. Changes occur in usual cycle. Periods may also be missed. There may be more frequent periods. Menstrual flow may be heavier or lighter than usual. These changes may persist for several months.

The most common indicator of irregular periods is a shorter than normal interval between periods, often as little as two weeks. In other cases, symptoms of irregular periods during menopause may consist of more widely spaced periods, including menstruation that comes every six weeks – or even less frequently. Some women will even miss a period - or several in a row - before resuming their regular menstrual cycle. Thus, a woman who had and regular monthly periods throughout her life may have a period in March, then miss it for 4-5 months and have an unpredicted period in August.

It is important to realize here that periods will eventually stop at menopause. Usually, this corresponds with decline or cessation of fertility. However, during perimenopause many women may still have periods. The periods may become irregular. Some women may even retain their fertility. So, at menopause when menstruation stops or its pattern changes, it is advisable to get a pregnancy test done to rule out conception, particularly among those who had not undergone tubectomy etc.

When menstrual pattern changes during perimnopause bleeding may last for as long as a week, or as little as 1-2 days. In some cases, the menstrual flow itself will vary - some women will experience lighter periods than what is normal for them, while other may have heavier flow.

Physical symptoms may also accompany irregular periods during perimenopause. These usually include severe painful cramping and blood clots. In fact, one more or a combination of range in pattern of menstrual period given below may occur in a woman:

- More frequent periods
- Shorter periods
- Longer periods
- Skipped periods
- Noticeable blood clots
- Bleeding in between periods
- Changes in menstrual flow
- Heavy cramping
- Breast tenderness
- Months without during menses
- Months without periods

Causes of irregular periods

Like most menopause symptoms, the primary cause of irregular periods is hormonal imbalance. During normal menstrual periods, in younger women estrogen is the hormone that causes the lining of the uterus to thicken in preparation for ovulation. Progesterone is the hormone that signals the uterus to shed that lining if there is no fertilized egg to make use of it.

During perimenopause, a woman may have a cycle in which no egg is produced. In that case, progesterone is not produced either, which leads to higher levels of estrogen. This build-up can result in heavier periods, since the uterine lining may have built up over several months. Further hormonal imbalances can lead to an irregular period duration, irregular heaviness in flow, and inconsistency in duration.

Some tips for relief from irregular periods

The basic resort to treating a heavy menstrual flow should be natural, non-invasive remedies, such as taking B-Complex vitamins, vitamin A and vitamin C, which are thought to regulate the body's estrogen levels. At this time, due to loss of blood, women may feel weak. They should add more of green leafy vegetables, juices fruits in their diet. In most cases the changes in pattern and flow of periods are tolerated well by women. Some cases may need hysterectomy if the bleeding is very severe or too heavy.

2. Hot flushes

Many women experience 'heat sensation' at meno-pause. It is called 'hot flushes.' It is a momentary sensation of heat that may be accompanied by a red, flushed face and sweating. The cause of hot flushes is not known. But it may be related to changes in blood circulation. Hot flushes occur when the blood vessels near the skin's surface dilate (open more). So, blood flow comes closer to outer skin surface. This produces the red, flushed look on the face. A woman may also perspire to cool down the body. In addition, some women experience a rapid heart rate or chills. Hot flushes accompanied with sweating can also occur at night("night sweats") All this interferes with sleep.

Some women report hot flushes in the upper body that may rise up from the abdomen. In some cases, it may emanate from the toes—into the chest, back, and head, and may be accompanied by perspiration. Hot flushes may last from about one to five minutes. Once the flushes are over, some women may also feel a cold sensation.

Reason for hot flushes

The reasons why women have hot flushes has not been fully explained. In the past, doctors said that it had everything to do with the decrease in estrogen as a woman approached menopause. However, not all women get hot flushes

How long hot flushes last?

The severity and duration of hot flushes varies among different women going through menopause. Some women have hot flushes for a very short time during menopause. Other women may have hot flushes— at least to some degree – for rest of their life. Generally, hot flushes become less severe as time passes.

Some tips to prevent hot flushes

- Physical and psychological symptoms of 'heat' can be tackled by drinking lots of water, *shikanjvi, lassi, amm pana* etc. Herbal teas can also help. Wear soft and loose clothing. Eat smaller meals, more often.
- **Stay cool:** Keep your bedroom cool at night. Use fans during the day. Wear light layers of clothes with natural fibers such as cotton. If possible, go to the bathroom and splash the face with cold water. This will quickly lower body temperature and alleviate the episode.
- **Breathing exercise:** Try deep, slow abdominal breathing (six to eight breaths per minute). Practice deep breathing for 15 minutes in the morning, 15 minutes in the evening. This can also be tried at the onset of hot flushes.
- **Exercise daily**: Walking, swimming, dancing, and yoga help women to stay fit.
- **Intake of more fluids:** Drink plenty of water. Drinking a glass of cold water help to reduce hot flushes. Cut down drinks with caffeine such as soda, tea, and coffee. Caffeine stimulates the body and worsens hot flushes. So, avoid these.
- **Diet:** Consume a diet rich in vitamins, minerals, and whole grains. Soya is also a food that is beneficial through menopause. It is wise to avoid alcohol and foods high in spices which increase hot flushes.
- **Fresh air**: Fresh air is great for reducing stress. Go for a short walk. If nothing else venture out in balcony or verandah. It is helpful for women with hot flushes. At the onset, breathe slowly and get some clean air.

3. Night sweats

This refers to excess sweating during the night. If severe, it can even drench bedding. It may also disturb sleep pattern. This is also caused by low levels of estrogen. Anxiety or depression can further aggravate night sweats.

Symptoms of night sweats

Sudden intense overheating, flushing and drenching perspiration are the primary symptoms of menopause. In addition, heart beat increases. Women may also experience irregular heartbeats. Night sweats may also cause nausea or headaches. As the profuse perspiration cools, women may also experience chills. In many women, rises in temperature and discomfort that accompany night sweats may also contribute to the development of insomnia or nightmares.

Most common night sweat symptoms are:

- Flushing
- Excessive perspiring
- Irregular heartbeats (arrhythmia)
- Rapid heart rate (tachycardia)
- Headaches
- Nausea
- Chills
- Panic attacks
- Bizarre or disturbing dreams
- Insomnia
- Exhaustion
- Difficulty in concentrating

Reasons that triggers night sweats: There are also many external triggers that can set off night sweats.

- **Environmental factors:** Warm weather or an overheated bedroom, are the two main causes.
- **Dietary factors:** Consuming hot or spicy foods, alcohol, caffeine and smoking are also likely to trigger night sweats.
- **Psychological factors**: Stress and anxiety can trigger the night sweats.
- **Addictions:** Alcohol, caffeine and smoking are also likely to trigger night sweats.

Basic tips to prevent night sweats

- Avoid doing anything that could stress out body or mind.
- Avoid spicy foods and caffeinated food/drink before bedtime.
- Avoid large meals before going to bed. Avoid official or physical household work before going to bed.
- Deep breathing exercise for 15 minutes every morning and night before sleep.
- Always wear light loose cotton clothes.
- Keep your bedroom cool when it's time to sleep.

4. Vaginal dryness

With the onset of menopause intercourse can become uncomfortable or painful. This is due to the thinning of the vaginal walls. There is also dryness and loss of elasticity in vagina. It leads to pain during intercourse. Menopause vaginal dryness occurs because of loss of moisture during menopause. There is loss of natural lubrication. Vaginal tissues get dehydrated. Skin in the genital region becomes itchy and dry.

Symptoms of menopause vaginal dryness

During menopause women can face symptoms such as itching, flaking of genital skin, and vaginal aching. Due to dehydration of the vaginal tissues that occurs during menopause, women may experience painful intercourse, leading to loss of libido and lowered sexual intimacy. Women may also experience irritation, stinging or burning sensations in the vagina and labia. In some cases, light bleeding may also occur as skin and surrounding tissues become irritated and broken.

Some tips to reduce vaginal dryness

Menopause vaginal dryness can be treated in many ways. Women may use specialized topical moisturizers or water-based lubricants in order to reduce the effects of vaginal dryness temporarily. Drinking plenty of water can also help keep vaginal tissues hydrated. Vitamin E oil also may be helpful for combating vaginal dryness in the short-term.

5. Aches and Pains

One peculiar symptom of menopause is an increase in frequency of normal aches, such as, headaches, neck, joint and back pains.

(a) Headaches: There may be persistent pain, pressure and tension in head due to hormonal imbalances. These symptoms are considered menopausal headaches.

Symptoms of menopause headaches

These may vary by the type of headache that occurs. Common symptoms include a surging, pulsating pain in the head and throbbing in the forehead or temples. Different women may face or experience one or more of following types of headache.

- Throbbing headache
- Tension
- Neck pain
- Nausea
- Sensitivity to sound - one feels irritated by noise (may want to put off TV)
- Light sensitivity – one feels uncomfortable in light (may like to turn off the light)
- Vomiting
- Sweating palms
- Visual distortion
- Sinus pressure

(b) Joint pains: This occurs when the joints become swollen, stiff or painful during menopause. This is also known as "menopausal arthritis." There may be pain and soreness in the back, knee joints and hips. However, many women also experience pain throughout the other joints in the body during menopause. Women may find that fingers and wrists become especially sore during menopause, particularly with repetitive motion. Some women may find that joint stiffness becomes worse in the morning, with swelling occurring around joints at the end of the day.

Symptoms of menopause joint pains

- Stiff joints
- High impact pain
- Swelling around joints
- Limited range of motion
- "Creaking" knees
- Finger and wrist pain
- Pain that subsides with rest
- Difficulty walking or running
- Painful joints
- Burning sensations
- Numbness
- Back pain
- Swollen ankles

Some tips to prevent aches and pains during menopause

While the underlying cause of menopause aches and pains is the hormonal imbalances that occur with age, self help measures may help to provide relief temporarily. Physical therapy, exercise, stretching, and muscle building can all help prevent aches and pains during midlife. Plenty of Vitamin D and calcium should be taken as part of a balanced menopause diet.

6. Bladder problems (menopausal urinary incontinence)

Menopausal urinary incontinence is simply defined as the **loss of bladder control**. There are two primary types of urinary incontinence related to menopause:

i. **Stress urinary incontinence** is most common. It occurs when there is increased pressure on the bladder by laughing, sneezing, coughing or lifting a heavy object.

ii. **Urge urinary incontinence** is a sudden need to urinate, often leading to uncontrollable release of urine.

Both stress urinary and urge urinary incontinence can occur as a result of the hormonal imbalance of menopause.

Causes of menopausal urinary incontinence

Primary cause of urinary incontinence among women experiencing menopause is lack of estrogen. One of the functions of estrogen is to maintain the lining of the bladder and urethra. These linings can deteriorate when estrogen is lacking. In addition, the bladder muscles tend to weaken during menopause. All this leads to urinary incontinence.

How to prevent bladder problems

- Kegel exercises help to strengthen the muscles of the pelvic floor (Overall 80% relief has been observed in women who do the kegel exercises).
- Reduce intake of foods or beverages that increase urination or may irritate the bladder (e.g., coffee, tea, alcohol).
- Drink plenty of fluids during the day; limit it 2 to 3 hours before going to sleep.
- Empty the bladder completely when you urinate. Bladder training also helps.

  (For details read books on urinary leakage and prolapse by the authors)

7. Skin problems

Skin also becomes thinner at menopause. So, dryness of skin is reported after menopause. Without estrogen, skin finds it difficult to retain moisture. During menopause, levels of hormone estrogen decline. This leads to reduction in the thickness of the skin. This is because there is reduction in collagen production that makes the skin more cushioned and flexible. This increases the appearance of wrinkles and lines around the face (particularly around the eyes and mouth). Menopausal changes also affect the body's ability to retain moisture. This in turn results in itchy skin.

Itching during the menopause may also occur in secondary situations, accompanied by rashes, skin flushing, eczema or other skin problems. Women may experience itches throughout the body, especially on their elbows. On the face, the "T-Zone," the skin along the forehead, nose and chin, can also be susceptible to itching and flaking. Menopause itching can also affect the rest of the body, such as the chest, abdomen, extremities and back. In some cases, women can even experience itching under their fingernails at menopause.

Some tips to avoid skin problems and itching

- Consumption of fatty acids, vitamins and minerals (particularly vitamin B, D and E) and proteins.
- Avoid harsh soaps.
- Avoid itching.
- The use of moisturizing creams that can replenish the skin's lost moisture.
- Drink plenty of water.
- Good hygiene.

8. Weight gain

About 90% of menopausal women experience some amount of weight gain. It is a natural and common aspect of getting older. It occurs because the body mass increases, as a result of fat deposits. However, weight gain associated with menopause typically involves increased amounts of fat around the abdomen. On an average, women gain between 8-10 kilogram between the ages of 45 and 55, the stage in life when menopause occurs. This extra weight generally does not evenly distribute itself throughout a woman's body. The weight tends instead to accumulate around the abdomen or thighs.

Beginning at about age 30, an individual's physical abilities begin to decrease and continue deteriorating until about age 60 or 70. The body's abilities then level off and decline at a slower rate. The rate of decline depends largely on an individual's physical activity and particular lifestyle. This decreasing physical ability affects weight because a person becomes less able to engage in physical activities that help to maintain a stable weight by burning calories. Even though physical changes are an unavoidable part of getting older that leads to weight gain, a woman's lifestyle is also a hugely important variable that can lead to put extra weight gain. Stress, reduced physical activity, change in eating habit, certain medication may also lead to weight gain. This can itself lead to very serious health conditions, e.g; Heart disease, stroke, high blood pressure, osteo-arthritis, breast cancer, high cholesterol, kidney disease, sleep apnea, insulin resistance (increasing diabetes risks),or more severe menopausal symptoms.

Some tips to control weight:

Simple changes in lifestyle can give good results in reducing weight gain.

- Regular exercise go for a walk and do yoga.
- Eat Balanced diet.
- Avoid potato, sweets, rice, fried food, *maida* based food, etc.
- Get sleep of 7-8 hours daily.
- Avoid alcohol, tea, coffee, soda/cola products.
- Drink a plenty of water.

9. Mood swings

Mood swings are defined as extreme or abrupt fluctuations in mood. During mood swings, people often experience drastic shifts in their emotional state. The term "mood swing" is often used to describe an emotional reaction that is inappropriate to its cause or trigger. Because each woman has her own unique way of managing her emotions, stress, and her environment, all women experience the symptoms of mood swings differently. However, many symptoms of mood swings are common among women going through menopause. Frequent mood changes are:

- Unexplainable emotions
- Sadness
- Aggression
- Increased stress
- Nervousness
- Depression
- Lack of motivation
- Irritability
- Decreased patience
- Anxiety

Mood swings during menopause are caused largely by the hormonal transitions women go through during this time. Hormones, such as estrogen influence the production of serotonin, which is a mood regulating neuro-transmitter. However, there are other causes of mood swings. Other menopause symptoms such as hot flushes, night sweats, physical changes, and fatigue can cause or intensify mood swings. But these symptoms are generally caused by hormonal imbalance as well.

Risk factors for mood swings

Psychological Factors	*Behavioral Factors*	*Health Factors*
• Past mental illness	• Smoking	• Diabetes
• Stress	• Alcohol	• Early menopause
• Past trauma	• Poor diet	• Heart disease
• Relationship issues	• Inadequate exercise	• Sleep disorders
• Coping with change		• Cancer
		• Thyroid disease

Simple changes in lifestyle can give good results in fighting mood swings, and achieving a higher overall level of health. For reducing stress; yoga or meditation, combined with regular exercise and an improved diet can do women a great help. Diet, in particular is critical in regulating mood swings. Eating a balanced diet and avoiding sugary foods or excessive amounts of caffeine, stabilizes mood levels.

10. Sleep disturbance

On an average, a healthy adult needs approximately 7-8 hours of undisturbed sleep per night. Yet, many women do not receive the proper sleep. Women with sleep disturbances, experience the persistent problem of going without the recommended amount of uninterrupted sleep, leading to a weakened immune system find increased anxiety. This may also have a strain on her professional business or personal relationships, and cause emotional disturbances. Women who wake up more often during the night get tired and can't concentrate on work during the day. For menopausal women, the most commonly reported sleep disorders are insomnia, sleep apnea, snoring, and restless leg syndrome.

Symptoms related to sleep disorders

The symptoms caused by sleep disorders are often closely correlated to other symptoms of menopause. For example, night sweats, the night time version of hot flushes, can disrupt sleep patterns by causing a woman to awaken several times during the night. Sleep disorders can also lead to further depression and anxiety, which may make sleep difficult. This can cause a vicious circle of lack of sleep, fatigue, and other unpleasant symptoms of menopause.During the years leading up to menopause, a woman undergoes a great deal of changes involving her body which can lead to feelings of anxiety, depression, and stress. Anxiety is linked to an inability to fall asleep, while depression has been known to cause early morning awakening. Problems at work or issue in interpersonal relationships can add to stress levels and make it difficult to relax to obtain a full night rest. This can cause insomnia or other sleep disorders.

Other risk factors for sleep disorders

Some women are more prone to sleep disorders than others. Below is a list of risk factors that can make a woman more susceptible to sleep disorders:-

- Obesity
- Age
- Use of drugs/alcohol
- A job with rotating/night shifts
- High blood pressure
- Use of caffeine/nicotine
- Inactivity/lack of exercise

Effects of sleep disorders

Women may also suffer from sleep disorders such as sleep apnea at menopause. These interruptions in a woman's sleeping patterns surely have a noticeable effect on her daily life. Below is a list of common effects of sleep disorders:

- Reduced capacity for learning, speech, and memory.
- Inability to concentrate on daily tasks.
- Higher chance of car accidents.
- Tendency towards weight gain.
- Weakened immune system.
- Damage to professional and personal relationships.
- Increased irritability.
- Depression/fatigue.

Some tips for a good night sleep

- Go to bed only when sleepy.
- Sleep only in the bedroom.
- Get up at the same time each morning.
- Discontinue caffeine and nicotine.
- Exercise daily.
- Avoid alcohol.
- Limit fluid intake in the evening.
- Practice relaxation techniques

11. Other symptoms

Irritability, depression, personality changes and anxiety are very common during this phase. These changes can lead to a loss of sexual desire. Women also report many emotional problems at menopause. Although these problems are related to the shortage of estrogen, some may be caused by the inability to cope with the psychological impact caused by all the other symptoms. Added to all this is the fact that, in many cases, women going through menopause might also be under a number of other stressful situations. Things like problems associated with teenage children, children moving out for job or higher education, problems related to care of aging parents and spouse's mid-life crisis can also influence the state of mind of menopausal women. Many symptoms are simply due to aging. It is often difficult to differentiate between purely menopausal (hormone related) symptoms and those due to aging or family problems. Studies by authors on menopausal women in Chandigarh showed that the combined prevalence of hot flushes and nights sweats (54% to 63%) was very high (Parashar, 2009). Hot flushes, excessive sweating and diminished acuity of vision were the most common symptoms of the rural north Indian women (Singh and Arora, 2005). A research conducted on the women of Dhanas village near Chandigarh showed that the diminished vision, joint pain/bodyaches/headaches and hot flushes were the most common symptoms after menopause (Kaur and Singh, 2005).

4. An Approach to Deal with Problems of Menopause

Menopause is only the end of fertility, not the end of the life or productivity. In fact, for adult women, often life can, in real sense, begin at menopause. They can live at least a good 30-40 years after menopause with new found independence (family settled, don't have to bother about menstruation and pregnancy and so on). It is up to the women to accept this natural event positively. They can make the non-reproductive years the most powerful, productive years of their lives.

We suggest following approaches and strategies to tackle the problems of menopause -

1. Having a positive attitude towards life: All women will benefit if they decide to have a positive attitude towards life. It will help them to accept menopause as a natural event. They should feel empowered enough to overcome the menopausal symptoms on their own naturally as far as possible. Usually by the time a woman attains menopause her family is settled. Thereafter, she need not remember the menstrual cycle date every month. There is no hassles of monthly menstruation. There is rather a feeling of independence. They should now yearn for a better quality of life. They are free to do what they like. They should think about a new role they can play in society and in their families.

2. Cultivate a hobby: Having spare time with nothing to do will aggravate menopausal symptom. Concentrate upon your 'purpose of life'. Menopause might be a good time to utilize for the things a woman really wants to do. Being active in new hobbies (or hobbies we put aside years ago) keeps our mind and body engaged. Such engagement can provide the natural menopause solution women are seeking. Engaging hobbies help a woman cope with menopause symptoms. They can focus on other, more enjoyable, things. Hobbies keep a woman active. These boost her mood and help keep her mind sharp.

At menopause, women may recollect something that women always talked about doing but have never actually done because of her busy schedule. They may join for a singing class or go to an art store and buy small things of your favorite materials. As you begin to focus on your hobbies, you'll notice that your menopause symptoms aren't as big a part of your life as they were before and that your hobbies have become a healthy and natural part of the solution. Once women choose their hobbies they have to learn how to work these into their schedule. At menopause, there is sufficient time. So set aside time every day or at least three times a week to engage in hobbies. Put them in your calendar. If you take a class or join a group, that's a good way to create an obligation for yourself that you won't discard. With hobbies worked into your lifestyle, menopause symptoms won't be as much of a burden.

Pursuing hobbies that keep women in menopausal age group engaged in any area of deep interest. This will help them to cope with menopause symptoms in a constructive, healthy and natural way. Hobbies remind women that they are active, interested and alive. They keep their mind and body occupied so that they are focused on doing the things they enjoy rather than suffer menopause symptoms. Many women find that once they become deeply engaged in various hobbies or interests, many of their symptoms disappear or are significantly reduced. In fact, once they get deeply engaged in doing something that really interests them, they may realize that they experienced hot flushes only after they have come and gone. This level of engagement helps make symptoms invisible. So, menopausal women may make a list of hobbies and interests. Rather they should treat this phase of their lives as freedom from monthly botheration of bleeding episode should be seen as a BOON. A change of outlook is required. This is an exciting time, so get out there and explore life more. Think about it.

3. Being religious may help women deal with menopause: Religion is a set of beliefs concerning the cause, nature, and purpose of the universe, especially when it is considered as the creation of a superhuman agency. It usually involves devotional and ritual observances, and often contains a moral code governing the conduct of human affairs. Religion gives a positive sense of self in terms of: Hope, Comfort, Meaning of life, Enjoyment of life, Love, Compassion, Self respect, Self confidence and Quality of life.

Often, in India, women do not offer prayers or go to temples, gurudwara etc., during menstruation. They consider themselves IMPURE during menses. After menopause, women are free from all bindings of monthly problems of menstruation. They can devote more time in *puja-paath.* This may give them a freedom of devoting more time to religious activities. This can also enhance psychological health and social interactions. Religious factors may improve physical health as well, by reducing psychological stress, increasing social support, and encouraging positive health behaviors.

Being religious improves some of the health behaviors of people (through prescribing a certain diet and/or discouraging the abuse of alcoholic beverages, smoking, etc). Religious people have also been seen to display more optimism and faith. Here it needs to be clarified that we do not advocate anything for or against "being religious "or "practicing religion" through this book. We feel that religion is a personal matter. Readers have to decide on their own about this issue. Of course, it gives us identity. Our opinion is that being religious or practicing a particular religion gives us something to hold on to; something which fills up a "void" in our life; it gives us a sense of purpose of life and guides us to do good deeds.

4. Spirituality and Menopause: At the age of menopause women may find themselves relatively free to pursue and explore hitherto untouched aspects of life. In modern era, leisure time is often the major dilemma for people. They do not know what to do with their spare time. Our view is that this phase of life can be gainfully utilized by venturing into the area of 'spirituality'. This does not necessarily mean renunciation of material wealth. It does not mean shunning relationships or abandoning the pleasures of the world and adopting the life of a saint. As a bird needs two wings to fly, man also needs the two wings of existence, the spiritual and the material, to lead a natural and harmonious life. If either is neglected for the other, our life becomes imbalanced. Spirituality provides the way to restore this balance within our own self. Material life may be fulfilling to a certain extent, but it often leaves us with a feeling of emptiness. Spirituality teaches us that real joy, happiness and peace, come from within. Spirituality teaches us to balance our aspirations.

Religion and spirituality are often used as synonyms. While religion is a specific set of organized beliefs and practices, spirituality is the way you find meaning, hope, comfort and inner peace in your life. Many people find spirituality through religion. Some find it through music, art or a connection with nature. Others find it in their values and principles. These are not opposed, but stem from one another. Religion is more organized & includes public rituals, spirituality is more private and personal.

Although, there is no way to actually measure spiritual health, it can be defined as consisting of following characteristics -

(1) Sense of inner peace
(2) Ability to find comfort and or strength in one's spiritual beliefs & values.
(3) Belief in one's own worth & goodness
(4) Ability to receive and offer love & care
(5) Strong connection with people
(6) Sense of purpose in world
(7) Ability to forgive self and others
(8) Hopefulness in future
(9) Sense of some control over one's own life
(10) A feeling and capacity of self realization (Who am I?)

Health and spirituality are generally looked upon as different from each other. But on examining the deeper aspects of both, we find that they are interdependent and almost merge with each other. Spirituality can be taken as the search for inner peace or foundation of happiness. Many techniques developed in this context such as meditation, prayer etc. are immensely valuable in themselves as the skills for managing various aspects of inner life.

Tips for spiritual growth

1. Read spiritual and uplifting books. Think about what you read, and find out how you can use the information in your life.
2. Meditate for at least 15 minutes every day. If you do not know how to meditate, it is easy to find books, websites or teachers who can teach you meditation.

3. Learn to make your mind quiet through concentration exercises and meditation.
4. Think positive. If you find yourself thinking negatively, immediately switch to thinking positively. Be in control of what enters your mind. Open the door for the positive and close it for the negative.
5. Develop the happiness habit, by always looking at the bright side of life and endeavoring to be happy. Happiness comes from within. Do not let your outer circumstances decide your happiness for you.
6. Exercise often will increase your will power and decision making ability. This strengthens you and gives you control over your mind.

5. Try meditation for menopause related problems: The practice of meditation is central to spiritual path. Meditation is the process of allowing and even embracing everything we are experiencing and feeling. It's the process of being receptive and open to vision and insight. It is the process of discovering *"who I really am."* Meditation is a key to good health. It can help us open the doors to our healing power that lie within us.

Meditation is a technique that we can use at any time and place to quite the mind and restore peace and harmony within ourselves. This subsequently gets manifested in our outward life as well. Meditation is intended not to stop us thinking but to help us to produce order in the midst of our confusion. By relaxing our mind through meditation, we can clear the chatter for a time and experience a renewed sense of energy. This enables us to bring identity, clarity and freedom to take control over our lives to become healthier and happier.

In fact, accumulated stress is the root cause of a high proportion of illnesses, including many common and serious conditions. By eliminating stress, meditation offers important benefits for the cure and prevention of a wide range of health problems and allows the mind and body to function with maximum effectiveness. This leads to good health and longevity.

Transcendental Meditation (TM), a type of meditation, is another way to attain inner peace and harmony. TM is a technique for gaining deep rest that brings balance to the body and mind. Benefits are gained through the natural self- healing processes that are enlivened by release of stress through transcending; practicing the TM technique will reduce stress, lower your blood pressure, enable you to tap into your inner intelligence, calm your mind, open up your creativity and improve your relationships. Many medical studies have been proved the beneficial effects of meditation.

TM can be learned easily from any guru or trainer in few days. After that it depends on you whether to continue with it or not. Only practice is involved. Basically, TM involves 20 minutes of meditation once or twice a day in sitting posture with eyes closed. Broadly speaking, a person doing TM has to start these 20 minutes with repeatedly chanting in one's heart a mantra (it may be a single word or a monosyllable like 'Shiva', Shiva', Shiva' or 'Rama', 'Rama', 'Rama'). It should not be spoken out. One keeps chanting this mantra. You will find that after sometime your mind wanders elsewhere. You subconsciously stop chanting the mantra. This is OK. The essence of TM is that 'you let you mind wander'. And when you again remember about mantra, you start chanting again. Your mind may wander again. Let it wander & let your mind go with flow of thoughts. Again go back to chanting the mantra when you remember what you were doing. And this may continue till 20 minutes.

Meditation is a ritual and a process of spiritual transformation. It is a learned skill and provides many physiological benefits, such as stress reduction. Also, it may lead to new insights about life issues, increased creativity, inspiration, greater compassion for others.During meditation, our attention and concentration are intentionally trained.

All meditative techniques involve conscious breathing and a focus on what is happening in each present moment until the mind becomes empty of thoughts, judgments and past and future concerns.

To enter into meditative state, the following methods may be helpful:-

- Breathing techniques
- Meditating with sound- mantras, chanting, audiotapes
- Meditating with visualization – picturing a sacred place, focusing on an external object. Visualizing sacred symbols
- The manifold benefits of meditation can be categorized as under:
- Improved hearing and mental performance
- Improved memory
- Improvements in psychosomatic and stress related disorders
- Improvement in heart disease
- Disorders of the nervous system can be improved
- Nose, throat and lung problems can be minimized
- Increased muscular tone and flexibility
- Posture gets corrected, allowing deep breathing
- Strengthening of the nervous system
- Bringing normalcy to the glandular secretions of the endocrine system
- Improving resistance to stress and diseases
- Deep relaxation
- Strengthens the body
- Improves concentration abilities.

Pranayama is another technique, which corrects basic faults within the body system, removes energy blockages and stress, improve blood circulation and enable higher level of oxygen intake. *Pranayama* helps us in removing symptoms of irritation, anger, and lack of energy through retention of breath, both inward and outward.

6. Doing exercise regularly: Often, women are told that their bones have become weak at menopause. Regular, moderate, weight bearing exercise is recommended because of its likely benefit to bones. Exercise increases muscle strength, co-ordination and flexibility. All other organ system in the body are also toned up. Physical exercise is generally beneficial for all age groups. In the elderly, exercise may improve physical fitness. Likelihood of falls and fractures is also reduced.

Simple stretching exercises are easy to start with. Deep breathing exercise may help. However, in Indian culture, women are not expected to do exercise. It is not an "in thing" for them. There is a need to grow out of such a mindset. When decision to do exercises is taken make a plan. One must start with an exercise regime slowly. It should suit one's routine. Start slowly. In the beginning, stretching exercises for 5 minutes will suffice. Gradually increase the duration and variety of exercises over a week. There should not be any abrupt change in your routine. For example, a woman who never did any exercises should not straight away start with 20-30 minutes exercise on the first day itself. These can be done in privacy of one's bedroom. Going for a walk in a group is also refreshing. Depending upon one's personality, family atmosphere or social set up, different approaches may be tried. Some will feel like doing exercise only in a group. Others may like to do it alone. There are some simple stretching exercises which women can perform. Some are given as below:

(a) **Knee-to-chest stretch:** The knee-to-chest stretch focuses on the muscles of your lower back. Don't do this stretch if you have osteoporosis because it may increase the risk of compression fractures in your vertebrae.

- Lie on your back on a bed with the backs of your heels flat on the bed.
- Gently pull one knee up to your chest (with both hands grasping the leg below the knee) until you feel a stretch in your lower back.
- Bring the knee as close to your chest as comfortably possible.
- Keep the opposite leg relaxed in a comfortable position, either with your knee bent or with your leg extended.
- Hold for about 10 seconds.

- Switch legs and repeat.
- Now do it with both knees together.

(b) Stretching side by side: This is the best workout to slim your waist. A perfect exercise for reducing belly fat.

- Stand erect with your feet together. Raise your hands above your head in a *Namaste.*
- Now keeping your legs grounded, bend your body to the right as much as possible till you feel a strain on your left waist. Stay for 5 seconds.
- Return back to the original position.
- Now bend left. Retain this position for another 5 seconds.
- Slowly you may increase the holding time to 10-15 seconds.
- Repeat it for 5-10 times.

(c) Toe-touch Exercise: This is the one of the best exercises which helps in reducing belly fat. This exercise also known as the standing forward bend pose. In this individual is required to stand straight with his hands stretched out overhead and then exhale and bend from the hips till his hands touch the toes. The knees have to be kept straight while performing this exercise. Return to standing position again. Repeat it 10 times. In the beginning one may not be able to touch the toes. Do not get disheartened. Try upto whatever level you can reach down with your hands. You will see that gradually over a period of 1-2 weeks you will be able to touch your toes. This toe touch exercise is very good for toning the abdominal muscles and also helps treat problems like indigestion, constipation, bloating and other stomach issues. Circulation within the body is improved and even the back muscles are strengthened by performing this exercise regularly.

(d) Toe-touch crossover: The exercise is almost similar to the above toe-touch exercise. When you start this exercise; start in a standing position, feet shoulder-width apart and arms held out to the sides at shoulder height. Then bend forward at the waist while twisting your body so you can touch the fingertips of your right hand to the toes of your left foot. Lift your torso back up, returning to the starting position, and repeat the move but twist to the right to touch the left fingertips to the right foot. Stand upright once more and repeat the movement, alternating sides as you go, for 30 seconds.

7. Try yoga: The practice of yoga makes the body strong and flexible. It also improves the functioning of the respiratory, circulatory, digestive, and hormonal systems. Yoga brings about emotional stability and clarity of mind. Practicing yoga is important. Yoga can have a huge beneficial effect on the entire body. Yogic poses not only strengthens and tones the muscles, tissues, ligaments, joints and nerves but also maintains the smooth functioning and health of all body systems like respiratory, circulatory, digestive, and hormonal. Yoga relaxes the body and mind allowing both to recover from fatigue and weakness, resulting from stresses of daily life. It also helps to re-energize your body and raises your everyday levels of enthusiasm.

You will find that your sleep also improves with yoga. You may even need less time to sleep as your rejuvenation levels and abilities improve. Yoga poses also boost the metabolism. It improves lymphatic and hormonal secretions. It also helps bring about a chemical balance within the body which is crucial for healthy living. It is important to keep practicing yoga. Try to incorporate this practice into your weekly schedule.

Please Note: *Yoga should always be learnt from an expert. First try to understand how different asanas are done. Then start practicing until you are absolutely comfortable with its dynamics and movements. Only then really start doing yoga independently. It is then that you will experience the full benefits of the yoga.*

Major role of yoga is to —

- Increase the flexibility of body and preventing formation of energy blocks. This helps in allowing a healthier body.
- Massage the internal organs of the body and the rarely stimulated parts such as the thyroid gland.
- Help obese people to loose extra fat and weight (a major causes of illness)
- Improve systemic circulation of blood throughout the body and thereby increase circulation of oxygen to the tissues
- Improve gastrointestinal tract functioning.
- Prevent protein load on kidney
- Improve psychology and help in developing more positive attitude towards life.

Yoga improves sleep and lowers depression. There are some Asanas which women can perform to get relief from menopausal symptoms. In the following pages, some important selected yoga Asanas have been described. However, advice from some yoga instructor should be taken before starting the actual sessions.

(a) *Padmasana* - The Lotus Pose

"Padma" means "lotus" in Sanskrit. "Padmasana" means sitting in the "Lotus Posture." This posture is called Padmasana because the arrangement of the hands and feet resemble a lotus when seen from a distance. The two feet placed upon the opposite thigh resemble the leaves while the two hands placed one over the other resembles the lotus in full bloom.

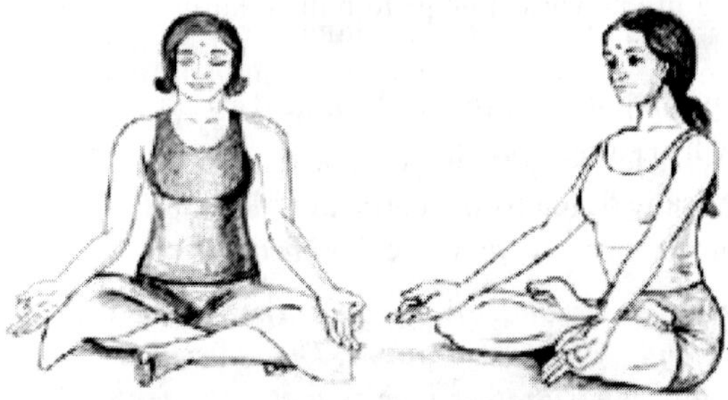

Figure 1 - Padmasana - The Lotus Pose

Sequence

- Sit erect.
- Stretch out your legs in front of you and keep the heels together.
- Hold the right ankle with the right hand and the right big toe with the left hand. Bending the right knee outwards, pull round the right foot towards your left groin line. Set the foot firmly at the root of the left upper thigh. The heel should lightly press the left side of the lower abdomen. The foot must lie fully stretched over the left thigh with its sole turned upwards. Keeps the right knee pressing the floor.
- Similarly, fold the left leg and place the foot firmly at the root of the right upper thigh. The foot must lie fully stretched over the right thigh with the sole turned upwards. Keep the left knee also pressing the floor.
- With both legs now interlocked, keep the spine, neck and head erect.
- Place one palm upon the other, both turned upward and cupped, and rest them on the upturned heels a little below the navel.
- Remain in this posture in perfect ease until you begin to be uncomfortable.
- Unlock the foot-lock. Stretch out your legs and return to the original sitting position.
- Practice alternating the legs.

Caution

- Do not sit in this posture while eating food or immediately after taking it.
- Persons having sciatica or varicose veins in the legs should attempt this posture cautiously.

Benefits

- Sitting in Padmasana helps to reduce fat in the abdomen, buttocks and thighs.
- This posture strengthens the thighs and calves and provides elasticity to the hamstring muscles.
- Padmasana develops the correct carriage of the body with perfect equilibrium since the spine has to be kept straight during the practice.
- The important muscles, ligaments and tendons of the lower extremities are extended and flexed while sitting in Padmasana and relaxed when it is released.
- This posture promotes a rich supply of blood to the organs in the pelvic and the abdomino-genital regions while the flow of blood to the lower extremities is limited. Since more blood is made to circulate in the lumbar region of the spine and the abdomen, the spine and the abdominal organs are toned up.
- It firms up the coccygeal and sacral regions of the spine and the sciatic nerve. It also tones up the colon.
- It limbers up stiff knees and ankles and improves the flexibility of the hip-joints. It relieves arthritic pain in these areas.
- Minor spinal deformities are set right.
- The erect spine prevents the compression of the abdominal viscera while sitting in this posture.

(b) Makarasana - The Crocodile Pose

"Makar" means "crocodile" in Sanskrit.

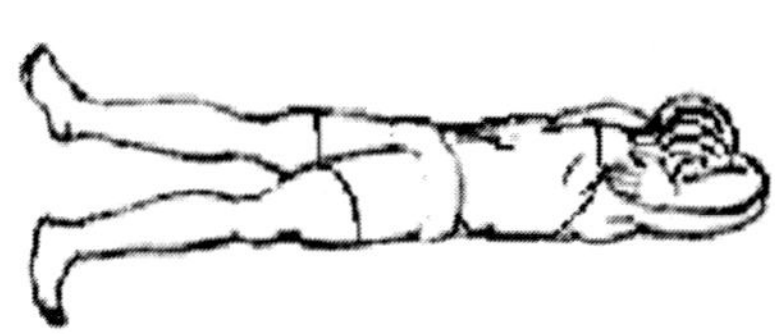

Figure 2: Makarasana - The Crocodile Pose.

Sequence

- Lie flat on the carpet with the chin, chest and abdomen touching the ground.
- Stretch out the legs together at full length.
- Keep the arms on their respective sides.
- Spread the legs comfortably apart and rest them on the floor.
- Heels must point towards each other and the edges of the feet must touch the floor.
- The feet should be at right angles to the legs and the toes pointing outward.
- Bring one hand beneath the opposite shoulder and grasp it lightly and place the other hand on the opposite shoulder and grasp it lightly. Do this in such a way that a 'double triangle is formed with the folded elbows resting exactly above one another and the forearms crossing the opposite upper arms.
- Rest your forehead on this 'double triangle' ; dip your face in the space in between.
- Close your eyes and relax.
- Do abdominal breathing and maintain this position as long as comfortable.
- Lie on your back and resume.

Benefits

- Makarasana induces a complete relaxation of the body and mind.
- It relaxes the muscles and relieves the fatigue after a strenuous asana.
- The asana relieves and helps correct many breathing troubles and disorders in the genito-urinary system.
- It helps to reduce high blood pressure.
- Makarasana stimulates the small intestines which, in helps the digestive processes.
- It prevents scoliosis and flatulence.
- This yoga pose helps to correct disorders of ovaries and uterus

(c) Bhujangasana

Cobra Pose: (Bhujanga = cobra). This asana is called 'Bhujangasana' as the raised trunk, neck and head while practicing it resemble a cobra rearing its hood and about to strike, while the joined and stretched legs resemble its tail.

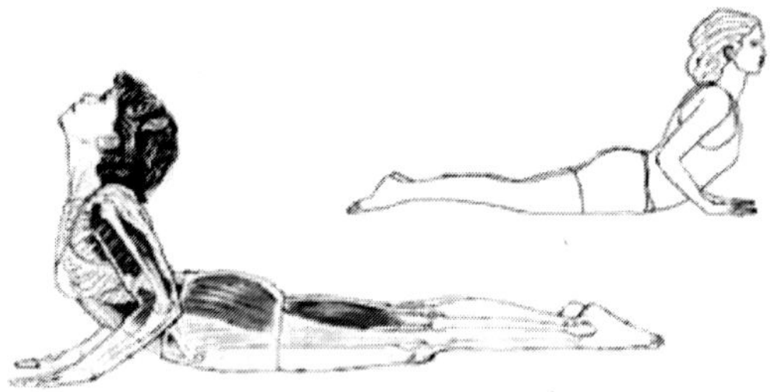

Figure 3: Bhujangasana - Cobra Pose

Sequence

- Lie flat on your abdomen at full length.
- Stretch your arms on the sides with the palms turned upwards.
- Rest the forehead and nose on the ground.
- Keep your legs and feet together and the whole body straight. Soles must be turned upwards.
- Relax the whole body.
- Place the palms flat on the floor exactly beneath the corresponding shoulders with fingers close together.
- Keep the elbows close to the sides.
- Place the chin on the ground.
- Slowly bend the neck and head backward as far as possible, keeping the chest close to the ground.
- Support yourself lightly on the hands and forearms and inhaling, raise slowly your head, shoulders, chest and upper abdomen(up to navel) in a smooth backward movement, tensing the muscles of the back and the nape of the neck.
- Bend the head and neck as far back as possible.
- Arch the back and bend the whole spine further back as far as you can, putting very little pressure on the hands.
- Gaze upwards.
- Maintain this position comfortably, holding your breath.
- Exhaling, return slowly to the starting position in the reverse order.

Caution

- Do this asana on an empty stomach.
- Persons with peptic ulcer, hernia or high blood pressure must not practice it.

Benefits

- It is very useful for removing excess fat in the abdomen and waist and reducing the hips.
- The practice of this asana after office work will dispel fatigue.
- The regular practice of Bhujangasana will help postpone old age and bring youthfulness by improving the elasticity of the spine.
- It relieves tension and stiffness in the neck and back.
- The alternate compression and stretching of the abdomen improves the digestive system and stimulates the appetite.
- This asana is especially beneficial to persons with a slight hump as the head, neck and back are bent in the reverse direction.
- It helps to cure low blood pressure.
- It strengthens the arms, wrists, shoulders and the posterior.

(d) Savasana - The Corpse Pose

"Sava" means "dead body" in Sanskrit. To practice this asana, one should lie motionless on the floor like as dead body in order to secure complete relaxation of all parts of his body and remove tensions, both physical and mental.

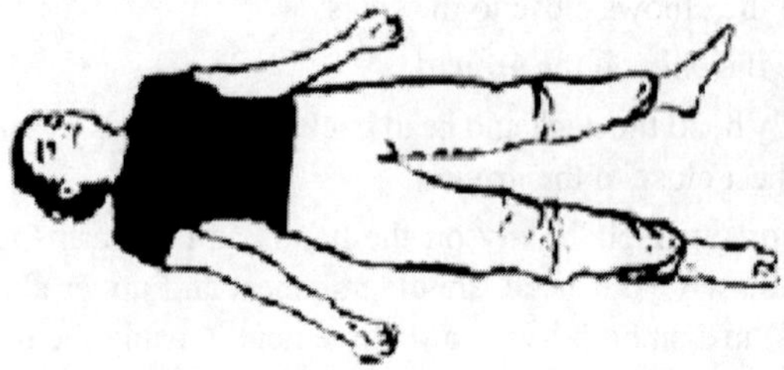

Figure 4: Savasana - The Corpse Pose

Sequence

1. Select a quiet and well-ventilated place.
2. Spread your carpet on a firm and flat surface.
3. Wear only minimum clothing.
4. Lie flat on your back at full length.
5. Rest your head in a comfortable position with the face turned upwards.
6. Stretch out your legs at full length.

7. Legs should be kept sufficiently apart.
8. Keep the knees slightly flexed. 368
9. Extend the arms fully and rest them lightly on their respective sides with the hands about a foot away from the thighs.
10. Palms should be turned upwards and fingers slightly curled.
11. Allow your mouth to fall open slightly.
12. Drop your chin and let your lower jaw sag a little.
13. Allow your teeth to part a little.
14. Close your eyes gently.
15. Breathe naturally through the nose and do not attempt to regulate your breathing.
16. Lie perfectly still like a corpse and persuade all your muscles to relax completely.
17. Relax your mind by freeing it from immediate cares, conflicts, worries and fears.
18. As you relax, allow your mind to run over every part and organ of your body from head to toe. Get a picture of each part in your mind and 'let go' without any conscious effort.
19. If there are any parts of your body that still feel tight, relax these.

Caution

- Do not practice under glaring light.
- Always relax on a firm and flat surface.
- Do not yawn at any stage of the practice.
- Do not keep your hands under your head or on your chest.

Benefits

- Relaxation in Savasana tames the mind and makes it calm and alert.
- It helps withdraw senses from their objects & makes concentration easy.

Daily practice of shavasana and deep breathing will help to combat insomnia and nervous anxiety in menopausal women. Yoga can also help reduce the tension that so often finds expression in emotional outburst. Women going through the menopause should have their blood pressure checked regularly. Practice of *shavasana* will help reduce blood pressure.

8. Generating family support-especially of the husband: An understanding husband can help the wife tremendously in this transitional phase of life. For this, the husband must know about menopause and expected symptoms. He also needs to be educated on this topic. Since menopause is still a little known subject, the members of the family cannot really understand the changes in a menopausal woman. Often, the common reaction of family members to a menopausal woman's verbalization of her symptoms is "she has gone mad; it is a sign of growing old."

Husband can help by going for walks together, by doing exercises together, by being patient when the wife is having mood swings. He can prove his good companionship by sharing household problems, going together for vacation and by being less demanding.

The children should also be told what their mother is going through. Otherwise, instead of helping their mother, they may create new problems for her. If the woman is living in a joint family with parents or in-laws, it is important to be open to them about menopausal problems. At this transitional period, if the family members can be understanding towards the lady of the house, they can really help her morally to sail through this rough patch of menopause smoothly.

9. Taking advice of a gynaecologist: Depending upon their financial situation and physical health menopausal women may need to consult a gynaecologist. Check-up may be requested as per the need. Sometimes, even by mere talking to a doctor about their symptoms and problems can make women mentally relaxed. A patient friendly doctor who gives sufficient time to listen to women will be quite helpful. A good doctor will make patients feel that their symptoms need attention.

10. Taking control of life style: This requires some self discipline among the women. Many a times, some simple changes in lifestyle can give good results in managing menopausal symptoms. Menopause signals a change in the hormone levels. It heralds changes in the reproductive system of a woman. Hence, this phase of 'change' needs to be tackled through 'changes' in lifestyle. Stress during menopause can be reduced by doing yoga or meditation. It can be combined with some light regular exercise. Involvement in religious activities may also help. Making lifestyle changes is an easy way to get rid of many problems associated with menopause. It is very simple to practice. Maintaining a healthy lifestyle can have an enormous impact on health. Controlling weight and managing stress are additional life style factors that contribute to optimal health.

5. Menopause in Housewives and Working Women

Menopause in housewives: It is often seen that impact of menopause on housewives is different from that of working women. This is partly because they stay at home. At the age of menopause they may have 'plenty of time to kill'. Their husbands will be at job. By the time they reach middle age their children are grown up. They may have shifted to other cities for studies and jobs etc. Idle sitting at home may aggravate their menopausal symptoms. Depression may set in their minds. This is an ideal time for housewives to pursue their hobbies. These days, because of small families women often get freed of family obligations by the age of menopause. The departure of her children can trigger depressive reactions. Most of them live in nuclear families. Grown-up children are settled outside. They may channelize their positive energies in a positive direction. They may even do some charitable activities. They can form a group of ladies, who do some social work, like teaching poor children. Women may learn some short term courses like stitching, knitting or join some cookery classes. At the menopause women may engage themselves more in household chores. They may now be able to devote more time to *puja-paath.*

Menopause in working women: They have to maintain a balance between their job, their families as well as their menopause related health issues. During menopausal transition they may be more irritable at work. They may have to take sick leave. There may not be anyone at home to share their problem with. Children may be away to other cities. Their husbands may be busy or not concerned at all. They may feel left out. So, for working women, getting themselves immersed in work can help them forget some of menopausal symptoms experience. A typical working woman in India at times has an extremely hectic schedule. She has to balance her family commitments along with multiple other responsibilities, which can lead to little time for sleep. The "turn of life" at menopause may represent a fundamental change in the life of working women. This period can lead to changes in a women's health. It may also lead to emotional changes. These can affect how a woman does her work. It can influence her relationship with her boss and colleagues. Unfortunately, at workplace, there is often very little understanding of the issues and very little support for women who are going through the menopause.

Employers have been slow to recognize that women of menopausal age may need special consideration. It is simply seen as a private matter. Many employers/managers will have no awareness of the issues involved. This means that many women feel that they have to hide their symptoms and will be less likely to ask for the adjustments that may help them. Many women consider themselves little prepared for the arrival of the menopause, and even less equipped to manage its symptoms at work. Studies on working women revealed that majority of the women felt they needed further advice and support. Workplaces and working practices are not designed with menopausal women in mind. Heavy and painful periods, hot flushes, mood disturbance, fatigue, and poor concentration pose significant and embarrassing problems for some women, leaving them feeling less confident. Where women had taken time off from work to deal with their symptoms, only half of them disclosed the real reason for absence to their employers/managers.

Office people also have a role to play towards women who are going through menopausal transition. Office representatives should raise the issue with their employers and ensure that the workplace meets the needs of menopausal women. For example, there may be specific issues in workplace (such as temperature or dress code) that make it even harder for women who are going through the menopause to cope up with daily hot flushes.

6. Additional Options for Dealing with Menopausal Symptoms

(a) Alternative medicine/home remedies: These can also be used to get relief from menopause symptoms in a safe and natural way. Alternative approaches involve little or no risk. This can be an extremely effective way to treat menopause symptoms.

(i) Applying **Henna (*mehndi*)** on to hands and feet, to get relief from symptoms like hot flushes. It gives relief from hot flushes due to its cooling effect.

(ii) **Liquorice (*mulethi*)** serves as an effective remedy for menopause, as it contains the natural female hormone estrogen. Thus, it helps in making up for the lost hormones.

(iii) Consume **"*Gundkatira*"** with water. It gives cooling effect during hot flushes.

(iv) For women who have symptoms related dryness in vagina. ***Shatavari,*** (*Asparagus racemosus)* use with ghee can be applied locally to enhance vaginal lubrication.

(v) **Cumin-coriander-fennel tea** contains natural phyto-estrogens that support healthy hormonal balance. Tea made from organic **Tulsi** will provide relief from stress during menopausal symptoms.

(vi) The mixture of bottle gourd ***(Lauki/Ghiya)*** and sesame ***(Til)*** oil is an effective medicine. Massage over the scalp every night, helps to treat insomnia.

(vii) Extract juice from green coriander (Dhaniya) and mix with water and sugar. Take it before sleeping. It provides a cooling effect. It provides respite from hot flushes and insomnia.

(viii) **Coconut water** gives cooling effect during hot flushes.

(ix) A glass of **Carrots and Beets juice** is advisable once a day. Freshly prepared fruit juices are also good for health.

(b) Dietary guidelines during menopause: Many of the menopausal symptoms can be managed by using appropriate diet. During menopause, eat a variety of food to get all the needed nutrients. Since women's diet are often low in iron and calcium, follow these guidelines:

- **Get enough calcium-** Eat and drink two to four servings of dairy products and calcium-rich foods a day. This will help to ensure that women are getting enough calcium in their daily diet. Calcium is found in dairy products, like *paneer*, milk, curd.
- **Get enough iron-** Eating at least three servings of iron-rich foods a day will help ensure that a woman is getting enough iron in her daily diet. This include leafy green vegetables, nuts, meat, fish, eggs, and enriched grain products.
- **Get enough fiber-** Get food high in fiber such as whole-grain breads, cereals, rice, fresh fruits, and vegetables.
- **Drink plenty of water.** This will help a woman stay hydrated. Drinking eight glasses of water every day fulfills the daily requirement. It will also help to get some relief from hot flushes.
- **Maintain a healthy weight.** Lose weight if you are overweight by cutting down on portion sizes and by reducing fatty food. But skipping meals is not a good solution.
- **Reduce foods high in fat.** Fat should provide 25% to 35% or less of total daily calories. Also, limit saturated fat to less than 7% of total daily calories. Saturated fat raises cholesterol and increases risk for heart disease. Saturated fat is found in fatty meats, whole milk, ice cream, and cheese.
- **Use salt in moderation.** Too much salt in the diet is linked to high blood pressure. Avoid food stuff having salt- bakery products, sauce, pickles, *papad*, tinned food etc.

Balanced diet is a good source to treat menopausal symptoms. Good diet in particular is key to all health problems. Diet rich in foods that promote estrogen levels such as, Soybeans, Garlic, Apples, Pumpkin, Wheat, cabbage, Oats and Cucumber are good sources to get relief from menopausal symptoms. Take foods rich in **Vitamin E** like raw sprouted pulses (dal) and milk.

Foods that need to be encouraged in the menopause diet are:

- Soya– Tofu paneer, soy milk (Protein): Soya food products have been said to be beneficial in menopausal women. Soybean has natural female hormones.
- Nuts– almonds (Omega 3, calcium)

- Seeds– sesame seeds (Omega 3, calcium)
- Whole grain (Vitamin B)
- Legumes– Soya beans, lentils, chickpeas (Vitamin B, Isoflavones)
- Low fat yoghurt (Calcium)
- Fat reduced cheese (Calcium)
- Vegetables– Dark leafy greens, bean sprouts (Calcium, Vitamin C, Minerals)
- Fruits (Potassium)

(c) Menopause and hormone replacement therapy (HRT): Recognize menopause as a natural process, just like the first periods (menarche). Realize that this is a time of change, not just in women's body, but also in her life. As described earlier, menopause occurs because of decline in hormone levels in body. Ovaries stops producing female hormones. This leads to development of many symptoms which women have to bear. Hence, Hormone Replacement Therapy (HRT) was evolved to "replace" women's depleting hormone levels to relieve associated symptoms. Starting in 1970s it was vigorously promoted by various pharmaceutical companies all over the world. Use of hormone to treat menopausal symptoms had become quite common in Western countries. In contrast, women in countries like India, view menopause rather positively and take menopausal symptoms in their stride. As documented by the authors in their studies, use of HRT is almost nil in rural India and is negligible in urban India.

Reason for such differential use of HRT is due to the difference in the way menopause is viewed in the two settings. In youth-oriented Western cultures, menopause is frequently intertwined with fears of ageing. Women associate menopause with a loss of their status in family and the society. However, women have been reported to welcome menopause in developing countries like India. As shown in many popular TV serials and in Indian movies the women get a status of power after middle age. Hence, it is not surprising that in India on attaining menopause women have been reported to say- '*Saari bimariyo se mukti mil gayi abb*' (I am now free from all illness), *'Saare paap kat gaye (*free from all sin)*', Abb puja path aaraam se kar sakti hoon' (*Now I can comfortably worship*), ' abb narak se mukti mil gayi'* (Now found salvation from hell). Still, some women may need HRT.HRT use is of two types.

Short-term HRT has a higher level of acceptance and compliance among women. Such use of HRT has been found to be effective in cases of vasomotor symptoms that appear in the early stages of menopause. The least expensive tablet for this condition available in India is Estriol. The cost of a 2mg tablet is Rs.3. The usual dosage is two tablets a day and one course runs for three months. Thus, the user spends Rs.540 per course. Success is usually assured. But often it needs to be continued for 2 years.

Long-term HRT This can extend for a period of 5-10 years. However, HRT does have its side effects. There are also strong contraindications for long term HRT use.

In fact, after a phase of widespread popularity over a period of time, a lot of problems have been attributed to HRT use. Recent research has found that HRT increases risk of breast cancer and ovarian/endometrial cancer. 377

Besides the risks associated with HRT use, there are following other hassles also associated with long term HRT use,

(i) HRT is costly. On a moderate estimate @Rs. 500/- per month x 12 months x 5 years Rs. 30000/- will be spent during 5 years HRT regime for a woman.

(ii) One needs to remember to take a pill daily.

(iii) Before starting HRT, baseline blood test, x-ray, pap smear etc. are required

(iv) Periodic check-ups are also needed. Both these require repeated visits of the women to hospitals. There are also problems like break through bleeding.

(v) All this may further increase the expenditure and botheration for the HRT users.

Thus, it is clear that HRT can provide relief from menopausal symptoms. However, it may be harmful also. Risk of cancer is likely to increase. Many hassles are also involved. So, there is a dilemma whether to use hormone therapy or not. One may think that it is safer to tolerate the symptoms for sometime rather than face the possible risk of cancer due to HRT. Many women may try home remedies for certain menopausal symptoms. Even these have been said to provide relief.

The decision whether to use or avoid HRT use is difficult. We leave this to the reader. However, our opinion is that hormone use should be avoided as far as possible. Only in rare cases, one may resort to hormone use. Even that too should be done with proper recommendations and counseling by a qualified doctor.

We are of the opinion that among menopausal women, it is better to tolerate minor symptoms. Suitable home remedies or supportive therapy may be tried. Non-medicinal approaches are safer. It should be remembered that use of HRT may require detailed check-up before starting the therapy. Even follow up may require regular tests and check-ups. Only in uncontrolled, persistent and severe symptoms, HRT may be tried after consulting a qualified doctor.

References

1. Singh A, Arora AK. 2005. Profile of menopausal women in rural north India. Climacteric 8(2):177-184.
2. Parashar P. 2009. Menopause among punjabi brahmin and khatri women of Chandigarh: a bio-social study. Ph.D Thesis, Department of Anthropology, Panjab University, Chandigarh, Unpublishesd.
3. Kaur S, Walia I, Singh A. 2004. How menopause affects the lives of women in suburban Chandigarh, India. Climacteric 7:175-180.
4. Devi, A. 2012. Ayurvedic Support for menopause. http://www.alandiashram. *org/school/school_html/articles/ menopause.html*
5. Nath GB, 1999. Menopause. Voluntary Health Association of Punjab. VHAI Press: New Delhi.
6. Singh A, Walia I and Dhaliwal L. 2010. Demedicalizing Women's Health Vol. II. Gyan Publishers: New Delhi.
7. Parihar M, 2009. Metabolic diseases in Menopause. Indian Menopause Society: New Delhi.
8. Singh, A. 2012. Mantras for healthy lifestyle – A Salutogenic Approach. Century Publications: New Delhi.
9. Pathak, R.K. and Prashar, P. 2010. Age at Menopause and associated bio-social factors of health in Punjabi women. The Open Anthropology Journal. Vol. 3 pp.172-180.

Chapter - 10

Dealing with therapy related issues of cervical cancer- A guide for patients/family caregivers

— Dr. Amudeep Singh, Dr. Vanita Suri,
Dr. Sushmita Ghoshal, Dr. Sukhpal Kaur,
Dr. Amarjeet Singh

Introduction

Our body parts continuously undergo wear and tear. Various organs are composed of thousands and lakhs of cells. These cells keep growing all the time. Cancer is one such a disease in which these normal body processes are deranged. Cell growth goes out of control. Abnormal cells are also formed. These can spread to other parts of the body from the cancerous organ.

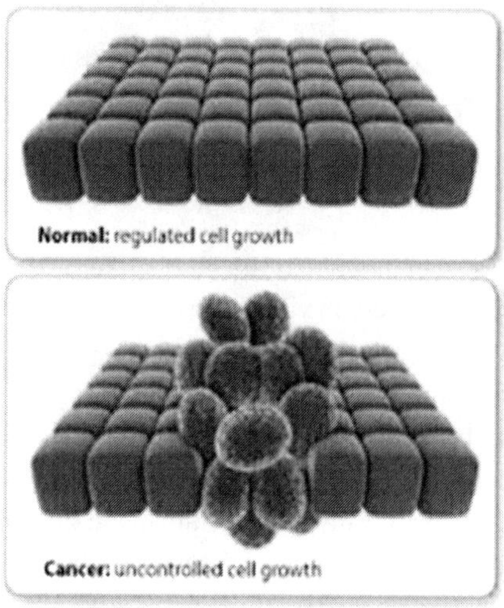

Cancer is usually named for the organ or part of the body where it starts, or the type of cell in which it starts. For example, cancer of mouth is called oral cancer, cancer of uterus is called uterine cancer, cancer that begins in the cervix is called cervix cancer.

Gynecologic Cancers

Gynecologic cancer is any cancer that starts in a woman's reproductive organs.

While they are often discussed as a group, each gynecologic cancer is unique. Each has different signs, symptoms, and risk factors (things that may increase the chance of getting each cancer).

The five main types of gynecologic cancer are (Figure 1):

- **Cervical Cancer:** Begins in the cervix, the lower part of the uterus (or womb) (Figure 2).

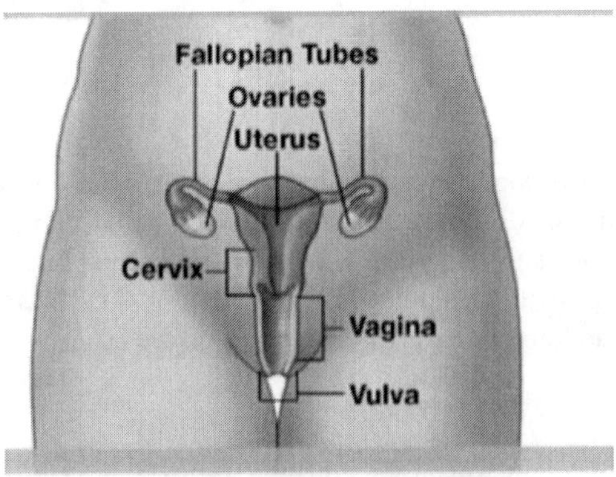

Figure I: Sites of gynaecological cancers

- **Ovarian Cancer:** Begins in the ovaries, located on each side of the uterus.
- **Uterine Cancer:** Begins in the uterus, the pear-shaped organ in a woman's pelvis where the baby grows when a woman is pregnant.
- **Vaginal Cancer:** Begins in the vagina, the hollow, tube-like channel between the bottom of the uterus and the outside of the body. It is also called the birth canal.
- **Vulvar Cancer:** Begins in the vulva, the outer part of the female genital organs, which includes the inner and outer lips of the vagina, the clitoris, and the opening of the vagina and its glands.

Extent of the Problem

There were 14.1 million new cases, 8.2 million cancer deaths and 32.6 million people living with cancer (within 5 year of diagnosis) in 2012 worldwide. Among women, the five most common incident sites of cancer were the breast (25.2% of the total), colorectum (9.2%), lung (8.7%), cervix (7.9%), and stomach (4.8%). Gynecological cancers like cervix uteri constitute 4.8% of all cancer cases. In 2012, India accounted to 23% of global total of cervical cancer new cases.

While all women are at risk for cervical cancer, this risk generally increases with age.

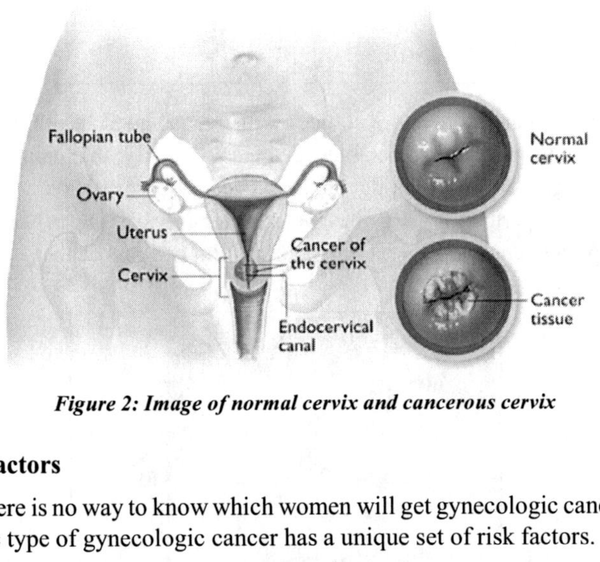

Figure 2: Image of normal cervix and cancerous cervix

Risk Factors

There is no way to know which women will get gynecologic cancer. Each specific type of gynecologic cancer has a unique set of risk factors.

- Human papillomavirus (HPV). It is a common sexually transmitted virus that can cause cervical, vaginal, and vulvar cancers.
- Obesity, smoking, hereditary, weakened immune system, taking DES (a hormone) while pregnant, having multiple sexual partners also increases the risk of acquiring cervical cancer.
- Cervical canceris more common among older women.

Prevention and early detection

While there is no known way to prevent cervical cancer, things can be done to help lower the chance of getting it or help to find it early. It is important to find cervical cancer early, when treatment is most effective.

- Pay attention to the body and know what is normal. If you have any abnormal vaginal bleeding, or any other symptoms of gynecologic cancer for two weeks or longer then you should talk to a doctor immediately. The symptoms may be caused by something other than cancer, but the only way to know is to see a doctor.

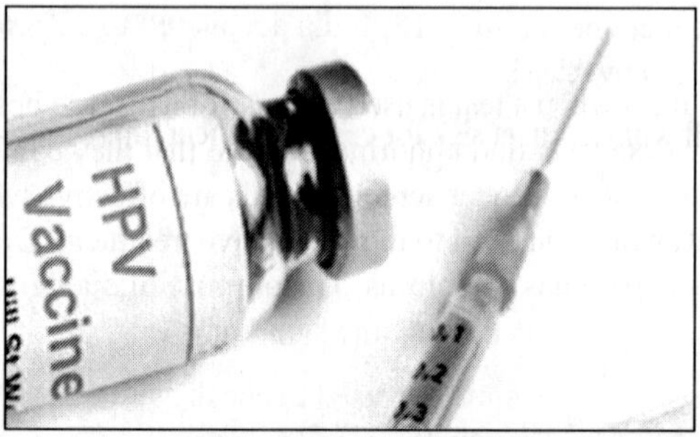

- Make healthy lifestyle choices. For overall good health, eat a diet rich in fruits and vegetables; exercise regularly; maintain a healthy weight; avoid smoking; and practice safe sex. Having multiple sexual partners is a definite risk factor for cervical cancer. Maintaining perineal/pelvic hygiene can help prevent cervical cancer.

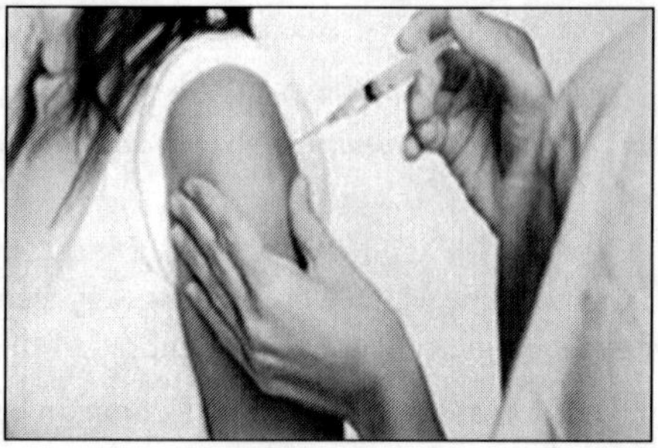

- **Know your family health history.** Share it with the doctor.
- **Get the HPV vaccine.** It protects against the types of HPV that most often cause cervical, vaginal, and vulvar cancers. It is given in a series of three shots. The vaccine is recommended for 11 to 12 year old girls. (Note: The vaccine can be given to girls beginning at age 9.) It also is recommended for girls and women aged 13 through 26 years who did not get any or all of the shots when they were younger.

- **Get regular *Pap* tests.** Pap tests (or Pap smears) are one of the most reliable and effective cancer screening tests available. It is a simple OPD procedure. Pap tests can find precancerous changes on the cervix that can be treated so that cervical cancer is prevented. A Pap test can also find cervical cancer early, when treatment is most effective.

Screening

Screening is when a test is used to look for a disease before there are any symptoms. These tests find abnormal cells so that they can be treated before they turn into cancer. Cancer screening tests are effective when they can find disease early, which can lead to more effective treatment. Diagnostic tests are used when a person has symptoms. The purpose of diagnostic tests is to find out, or diagnose, what is causing the symptoms.

Diagnostic tests also may be used to check a person who is considered at high risk for cancer. It is usually done for women aged 21 years or older.

- **Visual Inspection with acetic acid (VIA):** Visual Inspection with Acetic Acid, or VIA is a simple procedure. It allows doctors to directly see changes in the cervix that are large enough to, presumably, need treatment. The doctor simply swabs vinegar, i.e. acetic acid, on the cervix and looks for areas that change color. Normal cervical tissue remains unaffected by the acetic acid, but damaged tissue — such as that found in pre-cancerous or cancerous lesions turns white. Sometimes Lugol's iodine is used in place of acetic acid as a screening agent.
- **The Pap test:** Of all the gynecologic cancers, only cervical cancer has a screening test—the Pap test—that can find this cancer early, when treatment works best. The Pap test also helps prevent cervical cancer by finding precancers, cell changes on the cervix that might become cervical cancer if they are not treated appropriately.

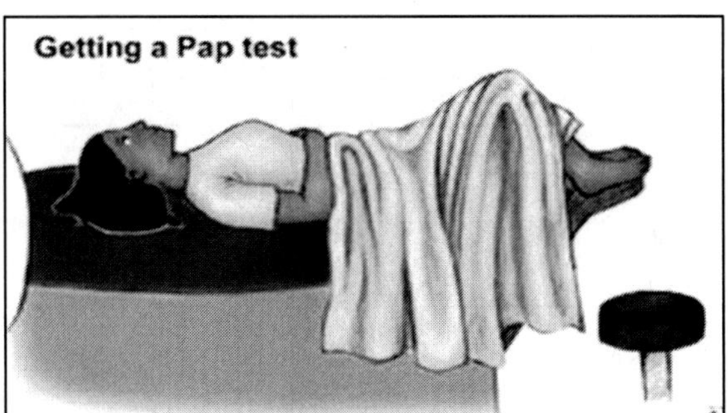

- **The HPV test:** In addition to the Pap test, which is the main screening test for cervical cancer, a test called the HPV test looks for HPV infection. It can be used along with the Pap test for screening women aged 30 years and older. It is especially important to recognize warning signsand to learn if there are things which can reduce the risk.

Symptoms of Cervical Cancer

Some symptoms specific to cervical cancer are:

- Post coital bleeding
- Foul smelling blood
- Irregular vaginal bleeding
- Stained vaginal discharge
- Post menopausal bleeding
- In later stages: Backache, weight loss and fatigue

The general symptoms that may appear in cancer are:

- Weight loss
- Loss of appetite (anorexia)
- Recurrent sore throat
- Prolonged fever
- Weakness
- Recurrent infections
- Frequent Diarrhoea/Constipation
- Blood in cough, vomit or urine

Table 1: Symptoms of Cervical Cancer.

SYMPTOM	*Cervical Cancer*	*Ovarian Cancer*	*Uterine Cancer*	*Vaginal Cancer*	*Vulvar Cancer*
Abnormal vaginal bleeding or discharge	Present	Present	Present	Present	-
Pelvic pain or pressure	-	Present	Present	-	Present
Abdominal or back pain	-	Present	-	-	-
Bloating	-	Present	-	-	-
Change in toilet habits	-	Present	-	Present	-
Itching or burning of vulva	-	-	-	-	Present
Changes in vulva color or skin such as rash, sores or warts	-	-	-	-	Present

If diagnosed with Cervical Cancer

If diagnosed with cervical cancer, the patient may feel scared, depressed, shocked, worried, angry, confused, and many other emotions. Everyone reacts differently to a cancer diagnosis. There is no one 'right' way to react.

As patient come to terms emotionally with the diagnosis, here are some practical things that can be done as care givers and doctor decide on the best medical course of action:

- Such patients may be referred to a gynecologic oncologist, a doctor who is trained to treat gynecologic cancers. Gynecologic oncologists may not be available at all places. If that is the case get referred to other types of doctors who help treat gynecologic cancer, such as gynecologists, medical oncologists, and radiation oncologists.
- Develop and bring a list of questions to ask.
- Take notes or use an audio recorder during your visit.
- Bring a family member or friend to help listen to and understand what the doctor says.

Preparing

Gynecologic oncology team needs a complete picture of the current health status and health history to plan care. Patient will be asked detailed questions bythe physician and nurse. Please make sure to get the copies of your records, biopsy slides, and X-rays to assist. Also patient should bring all medications currently taking.

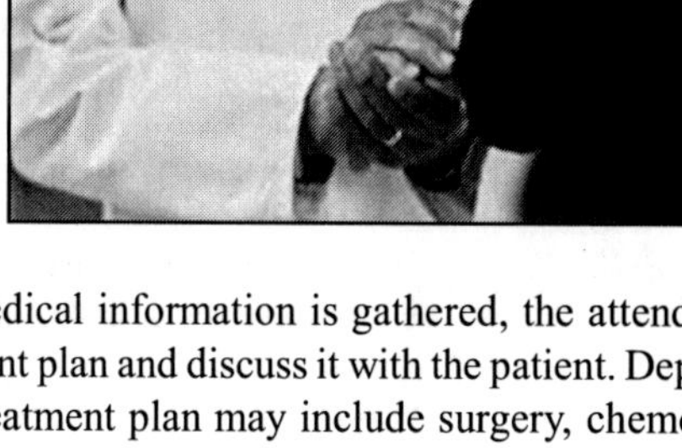

Once the medical information is gathered, the attending physician will prepare a treatment plan and discuss it with the patient. Depending on specific condition, the treatment plan may include surgery, chemotherapy, radiation therapy, hormone therapy, or a combination of treatments.

The Health Care Team

The goal of Gynecology Oncology program is to provide the best possible care while undergoing treatment for cancer.

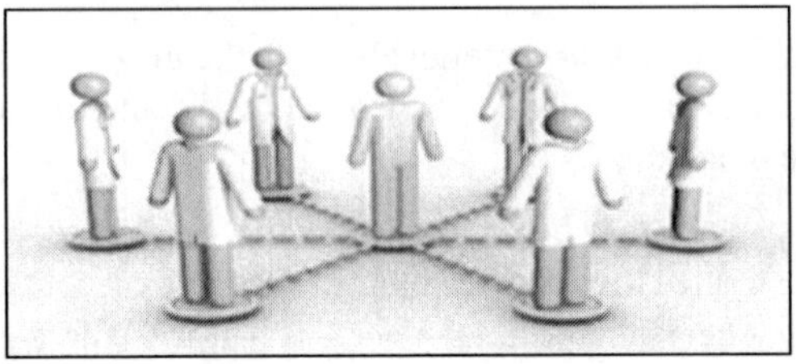

Physicians

While undergoing cancer treatment care will be provided by a team of doctors. Gynecologists and oncologists are trained physicians who are experts in cancer surgery, chemotherapy, and radiation therapy.

The goals include not only providing the best patient care, but also the education of students in health care related fields. Fellows and residents are medical students and will soon be specialists. They are part of the team and may participate in care giving under the guidance and supervision of the faculty ("attending") physician.

Nursing Staff

Nursing staff are part of the patient care team. They are available to talk about treatment and its side effects and to help answer any questions. Please bear in mind that the nurse may not know the specifics of the therapy, and thus treatment issues may be referred back for discussion with the physician.

Dietician

Dieticians are available to work with the patient to answer and address any nutritional concerns. Dietician works one-on-one with the patient and family to provide suggestions for appropriate nutritional intake. An inpatient dietitian is also available in the hospital.

Table 2: Some Tests done during treatment

S. No.	*Diagnostic tests*	*How these tests help*
1.	Biopsy	Removes a small piece of tissue or skin to see if cancer or pre-cancer is present.
2.	Blood Tests	Blood counts (i.e. CBC, liver and kidney tests) Tell how well you will be able to tolerate cancer treatment such as surgery or chemotherapy.

3.	CAT or CT Scan	Multiple X-rays are taken of a part of the body to produce pictures of internal organs. Injection of a dye is needed in some, but not all cases.
4.	Colposcopy	Use of a binocular microscope to evaluate the cervix in women with pre-cancer of the cervix.
5.	ECHO/ECG	These are different tests that determine how your heart is functioning.
6.	Pap Test	A gentle scraping of the cervix or vagina to see if cancer or pre-cancer (dysplasia) may be present.
7.	PET Scan	An imaging study in which a special sugar tagged with short acting radiation is injected into the body.
8.	Tumor Marker Blood Tests	A tumor marker is an indicator for the presence of cancer. The marker is a substance made by a cancer cell that can be measured in the blood and may go down in response to treatment. CA125 is an example, although other tumor markers are also utilized.
9.	Ultrasound	An imaging study that used sound waves to construct an image of internal organs.
10.	Urine culture	Checks for the presence of a urinary tract infection and assesses your kidney function.

Cancer Staging

Cancer slowly progresses from early to last stage when it may be difficult to save the life of patient. Staging describes the size and extent of the disease in the body. Staging also tells whether cancer has spread from its original site to other parts of the body. By knowing the stage of cancer chances of survival can be predicted.

It describes the size and extent of the disease in the body. Staging also tells whether cancer has spread from its original site to other parts of the body (Figure 3). To find out the stage of a gynecologic cancer, your doctor may perform several tests. These results:

- Will help the doctor develop the best possible treatment plan.
- Can be used to estimate the likely outcome or course of the disease.

Table 3: Staging of cervical cancer

Stage 0	Carcinoma in situ. Abnormal cells are found in the innermost lining of the cervix. These may become cancer and spread to other tissues.
Stage I	This is early stage where cancer is strictly confined to the cervix.
Stage II	This is early stage of the disease where the cancer has spread beyond the uterus but limited to upper two third of the vagina.
Stage III	This is advanced stage where the cancer has spread to the pelvic sidewall and lower third of the vagina.
Stage IV	This is advanced stage of disease where the cancer has spread beyond the true pelvis to the bladder and/or rectum

For good results of treatment, recognition of cervical cancer in its early stage is essential. At initial stages the cancer is easy to treat and patients can expect a good prognosis. At advanced stages chances of survival decrease and the treatment is more focused on palliative care measures.

Treatment

Different types and combinations of cancer treatment are possible. Treatment depends on several factors, including stage of cancer, size and location of cancer as well as age and general health of the patient. The aim is to remove the cancer affected part or to kill cancer cells and control spread of cancer. Possible treatments include:

- **Surgery:** A surgeon removes as much of the cancer as possible by operation. The extent or possibility of surgery depends on the type of cancer, the stage, and the patient's overall health.
- **Chemotherapy:** A doctor uses drugs to stop or slow the growth of cancer cells. These drugs also can harm healthy cells, which may cause side effects. Side effects usually get better or go away when chemotherapy is over.
- **Radiation Therapy:** A doctor uses high doses of radiation—high-energy rays—to kill cancer cells and stop them from spreading. Radiation therapy does not hurt while it is being given, but it can cause side effects.

Depending on stage of the disease surgery alone, surgery with chemotherapy, surgery with radiotherapy or surgery with both chemotherapy and radiotherapy may be used.

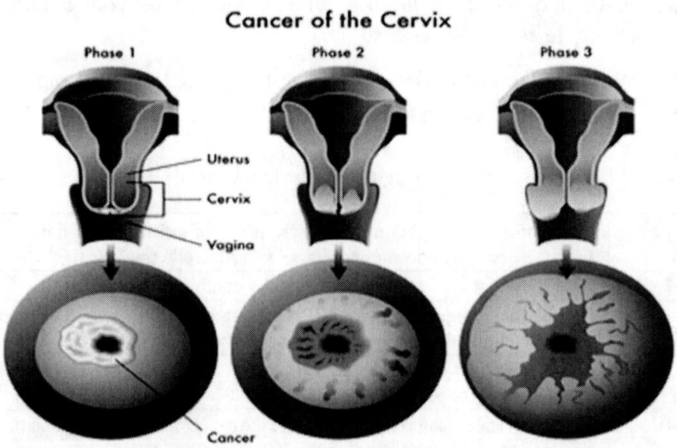

Figure 3: Staging of cervical cancer

When both chemotherapy and radiotherapy are required it is called **chemoradiation**.

Commonly all cervical cancer patients requiring chemoradiation are given External Beam Radiation Therapy. After this the response is assessed. Those found suitable may then undergo chemotherapy or brachytherapy.

All available treatment options for cervical cancer have some side effects. Most side effects can be managed or minimized. Some treatments may affect sexual function or ability to have children. The following chapters provide information on how to manage treatment related side effects on your own.

Care After Surgery

When used to treat cancer, surgery is a procedure where the surgeon removes cancer from your body. It is a local treatment, meaning that it treats only the part of your body affected with cancer.

Surgeons often use small, thin knives, called scalpels, and other sharp tools to cut your body during surgery. Surgery often requires cuts through skin, muscles, and sometimes bone. After surgery, these cuts are sutured. These may remain painful for a few days and you may need some time to recover from.

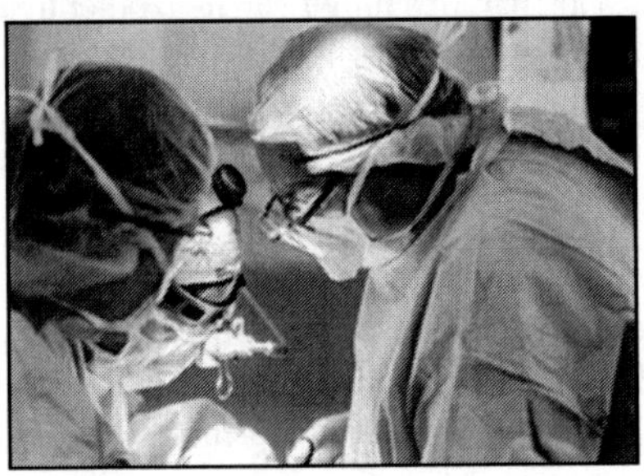

Anesthesia is given before surgery to keep you free from any pain. These are drugs that cause loss of sensation for desired time. Depending on the surgery patient may be given local, regional or general anesthesia.

- Local anesthesia ('Sunn karna') causes loss of feeling in one small area of the body.
- Regional anesthesia causes loss of feeling in a part of the body, such as an arm or leg.
- General anesthesia('Behosh karna') causes loss of feeling and a complete loss of awareness that seems like a very deep sleep.

Some surgeries like Laser, cryosurgery may not involve cuts with scalpels.

Types of surgery

Surgery may be open or minimally invasive.

- In open surgery, the surgeon makes a large cut to remove the tumor, some healthy tissue, and maybe some nearby lymph nodes.
- In minimally invasive surgery, the surgeon makes a few small cuts instead of one large one. A long, thin tube with a tiny camera is inserted into one of the small cuts. This tube is called a laparoscope. The camera projects images from the inside of the body onto a monitor, which allows the surgeon to see inside. Special surgery tools are inserted through the other small cuts to remove the tumor and some healthy tissue.

Goals of Surgery

Depending on your type of cancer and how advanced it is, surgery can be used to:

- Remove the entire tumor
  Surgery removes entire cancer tissue that is contained in one area.
- Debulk a tumor
  Surgery removes some, but not all, of a cancer tumor. Debulking is used when removing an entire tumor might damage an organ or the body. Removing part of a tumor can help other treatments work better.
- Ease cancer symptoms
  Surgery is used to remove tumors that are causing pain or pressure.

Role of Surgery

Surgery is used to remove the cancerous growth. Surgery is generally indicated in early stage of the disease and recurrent cancer which is resectable. Depending upon the stage of disease and weather fertility preservation is required the following surgeries may be performed.

- Radical trachelectomy (Cervicectomy): A surgery to remove the cervix, the upper part of the vagina and lymph nodes in the pelvis. As the uterine body is preserved, this type of surgery is a fertility preserving surgical procedure.
- Wertheim's hysterectomy: A radical operation involving removal of the entire uterus, the connective tissue and lymph nodes close to it, fallopian tubes, ovaries, and the upper part of the vagina.

Problems after Surgery

Common problems seen after surgery are:

- Pain
  After surgery, most people will have pain in the part of the body that

was operated on. Severity of painpatient feels depends on the extent of the surgery, the part of the body that had surgery, and how patient feels pain. (Refer section of pain in chapter 3)

- Infection

  Infection occurs due to contamination of the area where surgery was performed. To help prevent infection, follow your nurse's instructions about caring for the area where you had surgery. If you do develop an infection, your doctor can prescribe a medicine (called an antibiotic) to treat it.

Other risks of surgery include bleeding, damage to nearby tissues, and reactions to the anesthesia. Talk to your doctor about possible risks for the type of surgery you will have.

An informed consent is taken before undergoing surgery.

Wound Care

When patient comes home after surgery, she may have a dressing on the wound. Dressings do several things, including:

- Protect wound from germs
- Reduce the risk of infection
- Cover wound so that stitches do not catch on clothing
- Protect the area as it heals
- Soak up fluids leaking from wound

Key points regarding Bathing

The doctor will inform when it is OK to bathe after surgery. Keep in mind:

- Showers are better than baths because the wound doesn't soak in the water. Soaking the wound could cause it to reopen or become infected.
- Remove the dressing before bathing unless told otherwise. Some dressings are waterproof. Your doctor may suggest covering the wound with a plastic bag to keep it dry.
- If doctor gives the OK, gently rinse the wound with water as you bathe. Do not rub or scrub the wound.
- Do not use soaps, lotions, powders, cosmetics, or any other skin care products on the wound.
- Gently pat dry the area around the wound with a clean towel. Let the wound air dry.
- Apply a new dressing.

Key points regarding wound care

- Do not wear tight clothing that rubs against the incision while it is healing.
- Clean hands before touching the dressing. Wash hands with soap and warm water. Also clean under the nails. Rinse, then dry hands with a clean towel.
- Put on clean medical gloves if the wound is infected (red or oozing), or if changing the dressing for someone else. The gloves do not need to be sterile.
- Never touch the inside of the dressing.
- Do not apply antibiotic cream unless the doctor tells.
- Do not pull at your stitches or try to remove them.
- Call the doctor if there is pus discharge, swelling or redness around the wound or patient develops fever.

Nutritional guidelines for patients after surgery

A healthy, balanced diet is important for operated cervical cancer patients to maintain optimal health. It is suggested that following dietary recommendations should be followed:

1. Increase the intake of protein
2. Limit the fat intake
3. Prefer to take plant based diet
4. Include moderate amounts of soy foods in your diet
5. Have plenty of antioxidants
6. Eat fiber rich diet
7. Reduce or eliminate processed foods
8. Have adequate fluids in the diet
9. Be physically active to help achieve and maintain healthy weight

1. **Increase the intake of protein:** After cervical cancer surgery, the body needs more than its usual supply of proteins to repair cells, fight infection and heal incisions. After the surgery, the protein intake has to be increased as protein helps in healing. It will also help to regain the strength. If solid foods make you to feel sick consume liquid protein drinks like milk with almond and fruit shakes.

   Recommended intake: Intake of protein should be 1-1.5g/Kg body weight to maintain lean body mass and 1.5-2.0g/kg body weight to replete lean body mass.

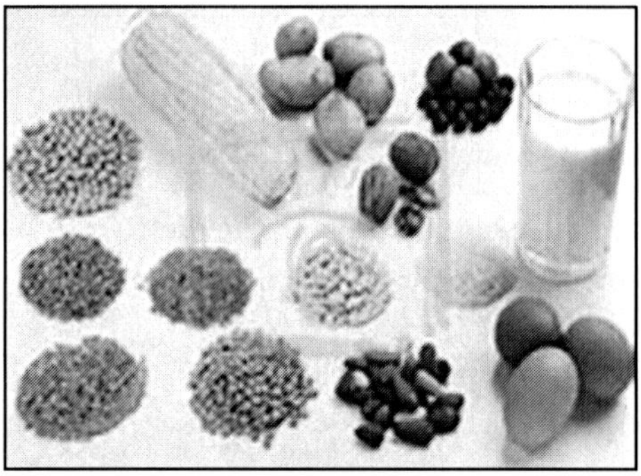

2. **Limit the fat intake:** A low-fat diet is linked to better health. Include more of healthy fats in your diet plan as these are essential to the functioning of your body. Healthy fats include omega-3 and omega-6 fatty acids, conjugated linoleic acid, monounsaturated fatty acids (MUFA) and polyunsaturated fatty acids (PUFA).Healthy fats are found in foods such as flaxseeds (Alsi), seafoods (cold-water fish, such as salmon, tuna, mackerel and trout), avocados and olive oil. Avoid unhealthy fats such as saturated fats (Desi ghee, Malai and Butter), trans fats and hydrogenated fats (cakes, pastries and bakery products etc.).

   Recommended intake: Intake of fat should be 20% of total calories with less than 7% of total calories from saturated fat. Total visible fat consumption should be 15gm/day.

Tips to reduce fat in the diet:

- Limit animal fats, saturated fatty acids, meat, chicken, baked foods and reduce whole milk dairy products, including butter, cheese and ice-cream.
- Avoid hydrogenated fats (margarine, fried foods, peanut butter, salad dressings, breads, crackers, cereals, bakery products like cakes, pastries and cookies etc.).
- Use common vegetable oils (corn oil, safflower oil, sunflower oil and cottonseed oil).
- Increase omega-3 fatty acids like flaxseeds, almonds, walnuts and pumpkin seeds.
- Replace fatty foods with fruits, vegetables, grains and beans.
- Eat smaller portions of higher-fat foods.
- Bake or boil foods instead of frying them.

(Contd...)

- Choose non-fat or low-fat milk and dairy products.
- Pick lean cuts of meat and keep servings small.
- Try beans, fish, and poultry instead of beef, pork and lamb.

Tips to increase the protein intake in the diet:

- Add protein powder or dry skimmed milk to dishes to boost their protein level.
- Add grated paneer to vegetables, potatoes, rice and salads.
- Include high-protein snacks such as almonds, peanuts and paneer in the diet.
- Include more of pulses in the menu like missi chapatti or besan or soya atta mixed with normal wheat flour.

3. Prefer to take plant based diet: Eating plenty of fruits and vegetables as a part of a healthy diet can help in reducing the risk of cancer. A plant based diet rich in fruits and vegetables provides an adequate intake of multiple constituents such as vitamins, fiber and various potentially beneficial biologically active compounds.

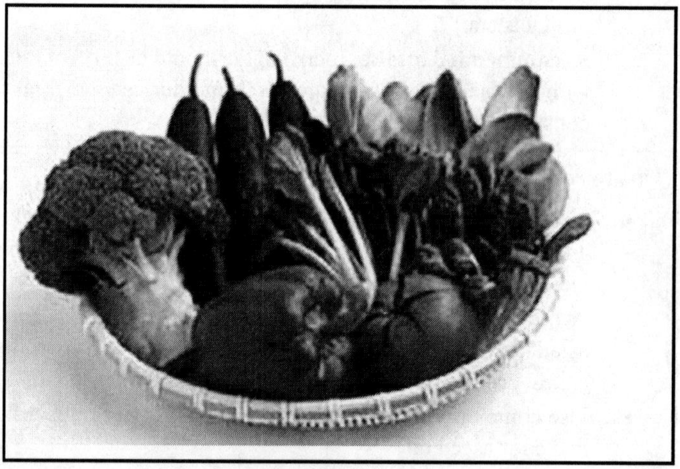

Beinglow in calories, high in fiber and high in water content plant-based diets can reduce excessive weight gain and help in weight maintenance.

Recommended intake: Eat at least 2 - 3 cups of vegetables and fruits each day.

Tips to Increase plant based diet:

- Choose vegetables, whole fruits and other low calorie foods instead of calorie-dense foods such as potato chips etc.
- Include vegetables and fruits at every meal and for snacks.
- Eat a variety of vegetables and fruits each day.
- Emphasize on eating whole vegetables and fruits. and soy milk all contain these phytoestrogens and proteins.

4. **Include moderate amounts of soy foods in diet:** Soy and soy-based foods contain weak estrogen-like compounds called phytoestrogens. Soy protein contains many chemicals.

   These can help regulate cell growth and help keep cholesterol levels low. Soy also contains important antioxidants that can help prevent DNA damage. Soybeans, tofu and soy milk all contain these phytoestrogens and proteins.

   Recommended Intake: One to three servings a day of soy food is advised.

5. **Have plenty of antioxidants:** Many vegetables, fruits, nuts and other foods contain antioxidants. Antioxidants protect the cells from damage by free radicals. Antioxidants include vitamin C, vitamin E and carotenoids (such as beta-carotene which is found in carrots, apricots, yams and other orange-colored vegetables and fruits). Beta-carotene is conver-ted to vitamin A, which is also helpful in prevention of cancer. An antioxidant called lycopene present in tomatoes and grapefruit also helps to prevent recurrence of cancer. Examples of specific foods with antioxidants include vegetables like broccoli, spinach, beets, eggplant, onions, red bell peppers and fruits like mangoes, strawberries, raspberries, apple and other products

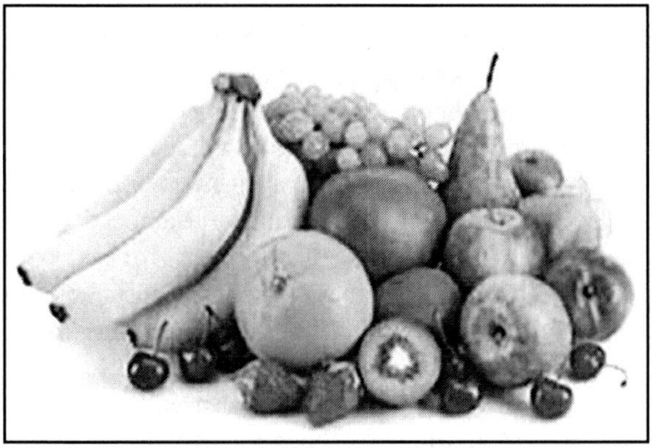

like cinnamon, oregano, ground cloves, red kidney beans etc.

Recommended intake: It is advised to eat a balanced diet with a variety of fresh foods to provide antioxidants.

Some tips for getting the most dietary punch from plant-based foods:

- Include fruits, vegetables and grains in every meal.
- Take fresh or dried fruits and raw vegetables in snacks.
- Try beans as an alternative to meat.
- Choose whole grains over refined ones.

6. **Eat fiber rich diet:** Dietary fiber includes a wide variety of plant carbohydrates that humans cannot digest. A plant-based diet is naturally high in fiber. Dietary fiber improves bowel function. Good sources of fiber are dried beans, whole grains, legumes, vegetables and fruits. Fibers are of two types soluble and insoluble. Soluble fibers are: oat bran, peas, beans, and Psyllium (isabgol). Insoluble fibers include: wheat bran, fruit peels and skins, nuts, seeds and cellulose.

   Recommended intake: Intake of fiber should be approximately 25 to 35 g daily.

Protective effects of dietary fiber:

- It increases fecal bulk and decreases intestinal transit time.
- Whole grains are rich in antioxidants, including trace minerals and phenolic compounds, which have been linked to disease prevention.
- It is associated with less obesity.
- It works to reduce hormone levels that are involved in the progression of cancer.

7. Reduce or eliminate processed foods: Food processing alters foods in many ways. Baked foods, such as white bread, croissants, chips, muffins and doughnuts should be avoided or limited because they contain hydrogenated oils. Many processed foods and beverages, including sugar-sweetened beverages, sweetened breakfast cereals, pastries, candies, and syrups, contain large amounts of added sugars. These added sugars come in many forms, such as high-fructose corn syrup, fruit juice concentrates and honey. Consuming products high in these added sugars adds little nutrient value to the diet and contributes to excess caloric intake which leads to increase in body weight. It is important for cervical cancer patients to maintain a healthy weight. Refining of grains and cereals lowers the amount of

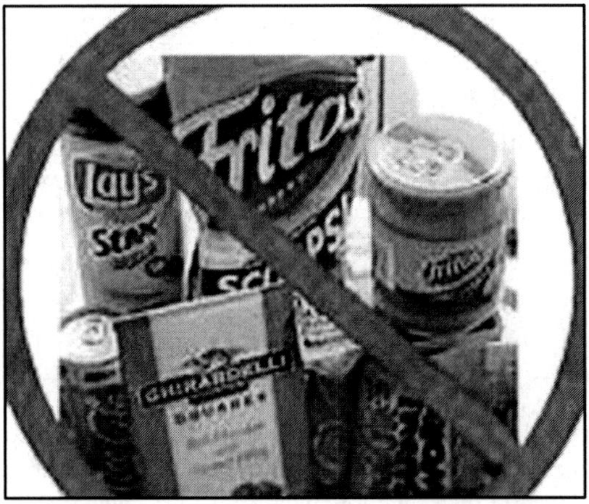

fiber. Various techniques of processing of meat increase the potential of these foods to cause cancer e.g. like by adding preservatives such as salt or sodium nitrite to prevent the growth of germs; smoking the meat to preserve or enhance color and flavor. Some food processing methods, such as freezing and canning vegetables and fruits, lower the content of some heat-sensitive vitamins e.g. Vitamin C and B.

Tips to avoid processed food:

- Limit intake of baked food and bakery products like biscuits, breads etc.
- Limit consumption of processed meats and red meats, sausage, luncheon meats and hot dogs.
- Choose fish, poultry, or beans as an alternative to red meat (beef, pork and lamb).
- Limit consumption of creamy sauces, dressings and dips.
- Prefer low calorie drinks like lemonade and buttermilk.

8. Have adequate fluids in the diet: Be sure not to overlook water as a part of the healthy eating plan. Water is especially important when you are going through chemotherapy, as it helps to rehydrate skin cells. It also flushes excess medicines and toxins from your system. Drink plenty of water daily to meet the fluid needs of your body. Limit consumption of sugar-sweetened beverages such as soft drinks, sports drinks and fruit-flavored drinks. Try to include lemon water (shikanji), buttermilk (lassi) and fruit shakes.

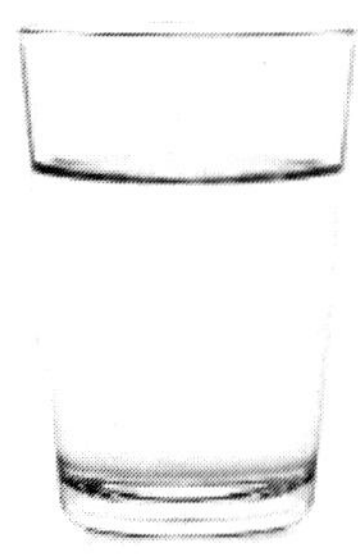

Recommended intake: Drink at least 10 - 12 glasses of water every day.

Functions of water in the body are:

- It carries nutrients and waste products.
- It participates in chemical reactions and maintains blood volume.
- It acts as a lubricant and cushion around joints.
- It acts as a shock absorber in the eyes and spinal cord.
- It aids in the body's temperature regulation.
- Increased fluid intake is needed for a high fiber diet.

9. Be physically active to help achieve and maintain a healthy weight: During and after cervical cancer treatment, on one hand it is important to get enough calories to nourish the body and on the other hand, it is also important to maintain a healthy weight. Exercise is an important preventive factor.

Tips to maintain a healthy body weight:

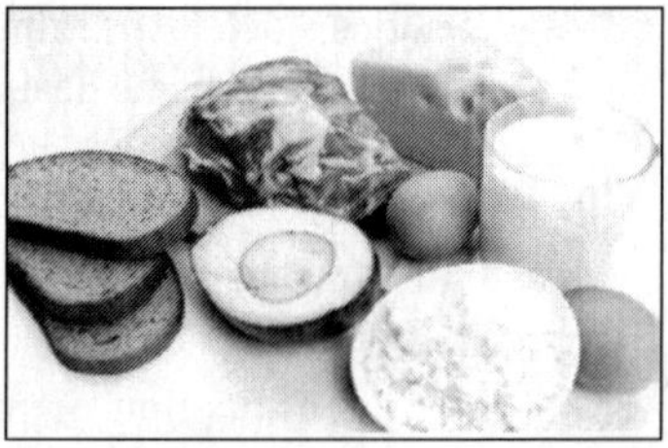

- Adopt a physically active lifestyle.
- Exercise as directed by doctor
- Consume a healthy diet with lots of fruits, vegetables and whole grains.
- Generally a diet with less fat and more of protein is recommended.
- Reduce the intake of sweets and high glycemic index foods like refined sugars etc.
- Caloric intake can also be reduced by decreasing the size of food portions and limiting snacks in between the meals.
- Limit the intake of foods and beverages that are high in calories, fat added sugars and that provide few nutrients (e.g. many fried foods, cookies, cakes, candy, ice cream and sugar-sweetened beverages). Such foods and beverages should be replaced with vegetables and fruits, beans, whole grains and lower calorie beverages.

Factors leading to obesity:

- Increasing portion size.
- The consumption of high-calorie convenience foods like: pizza, pastas and burgers; Sugar-sweetened beverages; Restaurant meals.

- Increased consumption of high-calorie foods outside the home.
- Declining levels of physical activity are contributing to obesity.
- Reduced leisure time and increased amounts of time spent sitting.
- Increased reliance on automobiles for transportation.
- Increased availability of electronic entertainment and communications media.
- Poor access to sidewalks, parks and recreation facilities.

Ways to achieve a healthy body weight:

- Balance energy intake (food and beverage intake) with energy expenditure (physical activity).
- Exercise regularly

Some important food handling tips: Patients who have undergone surgery and those receiving chemotherapy have compromised immune systems. To prevent oneself from any infection, always be careful in food handling in order to avoid food-borne illnesses.

- Wash hands before handling food.
- Make sure foods are refrigerated well.
- Fruits and vegetables should be rinsed well before eating.
- Do not use any type of raw food or cut fruit from the open market to avoid contamination of food.
- Make sure all meat/chicken products are cooked thoroughly.

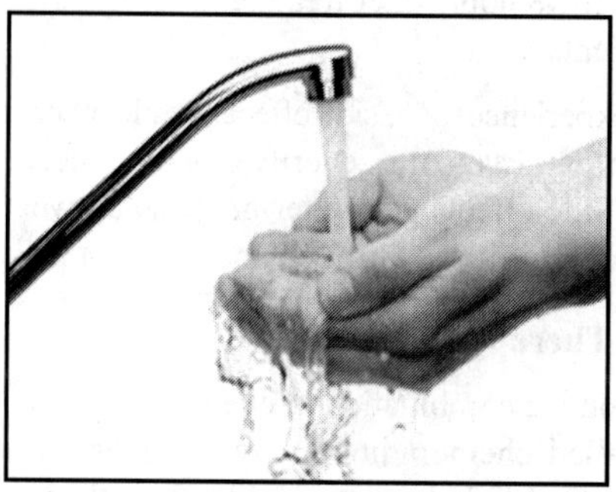

Managing nausea and vomiting: These are common in cervical cancer patients after surgery, chemotherapy or radiation therapy. Also, after surgery there is loss of appetite. Patients have less desire to eat. This may result in "wasting syndrome". In this there is reduction in muscles, organ tissues, and other lean body mass (LBM). There is weight loss and weakness also.

Tips to ease symptoms of nausea after gynaecological cancer treatment:

- Eat several smaller meals throughout the day instead of three regular big meals.
- Cold foods are better tolerated than hot foods.
- Use cold, clear fluids, carbonated beverages, ice creams, shakes and custards etc., as these are normally well tolerated.
- Vegetable soups, pureed foods and semisolid foods like khichri, thin dal and seera can also be included in the diet plan.

Care during and after chemotherapy

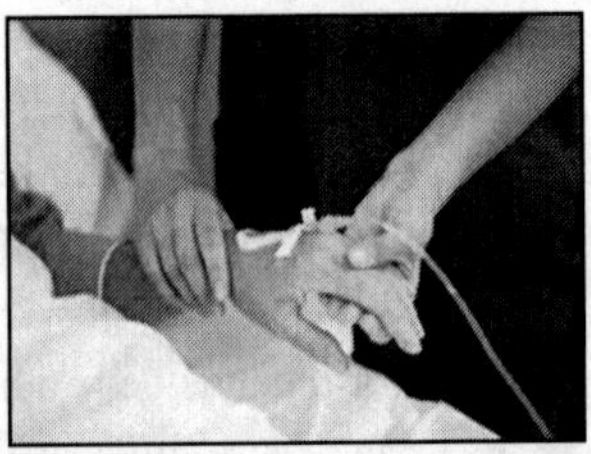

Chemotherapy is a kind of cancer treatment that uses drugs to destroy cancer cells. While surgery and radiation therapy focuses on the cancer bearing area, while chemotherapy works throughout the whole body. Chemotherapy can kill cancer cells that have spread to parts of the body far away from the primary (original) tumor. However, both radiotherapy and chemotherapy besides acting on cancer cells, can damage healthy cells that divide quickly like those which line the mouth, intestines and cause hair to grow. This causes side effects. Many people feel fine for the first few hours following chemotherapy. Usually, some reaction occurs about four to six hours later. However, some people do not show any symptoms until 12 or even 24 to 48 hours after treatment. Response depends on internal strength of the patients.

Some people experience more side effects, while others may not experience even a single symptom. Even, the severity of side effects varies greatly from person to person. Side effects get better or go away when chemotherapy is over. People commonly use the term 'chemo' in short for chemotherapy.

Chemoradiation Therapy

Chemoradiation is a combination of chemotherapy and radiotherapy. It is also sometimes called chemoradiotherapy. Chemoradiation may be given: before surgery to help shrink the cancer and reduce the risk of cancer coming back.

The chemotherapy helps the radiation work well. Options for concurrent chemoradiation include:

- Cisplatin given weekly during radiation. This drug is given into a vein (IV) about 4 hours before the radiation appointment.

- Cisplatin plus 5-fluorouracil (5-FU) given every 4 weeks during radiation.

Sometimes chemotherapy is also given (without radiation) before and/or after chemoradiation.

Goal of chemotherapy: Depending on the type of cancer and its stage (how far it has spread), chemotherapy can be used to:

- Cure cancer.
- Control cancer- Keep the cancer from spreading, slow the growth cancer cells.
- Ease cancer symptoms.

Using Chemotherapy

Sometimes, chemotherapy is used as the only cancer treatment. But more often, chemotherapy is given along with surgery orradiation therapy. Chemotherapy can:

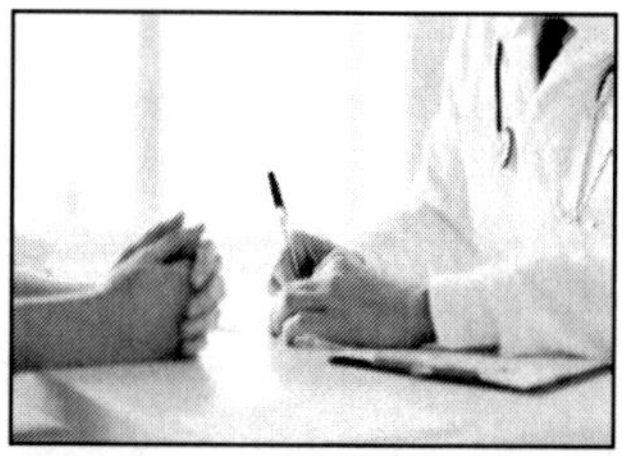

- Destroy cancer cells that may remain after surgery or radiation therapy. This is called **adjuvant chemotherapy.**
- Make a tumor smaller before surgery or radiation therapy. This is called **neo-adjuvant chemotherapy.**
- Destroy cancer cells that have come back (**recurrent** cancer) or spread to other parts of the body (**metastatic** cancer).
- Help radiation therapy and biological therapy work well.

Duration of Chemotherapy

Treatment schedules for chemotherapy vary widely. How often and how long the patient gets chemotherapy depends on:

- The type of cancer and stage of cancer
- The goals of therapy (whether chemotherapy is used to cure your cancer, control its growth, or ease the symptoms)
- The type of chemotherapy
- How the body reacts to chemotherapy

Chemotherapy is routinely given in cycles. A cycle is a period of chemotherapy treatment followed by a period of rest. For example, you might receive 1 week of chemotherapy followed by 3 weeks of rest. These 4 weeks make up one cycle. The rest period gives the body a chance to build new healthy cells.

Side effects of Chemotherapy

Chemotherapy is an individual experience. Every person experiences chemotherapy differently, both physically and emotionally. Even the side effects from chemotherapy are different for each individual. Different chemotherapy drugs cause different side effects. Fortunately, as the science of cancer treatment has advanced, so has the science of managing the side effects of treatment.

Cancer cells tend to grow fast. Chemotherapy drugs kill the fast-growing cells. These drugs travel throughout the body. These can also affect the fast growing normal, healthy cells of the body. Damage to healthy tissue causes side effects. Many people worry about the side effects of cancer treatment. Side effects are not always as bad as one might expect. The normal cells that are most likely to be damaged by chemotherapy are blood-forming cells in the bone marrow, hair follicles, cells in the mouth, digestive tract and reproductive system. Some chemotherapy drugs can damage cells in the heart, kidneys, bladder, lungs, and nervous system. Often other medicines are given along with the chemotherapy to the patients in order to protect the normal cells of the body. However, it is important to know the various side effects of chemotherapy and how these can be managed.

Duration of the side effects

Most side effects slowly go away after the treatment ends because the healthy cells recover over time. The time it takes to get over some side effects and regain energy varies from person to person and depends on many factors, including the overall health and the drugs given to the patient.

Many side effects go away fairly quickly, but some may take months or even years to completely go away. Sometimes the side effects can last a lifetime, such as when chemotherapy causes long-term damage to the heart, lungs, kidneys, or reproductive organs. Certain drugs sometimes cause delayed effects.

Before starting Chemotherapy

Before starting chemotherapy it is important that patient take care of some of the basic health needs. If time permits, have dental checkup before undergoing chemotherapy. If a major dental work is required, try to postpone it until after chemotherapy. Have a thorough exam of mouth and gums, dental x-rays and cleaning by a dental hygienist. Ask them how to take care of the mouth and teeth. Blood counts are also checked for any source of infection.

Ways of Chemotherapy

Chemotherapy can be given in many ways.

- **Injection:** The chemotherapy is given by a shot in a muscle in the arm, thigh, or hip, or right under the skin in the fatty part of arm, leg, or belly.
    - o Intra-arterial (IA): The chemotherapy is given into the artery that is feeding the cancer.
    - o Intravenous (IV): The chemotherapy is given into a vein. It is the most commonly used method.
    - o Intraperitoneal (IP): The chemotherapy is given into the peritoneal cavity (the area that contains organs such as the intestines, stomach, liver, and ovaries).

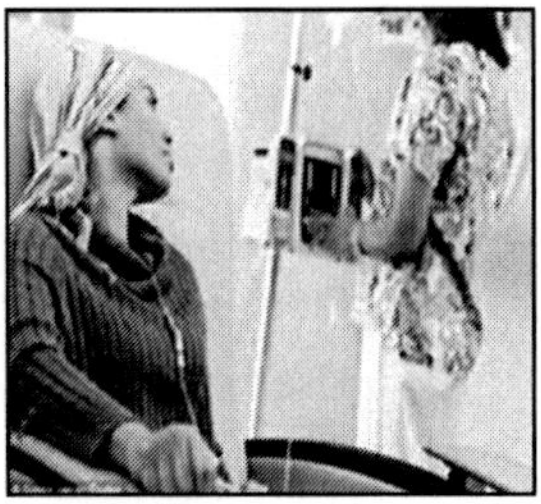

- **Topical:** The chemotherapy is given in a cream to rub on skin.
- **Oral:** The chemotherapy is given in pills, capsules, or liquids to swallow

Things to know about chemotherapy through injection

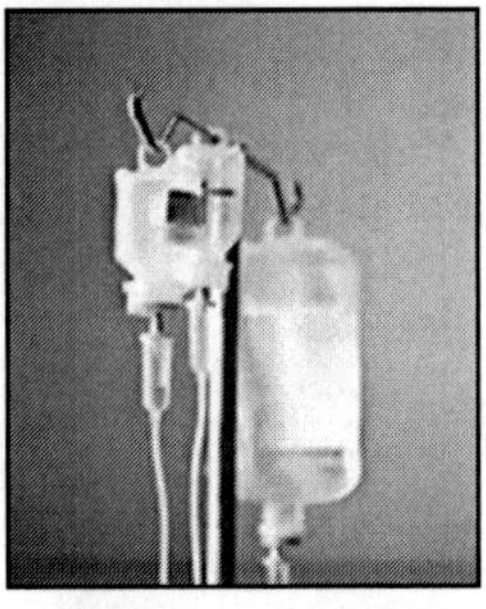

Often chemotherapy is given via a thin needle placed on hand or lower arm. This needle is put in at the start of each treatment and removed once treatment is over. Let the doctor or nurse know if pain or burning occurs while getting IV chemotherapy.

IV chemotherapy is often given through catheters or ports, sometimes with the help of a pump.

Catheters: A catheter is a soft, thin tube. Doctor places one end of the catheter in a large vein, often in chest area. The other end of the catheter stays outside the body. Most catheters stay in place until all chemotherapy treatments are done.

Ports: A port is a small, round disc made of plastic or metal that is placed under the skin. A catheter connects the port to a large vein, most often in the chest. A needle can be inserted into the port to give you chemotherapy or draw blood.

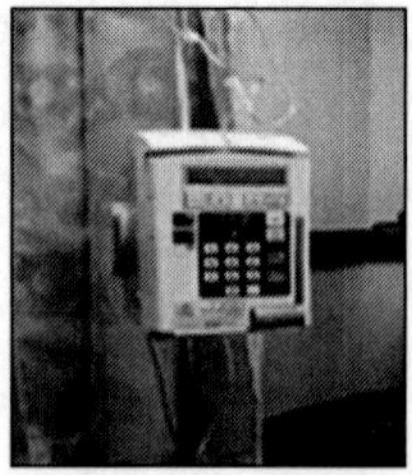

Pumps: Pumps are often attached to catheters or ports. They control how much and how fast chemotherapy goes into a catheter or port. Pumps can be internal or external. External pumps remain outside the body. Most people can carry these pumps with them. Internal pumps are placed under the skin during surgery.

Dos and Don'ts while undergoing Chemotherapy

Do's

- Practice good hand hygiene practices
- Use a mild moisturizer to treat dry skin that is common in chemotherapy patients, to avoid rashes and itchiness of the skin.
- Take bath or sponge yourself every day and take special care of the parts that are too sweaty like underarms, folds of the skin and private areas.
- Keep your nails trimmed.
- Sanitize hands before touching catheter or the area of treatment
- If possible try to use personal bathroom and toilet
- Flush the toilet twice after use
- Try to stay as active as possible
- Do light exercises
- Take adequate nutrition - include cooked seasonal vegetables, soups in your diet
- Prefer homemade diet
- Take medications on time

Don'ts

- Avoid crowded places like movie theaters, public transport etc
- Avoid meeting people who are ill
- Avoid contact with pets
- Avoid raw food items like uncooked meats or vegetables
- Avoid eating stale food or foods that have been refrigerated for more than five hours.
- Avoid packed food items
- Avoid having sex
- Avoid sharing your items with family

Care during and after radiotherapy

Radiotherapy

Radiation therapy (also called radiotherapy) is a cancer treatment that uses high doses of radiation to kill cancer cells and shrink tumors. Lay people often call it 'Bijlikisikai', 'garamsikai' or 'X – ray kisikai'. At low doses, radiation is used as an x-ray to see inside your body and take pictures, such as x-rays of your teeth or bones.

Radiotherapy works by killing tumor cells or inhibiting their growth and division. Other names for radiotherapy are radiation therapy, irradiation or x-ray therapy. Radiation can be given alone or can be used with other treatments, such as surgery or chemotherapy.

There are different ways to give radiation. Radiation therapy uses special equipment to deliver high doses of radiation to the cancer cells. This damages cancer cells and causes them to die.

Radiation works by breaking a piece of the DNA molecule inside the cancer cell, which keeps the cell from growing, dividing and spreading. When cure is not possible radiation may be used to treat pain and other symptoms of cancer. The nearby normal cells also may be affected by radiation, but most recover fully from the effects of the treatment and go back to normal condition in the way they are supposed to. Doctors try to protect healthy cells by using a low dose of radiation as possible, spreading out treatment over time and aiming radiation at a precise part of body only. Sometimes a patient gets more than one type of radiation treatment for the same cancer.

Types: There are 2 types of radiotherapies:

1. **External radiation therapy:** It is called external beam radiotherapy or tele therapy. In external radiation therapy, X-rays are delivered by a linear accelerator with the beam directed to the body through the skin. It is a type of local treatment where rays are directed only to a specific part of the body.
2. **Internal radiation therapy:** It is commonly called as Brachytherapy. It involves placing the radiation source inside the body in the area to be treated, thereby protecting the skin. Hollow tubes or a balloon are put in the body where tissue has been removed. Radioactive wires are inserted into these tubes or balloons which kill any cancer cells that may be left there. These hollow tubes or balloon may be left there in that same place for a few days or inserted for a few minutes each day.

External Beam Radiation Therapy

Duration: Most people have external beam radiation once a day, five times a week. Treatment may last from 2 – 10 weeks (more commonly for 5 weeks) depending on the type of cancer and goal of therapy. Most of the time external beam radiation does not require hospitalization i.e. patient remain as outpatient.

Preparing: Before starting with external beam radiation a nurse/doctor will explain about the benefits, potential side effects and ways to carefor yourself during and after therapy. Once ready for the therapy patient is asked to lie down very still while x-rays or scans are taken. Now a radiation oncologist will put marks on your skin to mark the treatment area. These marks are needed throughout the course of therapy. These ink markings will fade over time. Be careful not to remove these and inform the doctor if they fade away or loose colour.

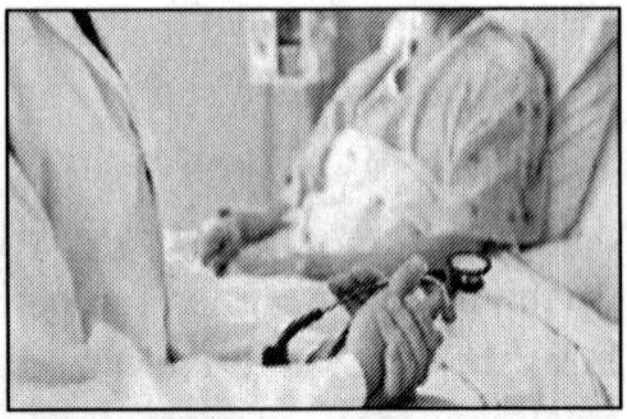

A body mould may also be made of the body part undergoing treatment. This may be of plastic/plaster that prevents one from moving during treatment. It helps to make sure that radiation is given on the same region each day.

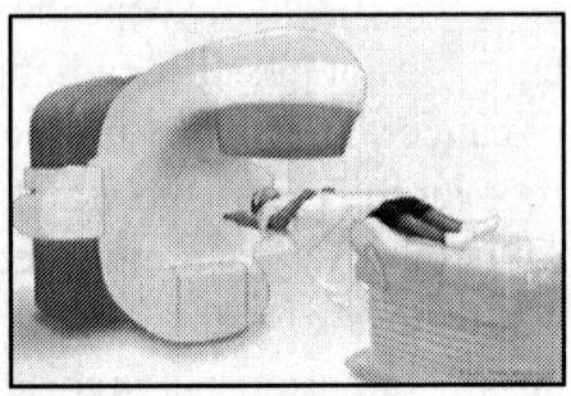

Wear comfortable and loose clothes on days of treatment. Choose clothes that are easy to take off as one may be asked either to remove them from treatment area or change to a hospital gown. Also do not wear jewelry or put powder on the treatment area.

Treatment Session: Patient is asked to lie down. The marks or body mould will help to get into correct position. One may see colored lights pointed at the skin marks. These lights are harmless and guide the therapist to set position for the treatment. Stay still so that radiation goes to the same place each time. Normally radiation is given one to five minutes. During the therapy one can breathe normally and there is no need to hold breath. The doctor will leave the room once one is ready for treatment. Doctor will go to a nearby room to control the radiation machine. The doctor can watch through a window or a TV screen and can talk to the patient with a speaker phone. Be sure to tell the doctor if feeling uncomfortable or sick. The radiation machine can be stopped anytime by the doctor. Radiation cannot be felt, seen, heard or smell.

The entire visit may last from 30 minutes to an hour. Only a certain type of radiations take longer. Visit may take longer if doctors need to review the reports.

Tips to relax during the treatment session:

- Try to remain busy in the waiting room. You can read a book, listen to music, do knitting or solve a crossword puzzle.
- You can meditate, breathe deeply and pray.

Internal Beam Radiation Therapy

Most brachytherapy is put in place through a catheter which is a small starchy tube. Sometimes a larger device called applicator may be used. The doctor will put the catheter or applicator into your body before beginning treatment. Now the radiation source is placed inside. The radiation source may be kept in place for a few minutes to many days depending on the type of treatment you are undergoing.

Types of Implants

Low-dose rate (LDR) implants. Here the radiation source stays in place for one to seven days. Patient is likely to be hospitalized during treatment. Once treatment is over, the doctor will remove the radiation source and the catheter or applicator.

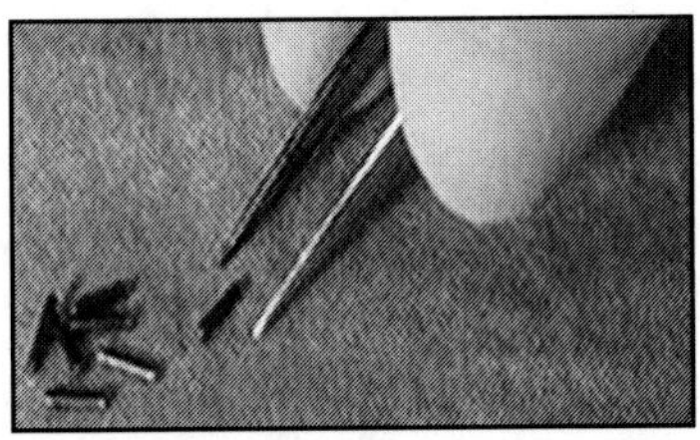

High-dose rate (HDR) implants. Here the radiation source is left in place for just 10 to 20 minutes at a time and then taken out. The treatment may last for twice a day for two to five days or once a week for two to five weeks. The schedule depends on the type of cancer. During the course of treatment, your catheter or applicator may stay in place, or it may be put in place before each treatment. Hospitalization may or may not be required during treatment depending on your condition. The catheter or applicator is removed once the treatment is over.

Permanent implants. These implants always stay in the body, but the radiation gets weaker each day. As time goes on, almost all radiation will go away. Initially one may need to limit the time around other people. Extra care should be taken while around with pregnant women or children.

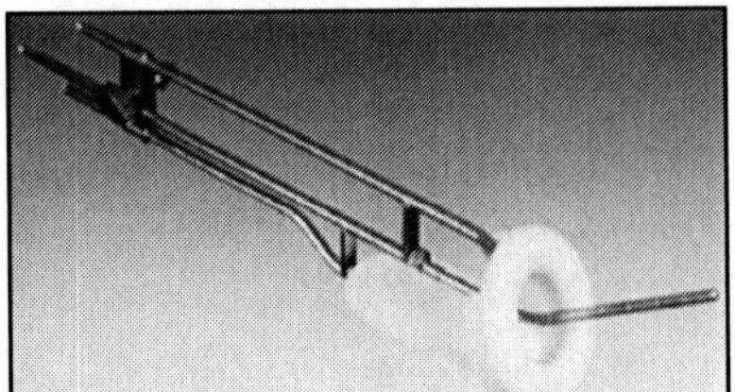

Removing the device: Before removing the catheter or applicator a medicine for pain is given to you. The area may remain tender for a few months.

After the device is removed there is no radiation in your body. Now it is safe for people including pregnant ladies and children to be around you. For a week or two you will be required to limit your activities which take a lot of effort.

Do's and don'ts for the patients undergoing radiotherapy:

DO's

- Take ample rest.
- Eat a balanced and nutritious diet.
- Take care of the skin in the treatment area. If you get external radiation therapy, the skin in the treatment area may become more sensitive and feel sun burned.
- Protect the treated area from the sun. Your skin may be extra sensitive to sunlight. If possible, cover the treated skin with dark-colored clothing before going outside.
- Tell your doctor about all medicines you are taking before treatment. Give your doctor a full list of all the medicines you take and how often you take it, Do not forget to list those you take only when you need them, such as aspirin, vitamins, sleeping herbs pills, antacids, headache remedies, antihistamines etc.

DONT's

- Do not wear tight clothes over the treatment area: Like girdle pants, pantyhose or close-fitting collars. Instead, wear loose and soft cotton clothing.
- Do not starch your clothes.
- Do not rub, scrub or use adhesive tape on treated skin.
- Do not put heat or cold packs (such as a heating pad or ice pack) on the treatment area.
- Do not get pregnant while having radiation therapy. Talk to your doctor if you want to have children in future.

Managing side effects of Chemotherapy and Radiotherapy

Common side effects of Chemo radiation therapy: Chemotherapy and Radiotherapy can damage normal parts of body also. It leads to side effects. Common side effects of cancer therapy are:

1. Nausea and vomiting
2. Fatigue
3. Hair loss
4. Anemia

5. Diarrhea
6. Constipation
7. Pain
8. Neuropathy
9. Skin problems
10. Appetite changes
11. Sexual changes
12. Infertility
13. Mouth changes
14. Throat changes
15. Urinary and bladder changes
16. Lower leg lymphedema
17. Fecal incontinence

A review of some of the more common side effects caused by chemotherapy and radiotherapy and some tips to manage them are discussed here:

1. **Nausea and vomiting:** These are the common and most dreaded side effects of chemotherapy and radiotherapy. Nausea is feeling of vomit. How often patient has these side effects and how bad they are, depends on the drugs/dose of radiation. Nausea and vomiting may start during treatment and last a few hours. Sometimes, but less often, severe nausea and vomiting can last for a few days. However, they can be controlled with different anti-emetics.

Key points for nausea and vomiting:

- Before therapy, eat a small and light meal. Most people do better if they have something in their stomach.
- Eat what sounds good to you. Generally starches such as rice, bread, potatoes, hot cereals and puddings are well tolerated.
- Try not to skip meals. An empty stomach will worsen all symptoms. If you do not feel like sitting down to a meal, try nibbling on something that appeals to you.

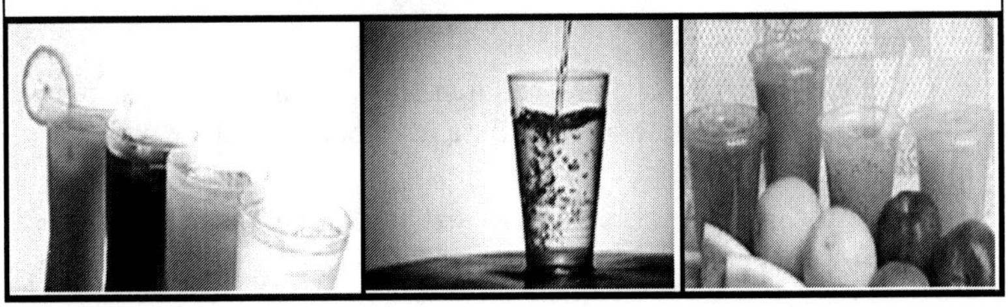

- Drink plenty of fluids. Herbal teas, water, lime juice, jaljeera, aampannaetc are recommended more than soda.
- Avoid foods with strong smells, very hot/cold, spicy, fatty, greasy or fried foods.
- Eat and drink slowly.
- Take (a Katorior glass) shikanji, fruit juice or glucose water every two hours.
- Avoid large meals. Eat five or six small meals and snacks each day.
- Avoid drinking beverages, with meals. Drink liquids at least an hour before or after meals
- Rest in a chair after eating. Do not lie flat for at least 2 hours after you have finished your meal.
- Rinse mouth with lemon water after eating.
- Suck on ice cubes, mints, or hard candies.
- Distractions such as TV, music, or reading may be helpful while eating.
- Wear loose-fitting clothes.
- Breathe deeply and slowly when you feel nauseated.

2. Fatigue: Chemotherapy and radiotherapy can make a patient feel tired. Fatigue is one of the most common side effects of cancer treatment. Fatigue is described as feeling tired, worn out and low. It can range from mild lethargy to feeling completely wiped out. Most people have to make some adjustment in work and family responsibilities. Try to balance activity and rest.

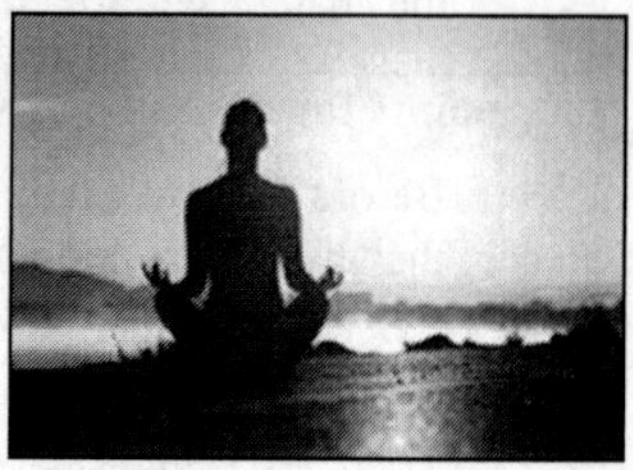

Try to maintain everyday activities. It can be very beneficial for physical as well as for emotional recovery. Fatigue may last six weeks to a year after your last radiotherapy session.

Key points for fatigue:

- If the patient has little children, rest when they are napping. Consider hiring a babysitter for a few hours so that the patient can relax or take a nap.
- Take naps early in the day so that you do not disturb your sleep pattern at night.

- Try to sleep at least for eight hours each night. This can be achieved by remaining active in the day, doing calming activities like reading, listening to music etc. before going to bed.
- Try not to do too much. Stay active but choose to do activities that are most important.
- Perform exercises as directed by the doctor.
- Include activities like swimming, walking, yoga etc.
- Try to relax. Meditation, prayer and yoga can ease relaxation.
- Get up slowly to help prevent dizziness after sitting or lying down.
- Keep track of the feelings each day. This will help in planning how to best use the time.
- Let other people around help in daily chores like cooking food.

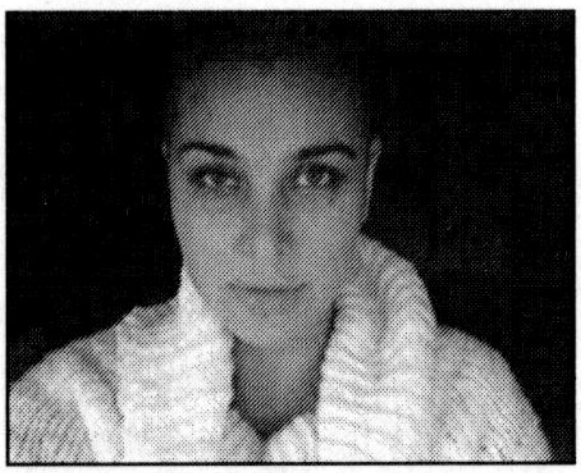

3. Hair Loss: Many people feel that hair loss is one of the most difficult aspects of chemotherapy. Not all chemotherapy drugs cause hair loss. Most often, hair loss begins about two to three weeks after starting chemotherapy. Some people will lose relatively little hair, while others may lose all the hair on their head, eyelashes and eyebrows, as well as other body hair.

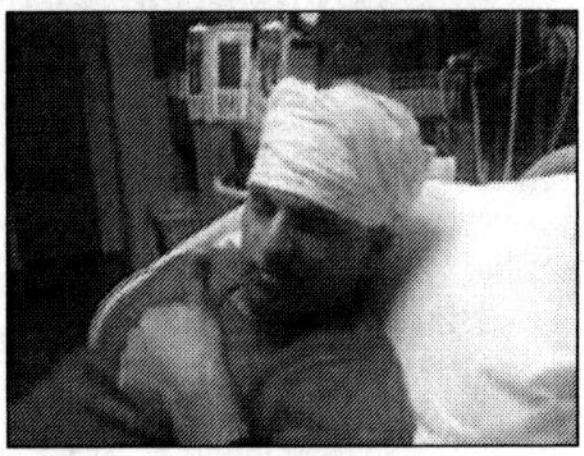

After hair loss: One may want to cover the head with a wig, scarf, hat or turban, or may not want to cover head at all. Do what makes one most comfortable. Many people choose different head coverings for different situations. If buying a wig, try to buy one while having hair because it can better match colour and style. After treatment scalp may be tender. Cover the head with a hat or scarf. This will be extremely useful in prevention of sun exposure. Also try to stay warm. Hair helps to stay warm therefore one may feel cold after losing hair.

The hair will begin to grow back after chemotherapy is over. It usually takes from two to three months to see the change from no hair to some hair. New hair may be slightly different in colour and texture than old hair. Often, the new hair will be baby soft and curly, but will generally return to its original texture after some time.

With radiotherapy hair loss occurs only in the treatment area.

Key points for hair Loss:

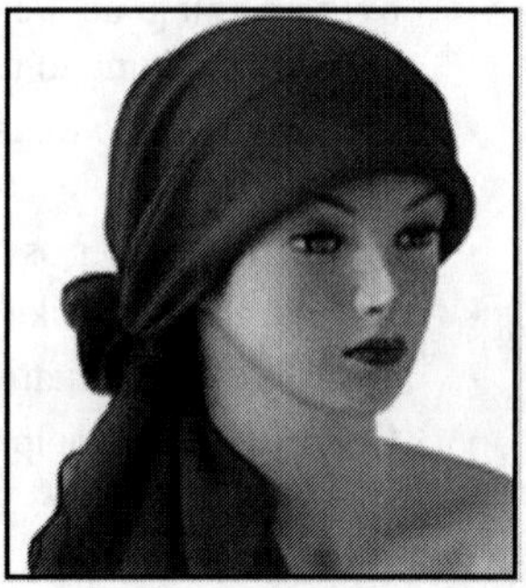

- Use mild shampoos. Also be gentle while washing hair.
- Use soft-bristle hair brushes.
- Do not use
- Straightening or curling irons
- Electric hair dryers
- Hair dyes
- Hairsprays
- Harsh hair products like hair colors, gels etc.
- It is not always necessary to buy a real wig. Synthetic wigs can look as good and are less expensive, easier to care for, lighter in weight and may be more comfortable to wear.
- Use hat, cap or scarf to cover head.
- Before possible hair loss, some people like to cut their hair short. The hair loss would not be so shocking if there is less hair to lose. A shorter style will make hair look thicker and fuller.
- Put a towel over pillow so that clean up in the morning will be easier while the hair shed.

4. Bleeding problems: Our bone marrow produces 3 important parts of blood: Red blood cells, White blood cells and Platelets

Platelets

These help blood to clot so that bleeding is prevented.

Platelet normal value: 1, 00,000-4, 50,000/mm3

Chemotherapy can affect the bone marrow's ability to make platelets. Platelet deficiency may lead to easy bleed or bruising, even from a minor injury. A shortage of platelets is called thrombocytopenia. Report these signs of thrombocytopenia to the doctor:

- Unexpected bruising
- Small red spots under the skin
- Red or pink urine
- Black or bloody stools
- Bloody sputum
- Any bleeding from gums or nose
- Bad headaches, dizziness

- An increase in weakness and
- Pain in joints and muscles etc.

Key points to avoid bleeding:

- Do not take any medicine without first checking with your doctor.
- Use an extra-soft bristle toothbrush to clean your teeth and talk to your doctor before using dental floss.
- Avoid constipation.
- If you have a running nose, blow gently into a soft tissue/ handkerchief.
- Take care not to cut or nick yourself when using scissors, needles, knives, or tools.
- Be careful not to burn yourself when ironing or cooking. Use a padded glove while touching any hot utensil.
- Avoid sports and other activities that might cause an injury.
- Drink plenty of fluids and eat enough fiber to reduce the chances of getting constipation.
- Do not use aspirin or related medicines unless prescribed by your doctor.

White Blood Cells

These help fight infection.

Normal values: Total WBC- 4000-10000/mm3

Neutrophils- 1400-7500/mm3

An infection is most likely to occur when the neutrophil count is low. Infections can begin in almost any part of the body and most often start in the mouth, skin, lungs, urinary tract and rectum. Report any signs of infection to doctor right away:

The symptoms of infection are-

- Fever of 100.5 C or above
- Sweating not related to work out
- Chills
- Diarrhea
- Fatigue
- Cough/sore throat
- Redness or swelling at site of incision
- Urinary burning or odor
- Vaginal itching

Key points regarding infection:

- Consult doctor immediately, if one has a fever of 101° Fahrenheit (38.3° Celsius), with or without chills, cough, sore throat, pain or burning sensation in urine.
- Keep a thermometer in home and know how to take temperature.

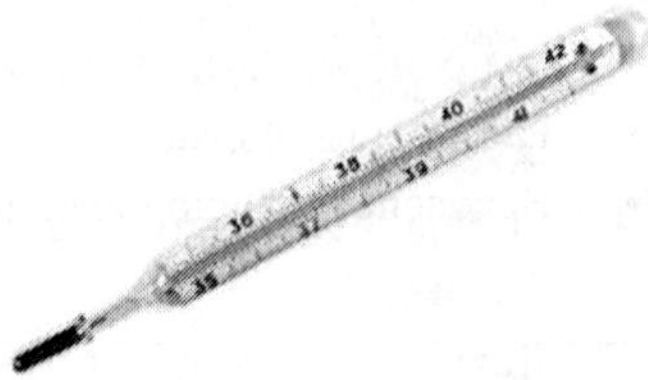

- Maintain personal hygiene like frequent hand washing and daily bathing
- Do not eat raw foods until one completes chemotherapy and blood counts have returned to adequate levels. Raw foods may carry bacteria that can lead to infection. Make sure to thoroughly wash any fruits and vegetables.
- Take a warm (not hot) bath, shower, or sponge bath every day. Pat skin dry using a light touch. Do not rub.
- Stay away from crowded places.
- Avoid sharing utensils and eating at public places

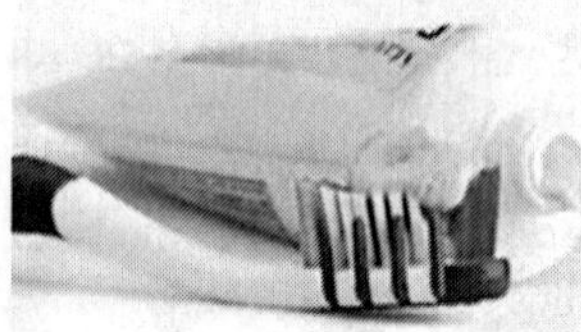

- Clean any cuts or wounds right away with suitable antiseptic
- Do not get any immunization shots (vaccines) without first checking with doctor.
- Clean rectal area very well but gently after each bowel movement. Ask doctor or nurse for advice if the area becomes sore or if hemorrhoids occur. Also, check with doctor before using enemas or suppositories.
- Carry out good mouth care practices.
- Periodically check the colour of urine for any Urinary tract infections.

In anemia one may have the following symptoms

Mild anemia

- Shortness of breath on exertion
- Weakness and/or fatigue

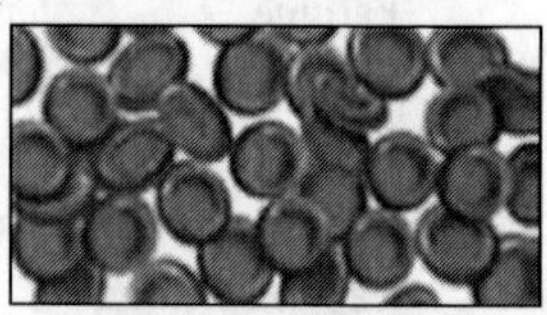

Normal RBC Count

Severe anemia

- Shortness of breath that interferes with normal daily activities like walking short distances
- Dizziness
- Pale color of skin
- Profound weakness/fatigue
- Palpitations of heart
- Headache or ringing in ears

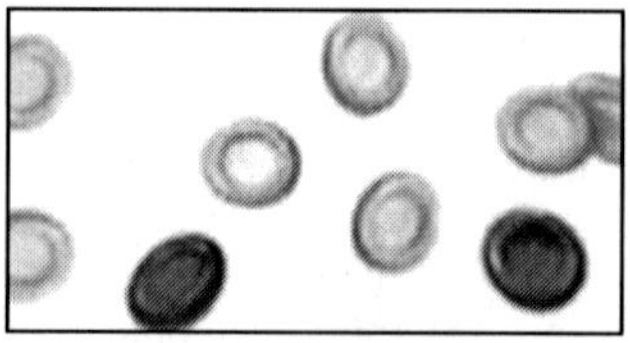

RBC Count in anemia

Key points regarding anemia:

- Rest frequently
- Eat high protein and high carbohydrate balanced diet
- Avoid strenuous activities
- Take an iron supplement as recommended by your doctor
- Eat iron rich fruits like pomegranates, carrots, spinach and green leafy vegetables.

5. Infertility: Some types of chemotherapy can cause infertility. For a woman, this means that one may not be able to get pregnant. In women, chemotherapy may damage the ovaries. This damage can lower the number of healthy eggs in the ovaries. It can also lower the hormones produced by them. The drop in hormones can lead to early menopause. Early menopause and fewer healthy eggs can cause infertility. Whether or not one becomes infertile depends on the type of chemotherapy, age, and other health problems. Infertility can last the rest of the life.

Talk with doctor or nurse about:

- Whether one wants to have children.
- Birth control: It is very important to not get pregnant while getting chemotherapy. These drugs can hurt the fetus, especially in the first 3 months of pregnancy. Talk with doctor or nurse about birth control and ways to keep from getting pregnant.

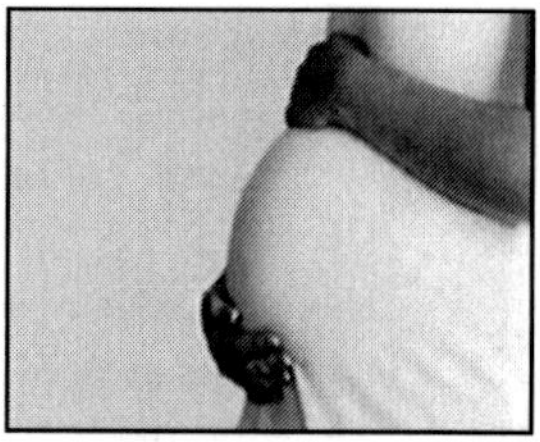

- Pregnancy: If one still has menstrual periods, doctor or nurse may ask to have a pregnancy test before starting chemotherapy. If found pregnant, doctor or nurse will talk with about other treatment options.

6. Sexual changes: Some types of chemotherapy and radiotherapy can cause sexual changes. These changes are different for women and men. In women, chemotherapy may damage the ovaries, which can cause changes in hormone levels. Hormone changes can lead to problems like vaginal dryness and early menopause. Most problems, such as loss of interest in sex, are likely to improve once treatment is over. But if undergone radiotherapy fertility changes may persist for rest of life. If one conceives after radiotherapy the fact that one had this treatment should not affect the health of the baby.

Problems for WOMEN include:

- Symptoms of menopause (for women not yet in menopause). These symptoms include:
    - Hot flashes
    - Vaginal dryness
    - Feeling irritable
    - Irregular or no menstrual periods
- Bladder or vaginal infections
- Vaginal discharge or itching
- Being too tired to have sex or not being interested in having sex
- Feeling too worried, stressed, or depressed to have sex

Radiation therapy to the pelvic area may additionally cause:

- Vaginal dryness, burning, itching or atrophy (vaginal muscles become weak and vaginal walls become thin)
- Vaginal stenosis (vagina becomes narrower, less elastic and may get shorter)
- Pain or discomfort on having sex
- Loss of fertility which means never being able to have children

Key points:

- Eat soy products to reduce hot flushes.
- Your doctor may recommend certain medications for hot flushes.
- Wear light cotton pyjamas to help prevent overheating when sleeping.
- Use vaginal moisturizers on a regular basis or other water-based lubricants as needed, especially during and before sexual activity. These products will help with vaginal dryness and irritation.
- Reducing stress- Try yoga, meditation, or other ways to relax.

Talk to your doctor about:

- Sex: Ask your doctor or nurse if it is okay for you to have sex during treatment. Most women can have sex, but it is a good idea to ask.

- Birth control: It is very important that you not get pregnant while having treatment for cancer. Both chemotherapy and radiotherapy may hurt the fetus, especially in the first 3 months of pregnancy. If you have not yet gone through menopause, talk with your doctor or nurse about birth control and ways to keep from getting pregnant.
- Medications: Talk with your doctor, nurse, or pharmacist about medications that help with sexual problems. These include products to relieve vaginal dryness or a vaginal cream or suppository to reduce the chance of infection.
- Stretching your vagina: Vaginal stenosis can make sex painful. You can help by stretching your vagina using a vaginal dilator which gently stretches the tissues of vagina. Ask your doctor where to find a dilator and how to use it.
- Muscle weakness: You can help strengthen muscles in your genital area by doing Kegel exercises.

7. Constipation: Constipation is when bowel movements become less frequent and stools are hard, dry and difficult to pass. One may pass a lot of gas, have abdominal cramps or feel pressure in the rectal area. Some people become constipated from chemotherapy. Others may become constipated because they are less active, eat less than usual, have diet changes, or because they are taking certain pain medicines. Consult the doctor, if one has not had a bowel movement in 2 or more days. Take a laxative or stool softener, after consulting the doctor, especially if the white blood cell count or platelet count is low.

Key points for constipation:

- Drink at least ten to twelve glasses of fluid a day.
- Stay as active as you can. Consistent regular exercise can reduce constipation. Walking, cycling and regular yoga can help ease constipation.

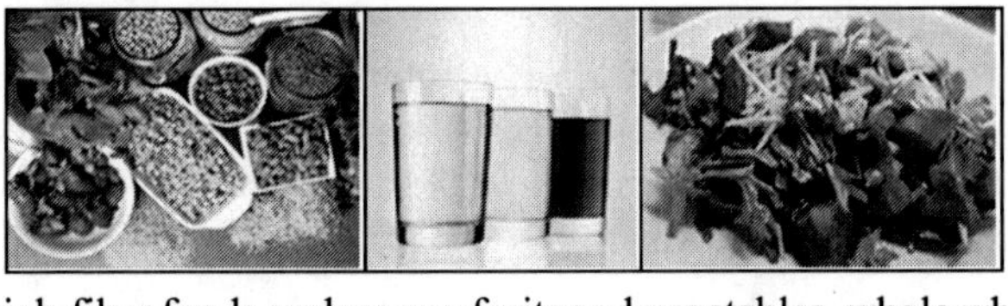

- Eat high-fiber foods such as raw fruits and vegetables, whole wheat breads and cereals and cooked dried beans and peas.
- Eat lot of salads before meals.
- Let your doctor know if you have not had a bowel movement for three or more days.
- Take a stool softener after consulting your doctor.

8. Diarrhoea: It refers to frequent bowel movements, which may be loose, watery or soft. Some chemotherapy drugs can cause diarrhoea. It can also occur any time while undergoing radiotherapy to the pelvis, stomach and abdomen. If one has more than three or four watery stools in 24 hours or blood in your stool, consult the doctor. Do not use over the counter anti-diarrhoea medications unless advised to do so by the doctor.

Key points for diarrhoea:

- To replenish lost fluids, drink eight to ten glasses of clear liquids per day like water, lemonade, soups, fruit juices etc.
- Eat small meals and snacks.

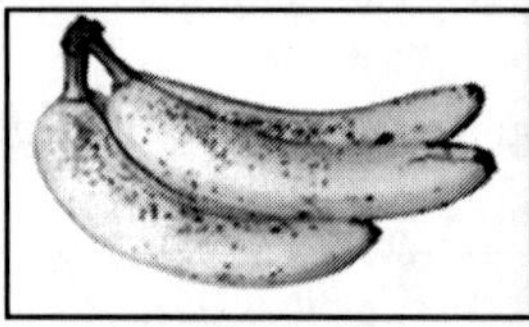
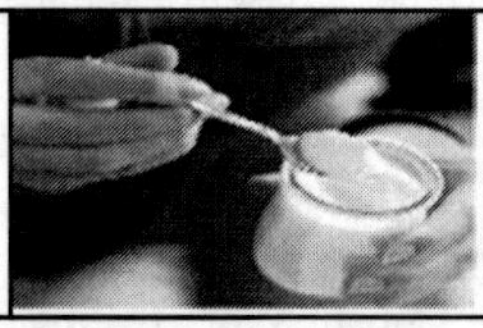
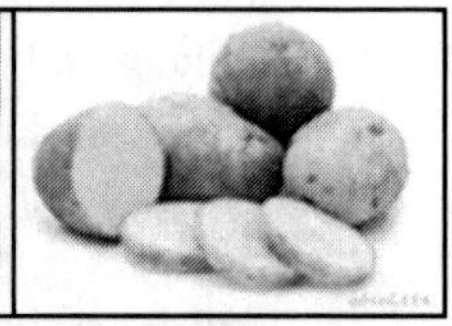

- Avoid hot, spicy, fatty, greasy, fried foods, foods from restaurants, caffeinated foods and drinks, high fibre foods as raw fruits and vegetables, whole cereals.
- Avoid milk and milk products if they make your diarrhoea worse.
- Eat foods high in salts as sodium and potassium. These include bananas, oranges, peaches, and apricot, boiled or mashed potatoes.
- Eat low fiber foods like bananas, white rice, yoghurt, white bread, mashed potatoes, and cooked refined cereals.
- Take care of your rectal area. If your rectum is sore, use baby wipe to clean.
- You can ask your doctor about taking sitz bath which is a warm water bath taken in a sitting position that covers only hips and buttocks.

9. Neuropathy: Certain chemotherapy drugs can cause peripheral neuropathy, a nerve problem that causes tingling, pins and needles, burning sensations, weakness, numbness in the hands and feet. One may feel any of these nerve-related symptoms:

- Tingling, burning, numbness or weakness in hands and feet
- Trouble picking up things
- Shaking or trembling
- Problems in walking
- Jaw pain
- Hearing loss

- Loss of balance
- Fatigue
- Confusion and memory problems
- Dizziness
- Vision changes etc.

Along with affecting the nerves, certain chemotherapy drugs can also affect the muscles and make them weak, tired or sore. Effects on the nerves and muscles are frustrating, yet in most cases they are not serious if caught early. Many problems get over within a year of completing chemotherapy but some may last for the rest of the life. Therefore it is important to tell the doctor about any nerve or muscle symptoms right away. They can get worse and become quite painful if left untreated. Consult doctor for specific treatments for this condition.

Key points for Neuropathy:

- Tight shoes and socks can worsen pain and tingling and may lead to sores that will not heal. Wear soft, loose cotton socks and padded shoes.
- Wear sneakers, sport shoes or shoes with rubber soles
- If you have burning pain, cool your feet or hands in cold, but not icy, water for 15 minutes twice a day.
- Massage your hands and feet or have someone massage them for you, to improve circulation, stimulate nerves and temporarily relieve pain.
- If your fingers become numb, be very careful when handling objects that are sharp, hot or otherwise dangerous like knives, scissors etc.
- Be extra careful while working in kitchen. You can wear gloves while washing utensils, cooking or gardening
- Steady yourself while walking by using a cane
- If your sense of balance is affected, move carefully, use handrails on stairs and use a bath mat in the tub or shower.

Pain: Pain can be caused by the cancer itself or by chemotherapy. These include burning, numbness, and tingling or shooting pains in the hands and feet. Mouth sores, headaches, muscle pains, and stomach pains can also occur.

10. Key points regarding pain

- Talk about pain with the doctor. Be specific and describe: where one feels pain, what the pain feels like (sharp, dull, or throbbing), does it come and go, or is it steady, how long the pain lasts etc.
- Lets your family and friends know about the pain.
- Practice pain control.
- Take pain medicine on a regular schedule (by the clock) even if not in pain. Do not skip doses of pain medicine.
- Try deep breathing, yoga, or other ways to relax. This can help reduce muscle tension, anxiety and pain.
- Meet with a pain or palliative care specialist.
- Let doctor, nurse, or pain specialist know if pain changes.

11. Appetite changes: Chemotherapy can cause appetite changes. Do not worry if not feeling hungry in the first few days or a week following chemotherapy; it is not unusual. One may lose appetite because of nausea (feeling like to throw up), mouth and throat problems that make it painful to eat, or drugs that cause taste changes. The changes can also come from feeling depressed or tired. Appetite loss may last for a day, a few weeks, or even months. Radiotherapy to the head and neck region may also cause appetite changes. Some cancer treatments cause weight gain or an increase in appetite.

Key points for appetite changes

- Eat 5 to 6 small meals or snacks each day instead of 3 big meals
- Drink milkshakes, smoothies, juice, or soup if one does not feel like eating solid foods
- Eat foods that are warm rather than hot
- Use plastic forks and spoons. Some types of chemotherapy give a metal taste in the mouth. Eating with plastic can help decrease the metal taste.
- Increase appetite by doing different activities like walking, cycling etc.
- Plan ahead - plan a daily menu in advance
- Make every bite count - choose high calorie and protein foods
- Pack snacks and keep them handy at all times
- Strive to eat at least 1/3 of calorie and protein needs at breakfast
- Do not be afraid to try something new, this might spark appetite
- Be sure to follow good mouth care practices

- After chemotherapy treatments, soft foods may improve swallowing problems
- Chew solid foods thoroughly
- Eat what appeals to one during this time
- Drink enough fluids i.e., 10 - 12 glasses per day and more if having fever or diarrhea
- Mix ½ teaspoon of salt or baking soda with a glass of water and rinse mouth 4-5 times daily or more often with this solution
- Eat with friends or family members. When eating alone, listen to the radio or watch TV
- Vary diet and try new foods and recipes

12. Mouth changes: Chemotherapy works by killing rapidly growing cells. The cells lining the oral cavity are fast growing cells and can be damaged by chemotherapy. The common problems seen with therapy:

- Mouth sores
- Dry mouth
- Tooth decay
- Infections of gums, teeth or tongue
- Jaw stiffness/ Bone changes
- Taste changes

These problems may go away when the treatment ends. Some problems like dry mouth may improve but never go away.

For dry mouth:

- Drink plenty of liquids
- Sip water often during the day
- Moisten dry foods with butter, gravy or sauces etc.
- Suck ice cubes or sugarless hard candy
- Eat soft foods
- Use lip balm if your lips become dry

For tooth decay:

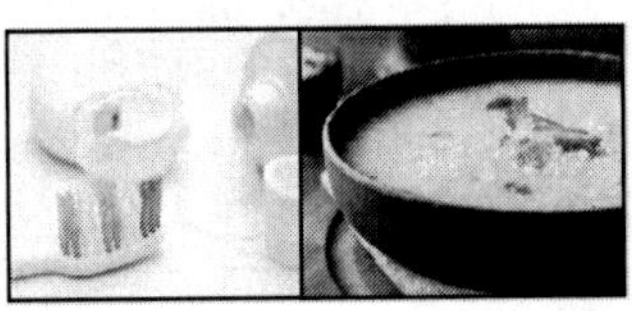

- Drink plenty of water
- Brush your teeth with a soft toothbrush three times daily
- Avoid sugary foods
- Use fluoride toothpaste
- If you wear dentures then make sure they are well fitting. Limit the time you wear the dentures. Also keep your dentures clean by brushing or soaking them every day.

For mouth sores:

- Rinse your mouth with a solution of one teaspoon baking soda and one teaspoon of salt, diluted in a glass of lukewarm water, three or four times daily.
- Turmeric based mouthwashes can be helpful.
- Avoid mouthwashes that contain alcohol.
- Avoid citrus and tomato based products.
- Eat soft, soothing foods, like ice cream, yoghurt, milk shakes, soft fruits (like bananas), mashed potatoes, cooked cereals, soft-boiled or scrambled eggs, paneer, macaroni, cheese, custards, puddings etc.
- Avoid food with sharp edges like chips and popcorns that could possibly scratch or cut the gums or inner lining of the mouth
- Avoid using toothpick and other sharp objects
- Avoid hot foods, tobacco and alcoholic drinks

13. Throat changes: Lining of throat may get sore or swollen in some cases. This problem is called esophagitis. Burning in your or chest may occur. Throat changes occur two to three weeks after starting radiation therapy. These symptoms go away four to six weeks after the therapy is over

Key points for throat changes:

- Eat small meals and snacks
  - Choose easy to swallow foods
  - Cut, blend or shred food items
  - Drink cool drinks
- Eat food with gravy, yoghurt, sauce or other liquids
- Eat high calories and high protein diet
- Avoid food items that can scrape or burn your throat
  - Hot foods/drinks Spicy foods
  - Sharp and crunchy foods as chips
  - Alcoholic drinks
  - Acidic fruits and juices like tomato and oranges

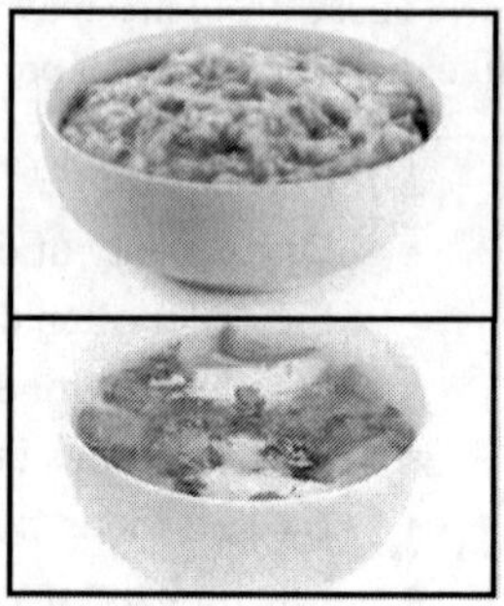

Consult with doctor if you choking, trouble swallowing or excessive coughing occurs.

14. Skin changes: When given through an intravenous (IV) drip, certain chemotherapy drugs may darken your skin along the vein. This discoloration usually fades over time after the treatment ends. Radiation therapy may also cause skin changes in the treatment area. The common skin problems associated with cancer therapy are:

- Redness in the treatment area
- Dry and peeling skin: Skin may become dry and start peeling. It may peel faster leading to sores and ulcers.
- Dry lips
- Severe itching: Skin in the treatment area may itch badly. It is very important that to avoid scratching as it may worsen the situation.

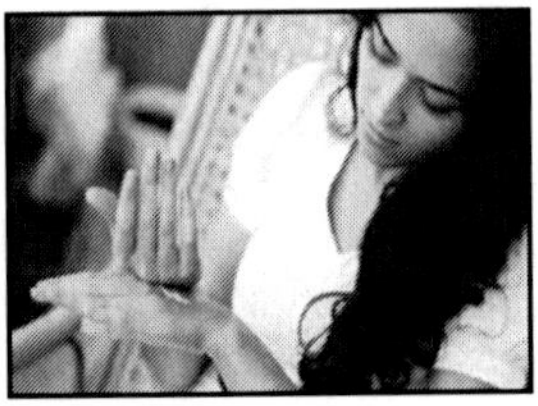

- Moist reaction: The skin may become wet, sore and infected. It usually occurs where skin has folds like behind the ears, buttocks, neck and under the breasts.
- Rashes and acne: Some chemo drugs may cause rashes and acne

Skin changes may start after a weeks of treatment. These problems usually fade away with time but some problems may persist forever. The skin in the treatment area may always look darker and blotchy. Also it may remain sensitive to the sun. Therefore one needs to take special care of skin for rest of the life.

Key points skin changes:

- Do not rub, scrub or scratch your skin in the treatment area. Use creams as suggested by your doctor.
- Do not apply anything too hot or cold on your skin.
- To help avoid dryness, take quick, warm showers rather than long, hot baths.
- Use mils soaps and do not soak in for too long.
- Apply creams or lotions after bathing, while your skin is still moist.
- Do not use perfume or deodorants. These products often contain alcohol, which can make your skin dry.
- Consult your doctor before using make up, sunscreen, hair removers, pre shave liquid, oil and other ointments.
- If you develop acne, try to keep your face clean and dry.
- Wear clothes and use bed sheets of soft fabrics only.
- Do not wear tight clothes in your treatment area like body shapers and panty hoses.
- Inspect the irradiated area daily and if you find any redness consult doctor immediately.

- Do not peel the dry lips. Apply any type of grease like Vaseline, oil, ghee, glycerin etc.
- Protect your skin from sun. Avoid going to beaches or sunbathing. Also try to cover your body fully when you need to go in the sun. You may need to protect your skin from sun even after the treatment is over.

15. Urinary and Bladder changes: Radiation therapy to the urinary and bladder area may damage the healthy cells of the urinary tract which can cause swelling, ulcers and infection. This is common with cervical cancer patients. These symptoms start three to five weeks after beginning of treatment and go away two to eight weeks after treatment is over. The symptoms include:

- Frequent, urgent need to urinate
- Cystitis, a swelling in the urinary tract
- Urinary incontinence i.e. when one cannot control urine especially while sneezing or coughing
- Trouble starting to urinate
- Trouble emptying bladder completely
- Blood in urine

Key points for Urinary and Bladder changes:

- Drink lots of fluids (3-4L water daily)
- Avoid coffee, black tea, alcohol, spicy food and tobacco products
- Take care of yourperinealarea .Keep it clean and dry.
- Wear cotton undergarments and change 2-3 times a day.

Talk to your doctor if you have incontinence. You may be referred to a physical therapist who can teach you exercise for bladder control

16. Fecal Incontinence: This might occur in advanced stages of the disease. It is frequent bowel movements sometimes immediately after having food. Local attention to hygiene and skincare is important to prevent any infections.

Key points for fecal incontinence

- Dietary changes
  - o Consult the doctor for diet modifications
- Wear a sanitary pad/brief
- Maintain perineal hygiene
- A physical therapist may advice exercises to strengthen sphincter muscles

17. Lower leg lymphedema: This is a common in late stage cervical cancer owing to low lymphatic blockage.Care focuses on reducing the swelling and controlling the pain.

Key points for lower leg lymphedema

Raising the leg

- Keep the leg raised by placing pillow below the feet

Exercises

- Light exercises in which you move your affected limb may encourage lymph fluid drainage and help prepare you for everyday tasks, such as carrying groceries.
- Exercises shouldn't be strenuous
- Focus on gentle contraction of the muscles in leg.

Wrapping the leg

- Bandaging the entire limb encourages lymph fluid to flow back toward the trunk.
- The bandage should be tightest around toes and loosen as it moves up your arm or leg.
- A lymphedema therapist can show you how to wrap limb.

Massage

- A special massage technique called manual lymph drainage may encourage the flow of lymph fluid out of the leg.
- Massage isn't for everyone.
- Avoid massage if you have a skin infection or blood clots.

Compression garments

- Long stockings made to compress the leg encourage the flow of the lymph fluid out of the affected limb.
- Wear a compression garment when exercising the affected limb.
- Obtain a correct fit for your compression garment by getting professional help.

Ask the doctor where you can buy compression garments.

Coping - During and after therapy

Cancer patients and their family caregivers face many diverse problems. Some such case studies are described here.

Case 1:

A 48 year old Ca Cervix patien.

"Ab pehle ki tarah kaam bhi ni kiya jaata…bacchon ka dhyan bhi ni rakha jaata….akelapan mehsoos hota he…bahar jaane ka mann nahi karta…darr lagta he…. neend bhi kam aati he…" Doctors ki salah se maine yoga aur meditation shuru ki. Ab farak he. Mann bi shaant rehta hai. ("Now I can't work like before. I am unable to look after kids…feel lonely…don't feel like going out….always feel afraid and sleep less…" I started on yoga and meditation as advised by doctors. It helped. I feel calm.)

Case 2:

Another 48 year old Ca cervix patient was accompanied by her daughter.

"Kisi se baat karne ka mann nahi karta…bachon ki chinta rehti hai…Baghwan ke upar chhod diya he…jo hua he bhagwan hi dekhega…" (" Don't feel like talking to anyone…always worry about kids…have left everything to God…He will look after…")

Caregiver (daughter)…."Hamare saath hi aisa kyon hua…Muje poora din kaam karna padta he…"(" Why did it Happen to us…I have to work all day…)

Doctors ne hume samjhaya and counselling ki. Usse bahut fark pada he. Mann se darr nikal gaya he. (Doctor counseled us. It helped us a lot. It dispelled all fears from within.)

Case 3:

A 66 yr old, Ca cervix patient

"Poora din dard rehta he…bahut darr lag ra he bimari ka….Bhookh hi nai lagti….1 roti bhi ni kha pati …..kamzori rehti hai…Logon se milne ka mann bhi nai karta…" Doctors ki salah se maine khane peene mai badlav kiya. Daily routine bhi change ki. Meditation bhi karti hun. Ab farak lag raha he. Khana ache se kha paati hun. Active feel hota he.

(" Feel Pain all day…Very much afraid of the disease… Don't feel like eating anything can't even take 1 chapati…feel weak…not in mood to meet people" On doctors advice I changed my diet. Also made changes in routine life. I also meditate. Now I feel better. I am able to eat well and feel active.)

Case 4:

A 55 year old, Ca cervix patient was accompanied by her daughter in law.

"Kamzori Lagti he. Ulti aane jaisa hota he….khana khane ka mann nahi karta….Shareer mai dard bhi hota he….Pata nahi ilaj kaise ho ga….paise bhi nahi hain…rehne ke liye jagah bhi nahi he….”Doctors ne khane peene ke parhez bataye . Counselling ki. Ab kamzori nai rehti aur ulti bhi nai aati. Ab dard mai bhi fark he. Doctors ne ilaj ke bare mai samjhaya. Ab confusion door hua he. (“ Feel weak. I remain nauseated. ..Don’t feel like taking meals… Full day I feel aches… Don’t know how treatment will be completed… We have no money… no place to stay…” Doctors told what to eat and what not to eat. They counseled us. Now I don’t feel weak anymore. Nausea is also gone. Pain is also less. Doctors explained about the treatment regime. Now I am not confused anymore.)

Emotional Concerns

Living with cancer and undergoing treatment can be very stressful. You may encounter many feelings while undergoing treatment. These include worrying about potential loss of relationships, job changes, changes in the ability to carry out certain responsibilities in private and professional lives, and many others. It is common to feel overwhelmed with all the information given. It is not unusual to have concerns related to life and death.

Here is list of feelings that one may encounter and ways to manage them:

Overwhelmed

At first when a person learns that one has cancer, one may feel as if life is out of control. Even if one feels out of control, there are ways to manage it. Try to learn as much as one can about cancer. Ask questions to the doctor and don’t be afraid to say when not clear. Try to stay busy. Indulge in activities such as music, crafts, reading, or learning something new.

Denial

Denial is trouble believing or accepting the fact that one has cancer. Usually by the time treatment begins, most people accept the fact that they have cancer and move forward. This is true for those with cancer as well as the people they love and care about.

Anger

It is not unusual to feel angry. The feeling of, “Why me?” and anger at the cancer is common. Anger or resentment towards doctor, friends and family may also occur. And if one is religious, one may even feel angry with God. Talk with family and friends. Or, ask the doctor to refer one to a counselor.

Fear and Worry

These are common in cancer patients. One may be afraid or worried about:

- Being in pain, either from the cancer or the treatment
- Feeling sick or looking different as a result of treatment

- Family and job
- Dying

Some fears about cancer are based on wrong information. To cope with fears and worries, one need to get informed. Learn about cancer and understand what one can do to be an active partner in care.

Hope

There are many reasons to feel hopeful. Millions of people who have had cancer are alive today. There are many success stories of people who have fought against cancer and lead a healthy life. And people with cancer can lead active lives, even during treatment. Here are some ways to build hope:

- Plan the days.
- Don't limit the things one like to do just because of cancer.
- Spend time in nature viz. take a walk, go to lakeside etc.
- Listen or read success stories (Refer chapter 9).

Stress and Anxiety

Both during and after treatment, it's normal to have stress over the life changes one is going through. Anxiety means one has extra worry, can't relax, and feel tense. Talk to doctor if such feelings develop.. Though they are common signs of stress, confirm they aren't due to medicines.

Sadness and Depression

Many people with cancer feel sad. One has little energy, feel tired, or not want to eat. These feelings may go away or lessen with time. If these do not get better it may lead to a medical condition called depression. Below are common signs of depression. If any of the following signs remain for more than 2 weeks, talk to doctor about treatment.

Emotional signs

- Feelings of sadness that don't go away
- Feeling emotionally numb
- Feeling nervous or shaky
- Having a sense of guilt or feeling unworthy
- Crying for long periods of time or many times each day
- Focusing on worries and problems
- No interest in the hobbies and activities one used to enjoy
- Feeling helpless or hopeless, as if life has no meaning
- Feeling short-tempered, moody
- Difficulty concentrating

- Finding it hard to enjoy everyday things, such as food or being with family and friends
- Thinking about hurting/killing one self

Body changes:

Unintended weight gain or loss not due to illness or treatment

Fatigue that doesn't go away

Recurrent headaches, other aches and pains

Sleep problems, such as not being able to sleep, having nightmares, or sleeping too much Racing heart, dry mouth, increased perspiration, upset stomach, diarrhea

If the doctor thinks that one is suffering from depression, medicines are given or one is refered to other experts. Don't feel that one should have to control these feelings on own. Getting the help is important for life and health.

Guilt

If feeling guilty, know that many people with cancer feel this way. One may blame oneself for upsetting the people, or worry that one is a burden in some way.These feelings are all very common. Share them with someone. Let the doctor know if one would like to talk with a counselor or go to a support group.

Loneliness

People with cancer often feel lonely or distant from others. Look for emotional support in different ways. Talk to other people who have cancer or join a support group. Or, one may feel better talking only to a close friend or family member, or counselor, or a member of one's faith or community. Do what feels right.

Gratitude

Some people see their cancer as a "wake-up call." They start enjoying the little things in life. They go to places they've never been, finish pending projects, spend more time with friends and family and more. Pay attention to the things that make one happy. They can be as simple as drinking a good cup of coffee or talking to a friend.

Ways to cope with emotions

During treatment:

- Write down questions that come to mind and prioritize them. Record the answers once received.

- Bring a family member or a friend to appointments to help remembering the information.
- Take one step at a time, focusing on one issue at a time. Looking down the road into the future can often seem overwhelming, but broken down into smaller pieces it can be easier to handle.

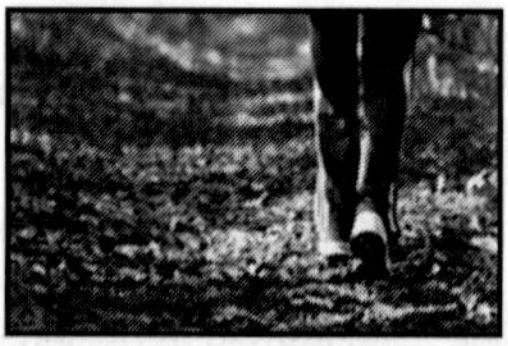

- Allow friends and family members to assist one in completing tasks that need to be done, i.e. cutting the lawn, doing laundry, getting groceries.
- Give one self permission to get what one need. For example, if one do or do not want people visiting, make it clear when and how often.
- If one is not feeling to go to a family get together, it is okay to limit time spent at an event or to not go.

After treatment

Living with cancer and going through treatment can be very stressful. It is normal to feel anxious, depressed, afraid, angry, frustrated, helpless, or alone at some point during radiation therapy. But there are ways one can learn to cope with these feelings.

- Many people find it helpful to talk with others who are going through the same thing. To meet others, think about joining support group. These groups meet in-person and online. Try yoga, relaxation or meditation exercises. Some people find prayer helpful.

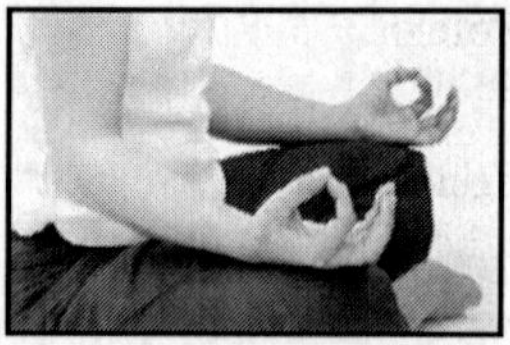

- Exercise can also boost mood. Try activities such as walking, yoga, or aerobics. Check with doctor or nurse about types of exercise that one can safely do during treatment.
- Join a support group (could be even on internet/Facebook) Cancer support groups are meetings for people with cancer. These groups allow meeting others facing the same problems. One will have a chance to talk about feelings and listen to other people and can learn how others cope with cancer, treatment and side effects. It helps immensely when one talks to people who understand what one is going through.

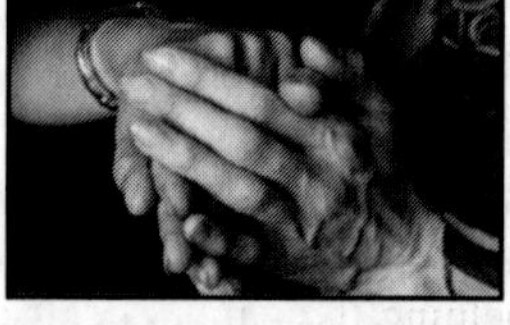

- Use distraction strategies to overcome stress and fatigue e.g. guided imagery, diverted therapy, reading, meditation, prayer, listening to music, painting, recreational activities etc.

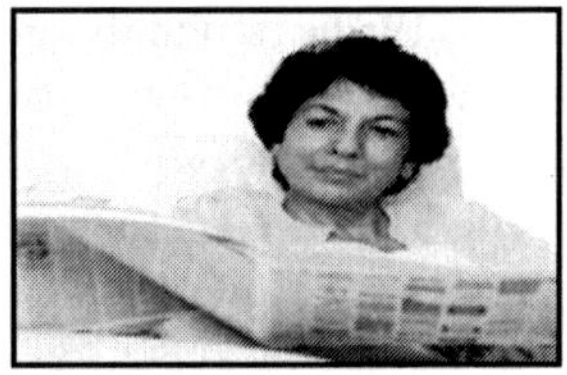

- Improve socialization with near and dear ones. Talk about feelings with some trusted person. One may choose a close friend, family member, nurse, social worker or psychologist. After treatment is completed, it is common to be uncertain about the future. Many women experience increased awareness of body sensations and may have fear related to follow-up appointments and exams. Transition back into the role of being well is often difficult, and family and friends may have different expectations than the patient herself. It is important to be frank when communicating needs to people around.

Fear of cancer recurrence is also common. Patients and family members may cope differently. It is also not uncommon to become uneasy when treatment ends and one is no longer seen by health care team as frequently.

Patients will continue seeing or talking with health care professionals after treatment is complete. Social workers support individuals while undergoing treatment and will often continue to do so after active treatment is completed. Counseling is available with professionals who specialize in the care of patients who are under treatment for cancer.

Role of Family

Love, care and support from the family is very important for a women fighting cervical cancer. Many cancer patients today receive part of their care at home. Hospital stays

> Family caregivers may be spouses, partners, children, relatives, or friends who help the patient with daily activities and health care needs at home.

have become shorter. These patients need to be cared for at home as much as possible. Cancer survivors may not be able to do things as they did earlier and need time to recover. Family caregivers are expected to help them in daily chores.

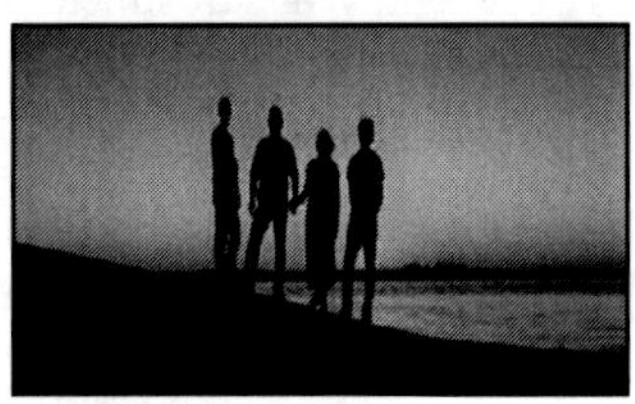

Caregiving also includes giving emotional and spiritualsupport, such as helping the patient deal with feelings and making hard decisions.

When treatment ends, families are often unprepared for the fact that recovery takes time. In general, recovery will take much longer than treatment did. Survivors often say that they didn't realize how much time they needed to recover. This can lead to disappointment, worry, and frustration for everyone. Some survivors say they would not have been able to cope without the help and love of their family members. And even though treatment has ended, they still need a lot of support.

Changes for the Family

Cancer affects family and friends, not just the person with the disease. The people in life may also feel worried, angry, or afraid. Family members may be very supportive, or they may start acting differently towards the patient.

Adjusting to the new situation

When someone in family has cancer, daily routines may change for everyone. Schedules may be focused around treatment. Caregivers may need to take time off from work to drive patient to treatment sessions.

Changing Roles

When someone has cancer, everyone in the family has to take on new roles and responsibilities. A child may have to do more chores, or a spouse may have to help shop or cook.

Money

Most people find it stressful to keep up with money matters. Cancer can reduce the amount of money family has to spend or save. If one is not able to work, someone else in family may need to get a job.

Living Arrangements

People with cancer sometimes need to change where they live or whom they live with. Caregiver may need to move in with someone else to get the care the patient needs.

Sexuality and related issues

It is common for people to have problems with sex because of cancer and its treatment. When treatment is over, one may feel like having sex again, but it may take some time. Sexual problems can last longer than other side effects of cancer treatment. It's important to seek help in learning how to adapt to these changes.

Treatment-Related Problems

Depending on the stage of cancer one may have short-term or long-term problems with sex after treatment. These changes result from chemotherapy, radiation, surgery, or certain medicines. Sexual function may be affected by several aspects of cancer care, including healing from surgery, vaginal dryness or other hormone affects, discomfort, changes in self-image, and the concerns of partner. Sometimes emotional issues such as anxiety, depression, worry, and stress may cause problems with sex.

Common concerns are:

- Worries about intimacy after treatment: Some may struggle with their body image after treatment. One may feel less attractive than before. Even thinking about being seen without clothes may be stressful. One may worry that having sex will hurt.
- Not being able to have sex as before: Some treatments may cause changes in vagina that also change your sex life. After cancer treatment, some women find it harder, or even painful, to have sex. Some women also have pain or numbness in their genital area.
- Having menopause symptoms: When women stop getting their periods, they can get hot flashes, dryness or tightness in the vagina, and/or other problems that can affect their desire to have sex.
- Losing the ability to have children. Some treatments can cause infertility, making it impossible for cancer survivors to have children. But keep in mind that:
    - o Depending on age, the type of treatment, and the length of time since treatment, one may still be able to have children.
    - o Families can come together in many ways. Some people choose adoption or surrogacy. Some people get involved in the lives of nieces or nephews, or in child mentoring programs.

Ways to Cope

Ask for Help

Even though one may feel awkward, let your doctor or nurse know if having problems with intimacy or sex. Some people also find it helpful to talk with other couples. Some solutions are:

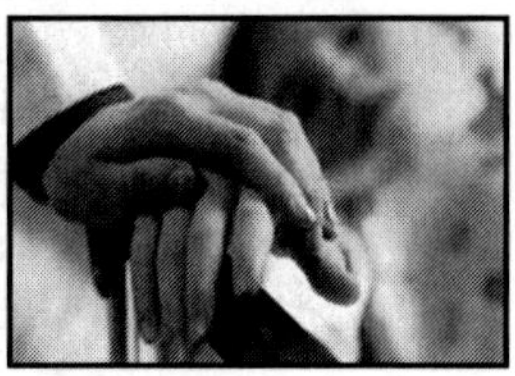

- **Talking with a counselor:** Some people find that sexual problems related to cancer start to strain their relationship with their partner. Talking to a counsellor alone, or with partner, may help.
- **Seeing a specialist:** A sex therapist may be able to help talk openly about one's problems, work through concerns, and come up with new ways to help.

Sharing with the partner

Talking to loved ones and sharing feelings and concerns is very important. Even for a couple that has been together a long time, it can be hard to stay connected.Let the partner know if one wants to have sex or not. The partner may be worried about hurting one or think that one is not feeling well. Talk with partner about any concerns one may have about sex life. Be open about feelings and stay positive to avoid blame.

Finding Ways to Be Intimate

One can still have an intimate relationship in spite of cancer. Intimacy is not just physical. It also involves feelings. Here are some ways to improve intimacy in a relationship:

- Focus on just talking and renewing connection.
- Find time together. Turn off the phone and TV. Ask someone to take care of the kids for a few hours.
- Try to be together without being physical. For example, one may want to listen to music, go for a movie or take a walk.
- Cancer treatment or surgery can change the body. Areas where touch used to feel good may now be numb or painful. Some of these changes will go away. Some will stay. Figure out together what kinds of touch feel good, such as holding, hugging, and cuddling.

Feeling Intimate after Treatment

Feeling close to partner is important. You can try the following:

- Being proud of the body
- Think of things that help one feel more attractive and confident
- Try to be positive and aware of thoughts
- Be open to change. One may find new ways to enjoy intimacy

Talking With Health Care Team

Prepare the visit by making a list of questions. Consider adding these questions to the list:

- Sexual and Sexuality-Related Questions
- What problems or changes I might have during treatment?
- How long will these problems last? Will any be permanent?
- Is there any treatment for these problems?

Fertility-Related Questions

- Will my fertility be affected by the treatment I receive?
- What are all of my options now if I would like to have children in the future?
- After treatment, how long should I use birth control?

Organizations providing financial assistance to cancer patients

Sahayta Charitable Welfare Society	Sahayata Cancer Kendra Sector 15/B, Chandigarh Website: www.cancersahayata.com
Can Support	Address: Kanak Durga Basti Vikash Kendra, Sec-12, R K Puram, New Delhi-110066 Tel:011-26102851/2859/2869 E-mail: cansup.india@hotmail.com Website: www.cansupport.org
Cancer Sahyog	Address: Q5A Jangpura Extension, New Delhi-110014 Contact: 011-24319572/4907 E-mail: incansocindia@vsnl.net.in
Cancer Patients Aid Association	Address: King Geoge V Memorial, Dr E. Moses Road, Mahalakshmi, Mumbai-400011 Email: webmaster@cpaaindia.org Web: www.cpaaindia.org
Karuna Care Foundation	Address: B/705. Ganesh Plaza. (opp. Navrangpura Bus Stop) Ahemdabad- 380009 Email: karunakare@hotmail.com
Care India Medical Society	Address: 4 / 22 Veer Bharat Society Bhavani Peth, Pune 411002 Tel: 020-26441808 Email: careindiamedicalsociety@gmail.com

Some cancer support groups in India

Global cancer concern India **www.globalcancer.org**

Courage India **www.courageindia.org**

Dream foundation **www.dreamfoundationcancercare.org**

Indian Cancer Society **brics@vsnl.com**

Cancer patients Aid Association **www.cpaaindia.org**

Can support **www.cansupport.org**

Some cancer support groups in Chandigarh

Sahayata **www.sahayta.org**

Tips to meet doctor or nurse

- Make a list of questions before each appointment

  Write down new questions every time meetingwith the doctor. Make sure to have space on this list so as to write down the answers from doctor or nurse.
- Ask all the doubts

- Bring a family member or friend along

  This will help in understanding what the doctor or nurse says. It will also help in reducing care giver anxiety and stress.
- Ask for printed information about type of cancer and chemotherapy Let doctor or nurse know how much information is needed Some people want to learn everything they can about cancer and its treatment. Others only want a little information.

Find out how to contact doctor or nurse in an emergency

This includes where to go and whom to call. Write all the important phone numbers in the spaces provided on the inside front cover of this book.

Questions to ask your doctor

Here is a list of questions you may want to ask your doctor:

About cancer:

What cancer do I have?

What is the stage of my cancer? How serious is my cancer?

What are the chances of my survival?

What are the chances that my cancer will come back?

About treatment:

Which treatments can I get?

Why do I need radiotherapy or chemotherapy or both? What is the goal of my treatment?

What are the benefits of therapy? What are the risks of therapy?

Are there any other ways to treat my type of cancer? What is the standard care for my type of cancer?

Are there any researches for my type of cancer?

Why do I have to come even after my treatment is completed? Can I leave the therapy in between?

What additional help is available for patients like me?

About chemotherapy:

How many cycles of chemotherapy will I get? How long is each treatment?

What types of chemotherapy will I get? How will these drugs be given?

Where do I go for this treatment?

Should someone come along with me to treatment sessions?

How long does each treatment session last?

About radiotherapy:

How will radiotherapy be given?

How long each session lasts?

About side effects:

What are the immediate side effects?

What are the long term side effects?

How serious are these side effects?

Will all the side effects go away when treatment is over?

How long will these side effects last?

How can I manage or ease these side effects?

When should I call my doctor or nurse about these side effects?

Frequently Asked Questions

Is getting a Pap test painful?

No, it doesn't pain, but it sometimes feels less than comfortable. You may feel some different sensations or some pressure in your pelvic area. Taking deep breaths helps to relax all of your muscles. It helps to have an empty bladder before the exam so you're more comfortable.

Can I be around my family and friends while I am undergoing treatment?

Only a few treatments require you to avoid close contact with family and friends. If this is something you will have to do, your doctor will tell you about it. It is important that you:

- Stay away from anyone who is sick.
- Washing your hands often, especially before touching your face, nose, mouth or eyes.
- Ask your family and friends to do the same when they are with you.

How can I protect myself and those I live with while I am getting chemotherapy?

There are many things you can do during and after chemo to keep yourself and your loved ones from being affected by the drugs while your body is getting rid of them. It takes about 48 hours for your body to break down and get rid of most chemotherapy drugs. Most of the waste comes out from your body fluids in the form of urine, stool, tears and vomit. The drugs are also found in your blood. When these drugs get outside your body, they can harm or irritate your skin or even skin of other people around you. Remember these important points:

- Flush the toilet twice after you use it. If using western toilet, put the lid down before flushing to avoid splashing. If possible, you may use a separate toilet during this time.
- Always wash your hands with warm water and soap after using the toilet. Use paper towels to dry your hands and throw them away.

- If you vomit into the toilet, clean off all the splashes and flush twice. If you vomit into a bucket, carefully empty it into the toilet without splashing the contents and flush twice. Wash out the bucket with hot soapy water and rinse it. Empty the wash and rinse water into the toilet and then flush it. Dry the bucket with paper towels and throw them away.
- Caregivers should wear disposable gloves if they need to touch any of your body fluids. They should always wash their hands with warm water and soap afterward even if they had gloves on.
- If a caregiver does come in contact with any of your body fluids, they should wash the area very well with warm soap and water. It is not likely to cause any harm, but try to take extra care to avoid this.
- Any clothes or sheets that have body fluids on them should be washed in the washing machine not by the hand. Wash them twice in hot water with regular laundry detergent. Do not wash them with other clothes. If they cannot be washed right away, seal them in a plastic bag.
- If using throw-away adult diapers, underwear, or sanitary pads, seal them in a plastic bag and throw them away with your regular trash.

Will my hair fall out and when does that occur?

The degree of alopecia or hair loss is highly variable from person to person and also depends on which chemotherapy drugs are in use. Hair loss caused by chemotherapy may become apparent over a 2-3 week period. After discontinuing chemotherapy, initial regrowth maybe seen in 4-6 weeks. If you are treated with radiation therapy, you will probably lose pubic hair, but you will not lose the hair on your head. Hair loss caused by radiation is usually permanent.

If my blood counts drop from chemotherapy what will be done?

Depending on your symptoms, you may receive medications to increase your white or red blood cells. Other medications such as antibiotics may also be prescribed. Occasionally, blood transfusion maybe necessary. If blood counts are very low, future chemotherapy doses may need to be reduced.

Will I be able to maintain the same level of activity? Can I go to work?

Whether you can continue work and other activities depends on your treatment and how it affects you. For some treatments, you may need to stay in a hospital for a week or more, but many people are able to keep working during treatment. It is normal to feel tired for the first few weeks after surgery. You may also be fatigued while undergoing chemotherapy or radiation treatments. Pay attention to the clues your body gives you and rest as needed, maintaining activity as you are able. It is a good idea to discuss fatigue with your doctor or nurse. If chemotherapy makes you tired, try to adjust your work schedule for a while. You may be able to arrange a part-time schedule or work from home.

Should my diet be any different before chemotherapy?

Some people find that it may be helpful to eat foods that are more easily tolerated such as bland foods, soups and tea, while avoiding spicy or fatty foods.

Can I drive?

It is not a good idea to drive if you are taking pain medications or medications for nausea that would impair your ability to react quickly in driving situations. Ask your physician when the best time is to beg in driving again.

Does radiotherapy hurt?

No, radiation therapy does not hurt when it is being given. But there are some side effects which may occur after you are done with the treatment.

Is radiotherapy expensive?

Yes radiotherapy may cost you a lot of money. It uses complex machines and involves services of many health care providers. The exact cost depends on the where and what kind of treatment you are undergoing. To find organizations providing financial assistance you can log in **www.globalcancer.org**

What does it mean to be treated in a research hospital?

Although we have made great strides in the treatment of cancer, many types of cancer are not yet easily cured. Our goal of being able to cure cancer will depend on continued research resulting in new surgical techniques, chemotherapy drugs, and radiation techniques in the years to come. We hope that totally new technologies such as gene therapy and immunotherapy, in addition to better technology for early detection or prevention of cancers may lessen the impact of cancer on each and every one of us. Breakthroughs such as these begin in the laboratory and eventually progress to clinical trials. A clinical trial is a research study conducted with cancer patients to evaluate a new treatment: if a new treatment is demonstrated to be effective in clinical trials, it is then adopted as standard therapy for cancer patients. Participation in a clinical trial is voluntary. To find out if you maybe eligible for participation in a clinical trial, you should ask your physician.

Research is subject to rules and regulations established by the ICMR and PGIMER.

These rules are designed to protect the safety of patients and to ensure that research is of the highest quality. A patient enrolled in a clinical trial is not a "guinea pig", but is instead contributing generously to our ability to understand how to best treat cancer patient.

Some success stories- People who won against cancer

"I know God will not give me anything I can't handle….."

MOTHER TERESA

Yuvraj Singh

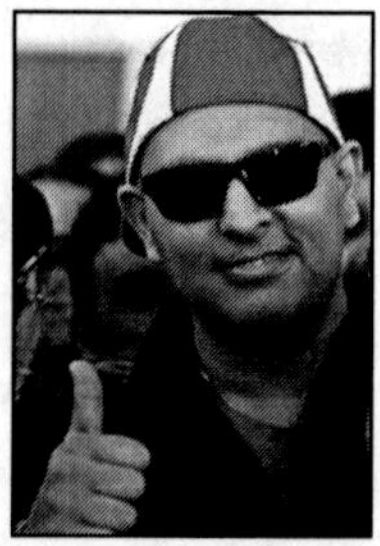

After winning the 2011 World Cup for India and being named the 'Player of the Tournament', Yuvraj Singh was diagnosed with Stage 1 Lung Cancer. He underwent chemotherapy in America and returned to India in March 2012. Yuvraj once said in his own words "At first I was in denial about it — playing for India was more important than my health and for a few months I chose to ignore the blood I spat out or my decline in stamina. It's only once I accepted cancer that I could beat it. When life knocks down you have a choice — to get up. So I thought to myself, 'get up and do it again.'" Yuvraj Singh was at the top of his game, winning titles and being in top form after the 2011 World Cup. India was delighted with his performance. However, no one knew was that Yuvi's health was deteriorating. He would often experience bouts of breathlessness, spit out gouts of blood, and experience a tremendous decline in stamina. A trip to the doctor confirmed his worst fears. He had cancer. A giant tumour was growing inside him and pressing against his lung and artery. The doctors told him that if he hadn't got it checked, he could have died of a heart attack because his artery was being squeezed – and no one would have known he had cancer. To Yuvi, this diagnosis meant taking an unpredictable break from cricket life. "I cried like a baby. When no one could see me or hear me. Not because I feared what cancer would do, but because I didn't want the disease. I wanted my life to be normal, which it could no longer be," he later said. However, he soon realized that he only had one option – to get up. Soon, he was undergoing rounds of chemotherapy. He had the determination to get better, forgetting the pain of long therapy sessions. He travelled to America in early 2012 for treatment. Three months later, he was back to his country and eager to get back on field. His sheer grit and determination made him win the toughest match of his life. He had won against cancer. Now Yuvraj is in best of health and plays for India.

Manisha Koirala

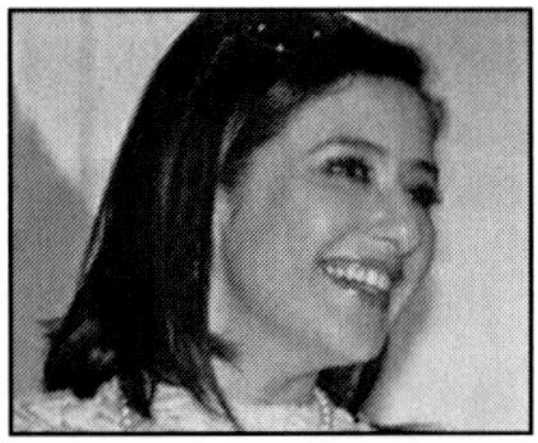

One of the leading actresses of the 1990s, Koirala had a dream debut with SubhashGhai's multi-starrer Saudagar. She went on to work in acclaimed projects from 1942: A Love Story, Bombay and Khamoshi: The Musical. Koirala came from Nepal to India and became a top actress; it seemed all her dreams were coming true. Later leading roles slowed down for Koirala but she continued working. Eventually, she shared she came to lose it all. "I had developed an unhealthy lifestyle which was attracting the wrong company. Restlessly, I was moving from one bad relationship to another. I was in a mess and I was in denial," Koirala admitted. In 2012, she was diagnosed with an aggressive form of ovarian cancer. Koirala continued living her life despite the diagnosis and thought about making a drastic change. She reconnected with her family, cultivated meaningful friendships and started to take care of herself, physically and spiritually. Since 2015, the gutsy actress has been cancer-free. 'There are two ways to recover: healthy diet and exercise. You have to revive yourself physically and mentally', she once said in an interview. She became a Goodwill Ambassador for the United Nations Population Fund in 2015, and came forward to help with the relief operations after the devastating Nepal earthquake the same year. She now lives a healthy life following her dreams.

Lisa Ray

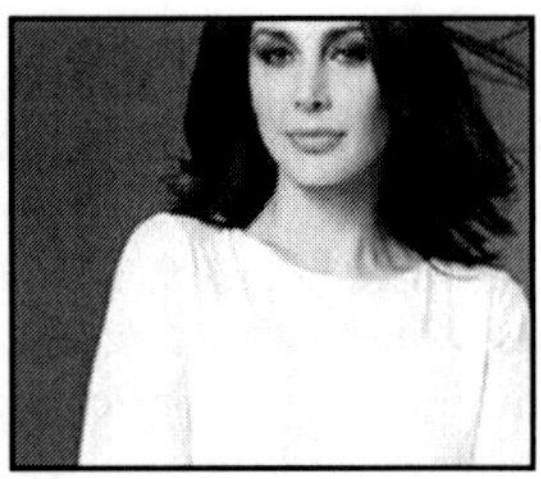

Lisa was raised in Canada by an Indian father and a Polish mother. She has had a successful career as a model and actor in Bollywood and Hollywood. She is an internationally acclaimed performer, philanthropist and actor with a reputation for taking on challenging issue-oriented films. At peak of her career, during the summer of 2009, Lisa scanned for multiple myeloma (a type of cancer). Initially she was in shock and denial. But she refused to bow before her dreaded illness and came out a survivor. "My father's love and support were unconditional and overwhelming." Lisa says. Love and support from the family and friends were her strengths which motivated her to overcome myeloma. "I believe in the power of prayers," she emphasises. "I worked hard – using meditation, positive affirmations and healers to reframe my cancer as an experience from which a lesson had to be learnt. I didn't think of it as a bout of bad karma or a death sentence," she says. In July 2010, Lisa was declared a survivor. Beating myeloma isn't easy but it is possible, stresses Lisa. Going through treatment was very tough at times but humour and writing helped. "And sometimes just crying and letting my grief out helped too," she adds. She also researched a lot about alternative therapies and approaches to healing as well as letting her grief out; all of which helped as well. She's now the global brand ambassador for Insight Vacations and promotes travel in India. Her national cancer campaign – Beauty Gives Back – has just been launched in Canada.

Mumtaz

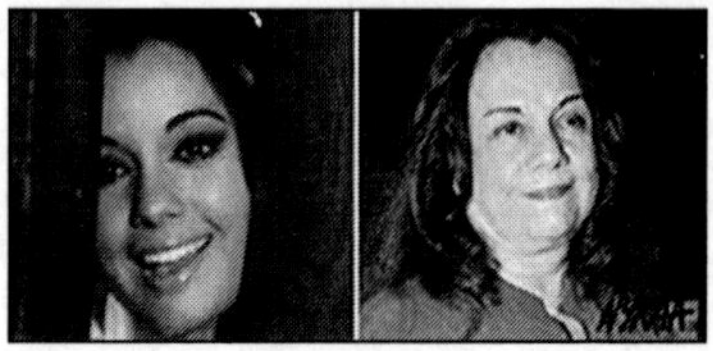

The legendary Bollywood actress had won many hearts with her performances in films such as Do Raaste, Chor Machaye Shor, Aag, Khilona, Aadmi aur Insaan, Upaasna and so on. But, she left all of her fans speechless when she fought against breast cancer at the age of 54. At the age of 54, Mumtaz, was diagnosed with a malignant lump in her breast in 2000, which turned out to be cancerous. She fought the disease for 11 years and made sure it did not get the better of her. Today, she openly shares her story and gives credit to the support she received from her family coupled with her own determination to survive the cancer. In an interview, she said, "I don't give up easily. Even death will have to fight me."

Angelina Jolie

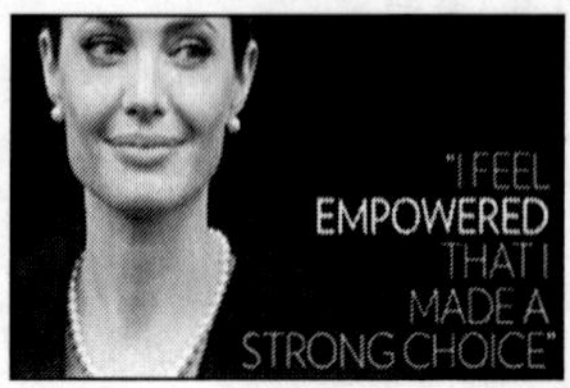

The acclaimed international actress has been privately fighting cancer for many years, and has undergone multiple procedures because of it. She showed signs of early ovarian cancer in 2015. The Oscar winner had already lost her mother, grandmother and aunt to the disease. But she didn't give up. She ended up getting her ovaries and fallopian tubes removed. She also had a preventative double mastectomy because she had an 87% risk of breast cancer. The procedure has changed her body, but she wrote in an open letter about how empowering the experience was. "I can tell my children that they don't need to fear they will lose me to breast cancer," wrote the actress in The New York Times. "It is reassuring that they see nothing that makes them uncomfortable. They can see my small scars and that's it. Everything else is just Mommy, the same as she always was. And they know that I love them and will do anything to be with them as long as I can. On a personal note, I do not feel any less of a woman. I feel empowered that I made a strong choice that in no way diminishes my femininity.

Annexures

ANNEXURE I - SOME DIET PLANS FOR CANCER PATIENTS

High Protein Normal Calorie Diet Chart (Vegetarian)

Calories – 1500, Protein 70 –80 g

S. No	Period/Time	Food Items	Quantity
1	Early Morning (07:00 AM)	Tea	1 Cup
		Biscuits	2 pcs
		Almonds	5 pcs
2	Breakfast (09:00 AM)	Toned Milk + Lamino HP (High protein supplement)	200 ml+ 1Tblsp
		Brown bread/*Paneer petties*/Stuffed *Chapatti (cauliflower/radish/methi/ paneer)/Missi chapatti*	1
		Curd	1/2 Katori
3	Midmorning (10:30 AM)	Low fat Buttermilk (Lassi)/Almond shake/ Fruit shake OR	1 to 2 glass
		Seasonal fruit with tinned juice	1 serving with 1 glass
4	Lunch (01:30 PM)	Thick vegetable soup	1
		Vegetable curry (1 leafy+1 other vegetable)	2 serving
		Curd/Raita (Potato/Ghia)	1 serving
		Missi Chapatti	2
		Paneer gravy/Soya bean wadi curry	1 serving
5	4:00 PM	High protein shake (boiled water + high protein powder)	15gm powder in 1 litre
6	Evening Tea (05:00 PM)	Tea	1 cup
		Mix vegetable *Poha*/Dalia/Boiled *channe*	1 serving
7	Pre-dinner (07:30 PM)	Thick vegetable soup/Dal soup	1 cup
8	Dinner (08:30 PM)	Vegetable Curry	1 serving
		Chapatti	1
		Whole Dal	1 serving
		Especially whole pulses and soya products/ *Paneer* curry	Twice a week
9	10:00 PM	Toned milk	1 cup

Paneer/skim-milk powder can be included in the diet plan to increase protein intake. Thick soups should be preferred, like vegetables, chicken or *channecan* be churned in the mixer and then mixed in the stock to increase protein in the diet. Fruits and vegetables are to be increased in the diet. Meals should be cooked in normal quantities of fat (15-20g/ day) Extra oil/butter to be avoided.

High Protein High Calorie Diet Chart (Non–Vegetarian)

Calories – 2000, Protein 70 – 80 g

S. No	Period/Time	Food Items	Quantity
1	Early Morning (07:00 AM)	Tea	1 Cup
		Biscuits	2 pcs
		Almonds	5 pcs
2	Breakfast (09:00 AM)	Toned Milk + Lamino HP (High protein supplement)	200 ml+ 1Tblsp
		Boiled egg whites/ Scrambled Eggs with Brown bread Or	1 to 2
		Stuffed Chapatti/Missi chapatti (cauliflower/radish/methi/omellete)	1 to 2
		Curd	1/2 Katori
3	Midmorning (10:30 AM)	Low fat Buttermilk (Lassi)/Almond shake/ Fruit shake OR	1 to 2 glass
		Seasonal fruit with tinned juice	1 serving with 1 glass
4	Lunch (01:30 PM)	Thick vegetable soup	1
		Vegetable curry (1 leafy+1 other vegetable)	2 serving
		Curd/Raita (Potato/Ghia)	1 serving
		Missi Chapatti	3 to 4
		Paneer gravy/Bhurjee	1 serving
5	4:00 PM	High protein shake (boiled water + high protein powder)	15gm powder in 1 cup
6	Evening Tea (05:00 PM)	Tea	1 cup
		Mix vegetable *Poha*/Dalia/Boiled *channe*	1 serving
7	Pre-dinner (07:30 PM)	Thick chicken soup/Dal soup	1 cup
8	Dinner (08:30 PM)	Vegetable Curry	1 serving
		Chapatti	3 to 4
		Whole Dal	1 serving
		Especially whole pulses and soya products/ *Paneer curry* or gravy fish/egg curry	Twice a week
9	10:00 PM	Sweet dish (custard/pudding/phirni/ paneer kheer)	1 serving

If eggs are taken in the breakfast, paneer can be taken later in the day, or vice versa. Thick soups should be preferred, like vegetables, chicken or channecan be churned in the mixer and then mixed in the stock to increase protein in the diet. Fruits and vegetables are to be increased in the diet. Meals should be cooked in normal quantities of fat Extra oil/butter to be avoided.

High Protein High Calorie Diet Chart (Vegetarian)

Calories – 2000, Protein 70 – 80 g

S. No	Period/Time	Food Items	Quantity
1	Early Morning (07:00 AM)	Tea	1 Cup
		Biscuits	2 pcs
		Almonds	6 to 8 pcs
2	Breakfast (09:00 AM)	Toned Milk + Lamino HP (High protein supplement)	200 ml+ 1Tblsp
		Brown bread/Paneerpetties/Stuffed Chapatti (cauliflower/radish/methi/ paneer)/Missi chapatti	1
		Curd	1/2 Katori
3	Midmorning (10:30 AM)	Low fat Buttermilk (Lassi)/ Almond shake/Fruit shake OR	1 to 2 glass
		Seasonal fruit with tinned juice	1 serving with 1 glass
4	Lunch (01:30 PM)	Thick vegetable soup	1
		Vegetable curry (1 leafy+1 other vegetable)	2 serving
		Curd/Raita (Potato/Ghia)	1 serving
		Missi Chapatti	3 to 4
		Paneer gravy/Bhurjee	1 serving
5	4:00 PM	High protein shake (boiled water + high protein powder)	15gm powder in 1 cup
6	Evening Tea (05:00 PM)	Tea	1 cup
		Mix vegetable *Poha*/Dalia/Boiled *channe*	1 serving
7	Pre-dinner (07:30 PM)	Thick chicken soup/Dal soup	1 cup
8	Dinner (08:30 PM)	Vegetable Curry	1 serving
		Chapatti	3 to 4
		Whole Dal	1 serving
		Especially whole pulses and soya products/ Paneer curry or paneer curry/tofu gravy	Twice a week
9	10:00 PM	Sweet dish (custard/pudding/phirni/ paneer kheer)	1 serving

Skim milk powder/paneer/tofu can be included in the diet plan to increase protein. Thick soups should be preferred, like vegetables, washed dal or channe can be churned in the mixer and then mixed in the stock to increase protein in the diet. Fruits and vegetables can be increased in the diet. Meals should be cooked in normal quantities of fat (15-20g/day) Extra oil/butter to be avoided.

High Protein Normal Calorie Diet Chart (Non-vegetarian)

Calories – 1500, Protein 70 –80 g

S. No	Period/Time	Food Items	Quantity
1	Early Morning (07:00 AM)	Tea	1 Cup
		Biscuits	2 pcs
		Almonds	5 pcs
2	Breakfast (09:00 AM)	Toned Milk + Lamino HP (High protein supplement)	200 ml+ 1Tblsp
		Brown bread/Egg petties Or	1 to 2
		Stuffed Chapatti/Missi chapatti (cauliflower/radish/methi/omellete)	1 to 2
		Curd	1/2 Katori
3	Midmorning (10:30 AM)	Low fat Buttermilk (*Lassi*)/Almond shake/ Fruit shake OR	1 to 2 glass
		Seasonal fruit with tinned juice	1 serving with 1 glass
4	Lunch (01:30 PM)	Thick vegetable soup	1
		Vegetable curry (1 leafy+1 other vegetable)	2 serving
		Curd/Raita (Potato/Ghia)	1 serving
		Missi Chapatti	2
		Chicken gravy/Fish curry	1 serving
5	4:00 PM	High protein shake (boiled water + high protein powder)	15gm powder in 1 cup
6	Evening Tea (05:00 PM)	Tea	1 cup
		Mix vegetable *Poha*/Dalia/Boiled *channe*	1 serving
7	Pre-dinner (07:30 PM)	Thick vegetable soup/Dal soup	1 cup
8	Dinner (08:30 PM)	Vegetable Curry	1 serving
		Chapatti	2
		Whole Dal	1 serving
		Especially whole pulses and soya products/ Paneer curry or egg curry	Twice a week
9	10:00 PM	Toned milk	1 cup

Paneer/egg white/skim-milk powder can be included in the diet plan to increase protein intake. Thick soups should be preferred, like vegetables, chicken or channe can be churned in the mixer and then mixed in the stock to increase protein in the diet. Fruits and vegetables are to be increased in the diet. Meals should be cooked in normal quantities of fat (15-20g/day) and extra oil/butter to be avoided.

ANNEXURE II

RATES OF COMMON TESTS AND PROCEDURES*

S. No	Test/Procedure	Private	General
1	Pap Smear	50	25
2	HPV Testing	1600	800
3	Cytopathology FNA	100	100
4	Biopsy (Histopathology)	250	100
5	Cone biopsy	1000	300
6	Cervical biopsy	250	100
7	Ultrasonography	250	100
8	CT Scan	2250	1125
9	MRI (Single Region)	4500	2500
10	Colposcopy	300	150
11	Colpotomy	500	150
12	Echo	100	100
13	ECG	250	Free
14	PET Scan	2000	1000
15	Tumor marker Blood Test	500	250
16	Urine Culture	300	150
17	Hysterectomy (abdominal)	2000	1000
18	Wertheim's hysterectomy nos.	5000	2500
19	External Radiation (Palliative Treatment)	3000	1500
20	External Radiation (Radical Treatment)	5000	2500
21	Medical Treatment of Cancer (Oncology)	1500	750
22	Radiotherapy by interstitial Brachytherapy	3000	1500

* Subject to changes

ANNEXURE III - RATES OF COMMON TESTS AND PROCEDURES*

Financial Aid & Resources Through The Central Government

- The Ministry of Health & Family Welfare has two schemes under which it offers financial assistance to poor patients.

  The Health Minister's Cancer Patient Fund (HMCPF) is available for patients living below the poverty line. This is admissible for treatment in 27 regional cancer centers in the country.

  The Health Minister's Discretionary Grants offers up to a maximum of Rs. 50,000 to poor patients to assist with a part of the hospitalisation/ treatment in government hospitals in cases where free medical facilities are not available.
- The Central Government Health Scheme (CGHS) is applicable for retired Central Government employees & dependents, which offers coverage for cancer treatment at approved rates from any hospital, apart from the hospitals set up under CGHS.
- Railways offers completely free travel to cancer patients and the attender/ bystander has to pay only 25% of Class II fare. And air concession of 50% is offered to patients traveling for treatment.

Health Minister's Cancer Patient Fund (HMCPF) under Rashtriya Arogya Nidhi (RAN) The "Health Minister's Cancer Patient Fund (HMCPF) within the Rashtriya Arogya Nidhi (RAN)" has been set up in 2009. In order to utilize the Health Minister's Cancer Patient Fund, the Revolving Fund as under RAN, has been established in 27 Regional Cancer Centres (RCCs).

Such step would ensure and speed up financial assistance to needy patients and help fulfil the objective of HMCPF under RAN. The financial assistance to a Cancer Patient up to Rs. 2,00,000/- (Rs. Two lakh only) [Rs. 5,00,000/- in emergency cases], would be processed by the RCC concerned, on whose disposal the Revolving Fund has been placed. Individual cases, which require assistance of more than Rs. 2.00 lakh is to be sent to the Ministry for processing. Revolving Funds have been created in all the 27 Regional Cancer Centres (RCCs) and funds upto Rs. 50 lakhs will be placed at their disposal. The Revolving Funds will be replenished on fulfilment of conditions regarding submission of utilization certificate and list of beneficiaries.

Eligibility for Health Minister's Cancer Patient Fund (HMCPF) within RAN:

1. The fund will provide financial assistance to patients, living below poverty line who is suffering from Cancer.
2. Assistance is admissible for treatment in 27 Regional Cancer Centre(s) (RCC) only.

3. Central Govt./State Govt. /PSU employees are not eligible for financial assistance from HMCPF.
4. Grant from HMCPF would not be used where treatment /facilities for cancer treatment are available free of cost.

List of 27 Regional Cancer Centers:

1. Kamala Nehru Memorial Hospital, Allahabad, Uttar Pradesh.
2. Chittaranjan National Cancer Institute, Kolkata, West Bengal
3. Kidwai Memorial Institute of Oncology, Bangalore, Karnataka.
4. Regional Cancer Institute (WIA), Adyar, Chennai, Tamil Nadu.
5. Acharya Harihar Regional Cancer, Centre for Cancer Research & Treatment, Cuttack, Orissa.
6. Regional Cancer Control Society, Shimla, Himachal Pradesh.
7. Cancer Hospital & Research Centre, Gwalior, Madhya Pradesh.
8. Indian Rotary Cancer Institute, (AIIMS), New Delhi.
9. R.S.T. Hospital & Research Centre, Nagpur, Maharashtra.
10. Pt. J.N.M. Medical College, Raipur, Chhatisgarh.
11. Post Graduate Institute of Medical Education & Research (PGIMER), Chandigarh.
12. Sher-I- Kashmir Institute of Medical Sciences, Soura, Srinagar.
13. Regional Institute of Medical Sciences, Manipur, Imphal.
14. Govt. Medical College & Associated Hospital, Bakshi Nagar, Jammu.
15. Regional Cancer Centre, Thiruvananthapuram, Kerala
16. Gujarat Cancer Research Institute, Ahmadabad, Gujarat.
17. MNJ Institute of Oncology, Hyderabad, Andhra Pradesh.
18. Pondicherry Regional Cancer Society, JIPMER, Pondicherry.
19. Dr. B.B. Cancer Institute, Guwahati, Assam.
20. Tata Memorial Hospital, Mumbai, Maharashtra.
21. Indira Gandhi Institute of Medical Sciences, Patna, Bihar.
22. Acharya Tulsi Regional Cancer Trust & Research Institute (RCC), Bikaner, Rajashtan.
23. Regional Cancer Centre, Pt. B.D.Sharma Post Graduate Institute of Medical Sciences, Rohtak, Haryana.
24. Civil Hospital, Aizawl, Mizoram.
25. Sanjay Gandhi Post Graduate Institute of Medical Sciences, Lucknow.
26. Government Arignar Anna Memorial Cancer Hospital, Kancheepuram,Tamil Nadu.
27. Cancer Hospital, Tripura, Agartala.

How to avail benefits

To avail financial assistance under HMCPF, the patient is required to submit :

1. Application form in prescribed proforma duly signed by the treating doctor and countersigned by the Medical Superintendent of the Government hospital/institute/ Regional Cancer Centre.
2. Copy of the income certificate.
3. Copy of the ration card.
4. Revolving Funds have been set up in 27 RCCs and funds upto 50 lakhs are placed at their disposal for providing treatment upto Rs. 2 lakh in each case.

Cases involving treatment beyond 2 lakh are referred to Ministry of Health & Family Welfare, Government of India for providing funds.

For Further Information, Please contact:
Ministry of Helath and Family Welfare
www.mohfw.gov.in | E-mail- so.grants-mhfw@nic.in

Initiatives by Punjab Government

- Financial assistance under State illness Fund through Punjab Nirogi Society is provided to cancer patients along with other life threatening diseases belonging to BPL families.
- Mukh Mantri Punjab Cancer Raahat Kosh Society – Under this scheme 50.00 crores has been made available by Govt. of Punjab, for treatment of all cancer patients except Govt. employees and those having health insurance cover. An amount of upto 1.50 lakhs is made available for treatment of every cancer patient.
- School children suffering from cancer are provided free treatment by Health Department.
- Regional Cancer Centre, PGI is connected to all districts of Punjab via Tele-Medicine facility.

For Further Information, Please contact:
Cancer Control Cell, Punjab
Phone No. 0172-5012356
www.pbhealth.gov.in
E-mail-cancercontrolcellpunjab@yahoo.com

ANNEXURE IV - WORDS TO KNOW

- **Alopecia-** Partial or complete loss of hair. This may result from radiation to the head, or from certain chemotherapy drugs.
- **Anemia-** A condition when there is a decrease in the number of red blood cells or in hemoglobin.
- **Anti-emetics-** Drugs given to prevent or minimize nausea and vomiting.
- **Ascites-** An abnormal fluid collection in the abdomen from cancer or other causes.
- **Biopsy-** The surgical removal of a small portion of tissue for diagnosis.
- **Brachytherapy-** The use of a radioactive "seed" temporarily implanted directly into a tumor. This allows a very high, localized dose of radiation to be given to a tumor, while limiting significant radiation exposure to other tissues.
- **Chemotherapy-** The treatment of cancer by drugs designed to kill cancer cells or stop them from growing.
- **Clinical trials-** The process by which new cancer treatments are tested in humans. Clinical trials are conducted after preliminary testing has shown that a new treatment might be effective.
- **Cone Biopsy-** The removal of a cone-shaped piece of tissue from around the opening of the cervix.
- **Complete Blood Count-** (CBC) A blood test that determines the number of red blood cells, white blood cells and platelets in the blood.
- **Debulking-** A surgical procedure that removes a significant part or most of a tumor. This may make future chemotherapy or radiation more effective.
- **Effusion-** A collection of fluid inside a body cavity, such as around the lungs, (pleural), intestines (peritoneal) or heart (pericardial).
- **Electrolytes-** Certain chemicals including sodium, potassium, chloride and bicarbonate found in the tissues and blood. They are often measured to monitor toxicities, effects of treatment, etc.
- **Emesis-** Vomiting.
- **Enteral feeding-** Administration of liquid food (nutrients) through a tube inserted into the stomach or intestine.
- **Epidural-** The space just outside the spinal cord. Catheters may be inserted into this space to deliver anesthetics or morphine for pain control.
- **Estrogen-** The female sex hormone produced by the ovaries. Estrogen controls the development of physical sexual characteristics, menstruation and pregnancy.

- **Extravasation-** Leakage into the surrounding tissues of intravenous chemotherapy drugs from the vein being used for the infusion or injection. Extravasation may damage tissues.
- **Frozen section-** A procedure done by the pathologist during an operation to give the surgeon an immediate answer as to whether a tissue is benign (non-cancerous) or malignant (cancerous).
- **Grade of Tumor-** A way of describing tumors by their appearance under the microscope. Low-grade tumors are slow to grow and spread, while high- grade tumors grow and spread rapidly.
- **Hematocrit-** A way of measuring the red blood cell content of the blood. A low hematocrit is a sign of anemia.
- **Hematuria-** Blood in the urine. This may be seen easily by the naked eye (gross hematuria) or it can be hidden (microscopic hematuria).
- **Hemoglobin-** A way of measuring the oxygen carrying ability of the blood.
- Immunosuppression-The state of having decreased immunity and thus being less able to fight off infection.
- **Intravenous (IV)-** Within or through a vein.
- **Laparoscopy-** A type of surgery using a very small camera and instruments that are inserted into the abdomen through small, band-aid sized incisions in order to perform complex surgeries.
- **Malaise-** The feeling of tiredness, lack of drive.
- **Metastasis-** The spread of cancer from one part of the body to another. Cells that spread are like those of the original cancer. .
- **Mucositis-** Inflammation and soreness of mucous membranes such as tissue lining the mouth or throat. This is sometimes a side effect of chemotherapy or radiation.
- **Nadir-** The lowest point at which the blood counts drop after chemotherapy.
- **Nephrotoxic-** Medications or drugs that are toxic to the kidneys.
- **Neuropathy-** This is a side effect caused bya few chemotherapy drugs that causes numbness and/or tingling in the fingers and toes.
- **Oophorectomy-** The surgical removal of one or both ovaries.
- **Paracentesis-** A procedure in which fluid is taken out of the abdomen by a very thin catheter.
- **Petechiae-** Small red spots under the skin caused by a low platelet count.
- **Port-** An implanted, reusable IV to administer chemotherapy. Once placed, an I.V. can be easily connected to the port again and again without having to start a new I.V. in the arm.

- **Residual Disease or Residual Tumor-** Cancer left behind after surgery or other treatment.
- **Stage-** Stage refers to the mapping of where cancer may or may not have spread.
- Determination of the stage is very important for planning the most effective treatment for a cancer by taking into account where the disease is located.
- **Stomatitis-** Inflammation and soreness of the mouth. This is sometimes a side effect of chemotherapy or radiation.
- **Transfusions-** The infusion of any blood cell product. Example: red blood cells, platelets.

References

1. WHO. World Cancer Report. Geneva, Switzerland. WHO.2014.
2. American Cancer Society. Global Cancer Facts & Figures 3rd Edition. Atlanta. American Cancer Society.2015.
3. Takiar R, Nadayil D, Nandakumar A. Projections of number of cancer cases in India (2010-2020) by cancer groups. Asian Pac J Cancer Prev. 2010;11(4):1045-9.
4. WHO. Fact Sheets Cancer. Geneva, Switzerland. WHO.2015.
5. India. Chandigarh. Cancer Incidence and Mortality in Chandigarh Union Territory, Post Graduate Institute of Medical Education and Research. 2013.
6. ICMR. Consolidated Report of the Hospital Based Cancer Registries. Bengaluru, India. ICMR.2016.
7. Foundation for Women's Cancer - [Internet]. Foundation for Women's Cancer. 2016 [cited 22 August 2016]. Available from: http://www.foundationforwomenscancer.org/.
8. TNM Classification of Malignant Tumor [Internet]. 7th ed. Union for International cancer Control; 2011 [cited 29 August 2016]. Available from: http://www.uicc.org/ sites/main/files/private/TNM_Classification_of_Malignant_Tumours_Website_15%20 MAy2011.pdf
9. Schofield P, Juraskova I, Bergin R, Gough K, Mileshkin L, Krishnasamy M et al. A nurse- and peer-led support program to assist women in gynaecological oncology receiving curative radiotherapy, the PeNTAGOn study (Peer and nurse support trial to assist women in gynaecological oncology): study protocol for a randomised controlled trial. Trials. 2013;14(1):39.
10. Reis N, Beji N, Coskun A. Quality of life and sexual functioning in gynecological cancer patients: Results from quantitative and qualitative data. Eur J OncolNurs. 2010;14(2):137-146.
11. Lutgendorf S, Anderson B, Ullrich P, Johnsen E, Buller R, Sood A et al. Quality of life and mood in women with gynecologic cancer. Cancer. 2001;94(1):131-140.

12. Rehse B, Pukrop R. Effects of psychosocial interventions on quality of life in adult cancer patients: meta analysis of 37 published controlled outcome studies. Patient EducCouns. 2003;50(2):179-186.
13. Given B, Given C, Kozachik S. Family Support in Advanced Cancer. CA: A Cancer J Clin. 2001;51(4):213-231.
14. Mellon S, Northouse L. Family survivorship and quality of life following a cancer diagnosis. Res Nurs Health. 2001;24(6):446-459.
15. Harter P, Schrof I, Karl L, Hils R, Kullmann V, Traut A et al. Sexual Function, Sexual Activity and Quality of Life in Women with Ovarian and Endometrial Cancer. Geburtshilfe und Frauenheilkunde. 2013; 73(05):428-432.
16. Vanlerenberghe E, Sedda A, Ait-Kaci F. The impact of gynaecological cancers on woman's sexuality and her couple. Bulletin du Cancer. 2015;102(5):454-462.
17. Aniebue U, Onyeka T. Ethical, Socioeconomic, and Cultural Considerations in Gynecologic Cancer Care in Developing Countries. J Palliative Care. 2014;2014:1-6.
18. Seven M, Yýlmaz S, ªahin E, Akyüz A. Evaluation of the Quality of Life of Caregivers in Gynecological Cancer Patients. J Cancer Educ.2014; 29(2):325-332.
19. Given B, Given C, Kozachik S. Family Support in Advanced Cancer. CA: A Cancer J Clin. 2001;51(4):213-231.
20. Northouse L, Katapodi M, Schafenacker A, Weiss D. The Impact of Caregiving on the Psychological Well-Being of Family Caregivers and Cancer Patients. SeminOncolNurs. 2012;28(4):236-245.
21. Courneya K, Karvinen K, Campbell K, Pearcey R, Dundas G, Capstick V et al. Associations among exercise, body weight, and quality of life in a population-based sample of endometrial cancer survivors. J Gynecol Oncol.2005;97(2):422-430.
22. Tahmasebi M, Yarandi F, Eftekhar Z, Montazeri A Namazi H. Quality of Life in Gynecologic Cancer Patients. Asian Pacific J Cancer Prev. 2007;8(1):591-592.
23. Kumbhaj P, Sharma R, Bhatnagar A. Quality of life and sexual functioning in cervical cancer survivors after surgery and radiotherapy. Fertil. Steril.2013;100(3):S67.
24. Satwe S, Salunkhe J, Satave V. Quality of Life (QOL) of Women with Radiation Therapy. International Journal of Science and Research (IJSR). 2014;3(3);14-8.
25. McCorkle R, Dowd M, Ercolano E, Schulman-Green D, Williams A, Siefert M et al. Effects of a nursing intervention on quality of life outcomes

in post-surgical women with gynecological cancers. Psychooncology. 2009;18(1):62-70.

26. von Gruenigen V, Frasure H, Kavanagh M, Janata J, Waggoner S, Rose P et al. Survivors of uterine cancer empowered by exercise and healthy diet (SUCCEED): A randomized controlled trial. J GynecolOncol. 2012; 125(3):699-704.
27. Petersen R, Quinlivan J. Preventing anxiety and depression in gynaecological cancer: a randomised controlled trial. BJOG: Int J ObstetGynaecol. 2002;109(4):386-394.
28. Gruenigen V, Courneya K, Gibbons H, Kavanagh M, Waggoner S, Lerner E. Feasibility and effectiveness of a lifestyle intervention program in obese endometrial cancer patients: A randomized trial. J GynecolOncol.2008;109(1):19-26.
29. Aranda S, Schofield P, Weih L, Milne D, Yates P, Faulkner R. Meeting the support and information needs of women with advanced breast cancer: a randomised controlled trial. Br J Cancer. 2006;95(6):667-673.
30. Pitceathly C, Maguire P, Fletcher I, Parle M, Tomenson B, Creed F. Can a brief psychological intervention prevent anxiety or depressive disorders in cancer patients? A randomised controlled trial. Annals of Oncology. 2009;20(5):928-934.
31. Korstjens I, May A, van Weert E, Mesters I, Tan F, Ros W et al. Quality of Life After Self-Management Cancer Rehabilitation: A Randomized Controlled Trial Comparing Physical and Cognitive-Behavioral Training Versus Physical Training. Psychosom. Med.2008;70(4):422-429.
32. Antoni M, Wimberly S, Lechner S, Kazi A, Sifre T, Urcuyo K et al. Reduction of Cancer- Specific Thought Intrusions and Anxiety Symptoms With a Stress Management Intervention Among Women Undergoing Treatment for Breast Cancer.Am J Psychiatry. 2006;163(10):1791-1797.
33. Lopez V, Copp G, Molassiotis A. Male Caregivers of Patients With Breast and Gynecologic Cancer. Cancer Nurs. 2012;35(6):402-410.
34. Scott J, Halford W, Ward B. United We Stand? The Effects of a Couple-Coping Intervention on Adjustment to Early Stage Breast or Gynecological Cancer. J. Consult. Clin. Psychol. 2004;72(6):1122-1135.
35. Schemes and Programmees: National Cancer Control Programme - Health & Family Welfare - Sectors: National Portal of India [Internet]. Archive.india.gov.in. 2016 [cited 22 August 2017]. Available from: http://www.archive.india.gov.in/sectors/health_ family/index.php?id=11.
36. National Cancer Control Programme (NCCP) [Internet]. www.aarogya.com. 2017 [cited 29 August 2017]. Available from: http://www.aarogya.com/health-resources/health- programs/national-cancer-control-programme-nccp.html?start=1.

37. Quality of life [Internet].www.eortc.com.2016 [cited 5 December 2016]. Available from: http://www.eortc.com/quality of life/quality of life modules/qol.html?start=1.
38. Quality of life [Internet].www.eortc.com.2016 [cited 5 December 2016]. Available from: http://www.eortc.com/quality of life/quality of life modules/qol.html?start

Chapter - 11

Dealing with diagnosis and therapy related issues of ovarian cancer - A guide for patients/family caregivers

— Dr. Janavi , Dr. Bhavana Rai,
Dr. Vanita Suri and Dr. Amarjeet Singh

What is cancer?

Cells are the body's basic building blocks. Our body constantly makes new cells to help us grow. New cells replace worn-out tissue and heal injuries. Normally, cells multiply and die in an orderly way.

Sometimes cells don't grow, divide and die in the usual way. This may cause blood or lymph fluid in the body to become abnormal. This may be in the form of a lump called a tumour (or cancer). A tumour can be benign or malignant.

Benign tumour – Cells are confined to one area and are not able to spread to other parts of the body. This is not real cancer.

Malignant tumour – This is made up of cancerous cells, which have the ability to spread to other parts of the body by travelling through the bloodstream or lymphatic system (lymph fluid).

STAGES OF MELANOMA CANCER

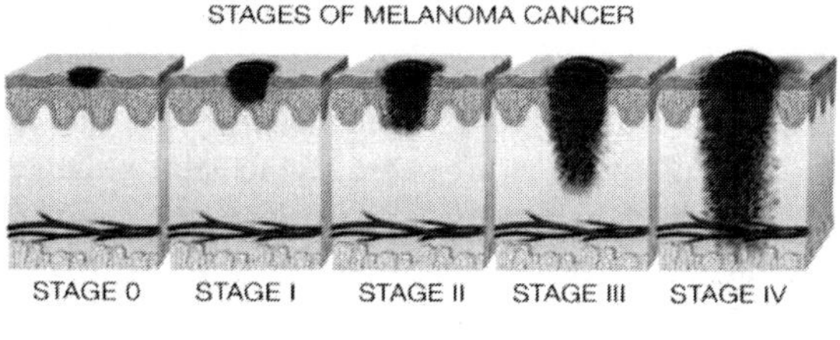

The cancer that first develops in a tissue or organ is called the primary cancer. A malignant tumour is usually named after the organ or type of cell affected.

A malignant tumour that has not spread to other parts of the body is called localised cancer. A tumour may grow deeper into surrounding tissue and can grow its own blood vessels in a process called angiogenesis.

If cancer cells grow and form another tumour at a new site, it is called a secondary cancer or metastasis. A metastasis keeps the name of the original cancer. For example, ovarian cancer that has spread to the abdomen is called metastatic ovarian cancer, even though the woman may be experiencing symptoms caused by problems in the abdomen.

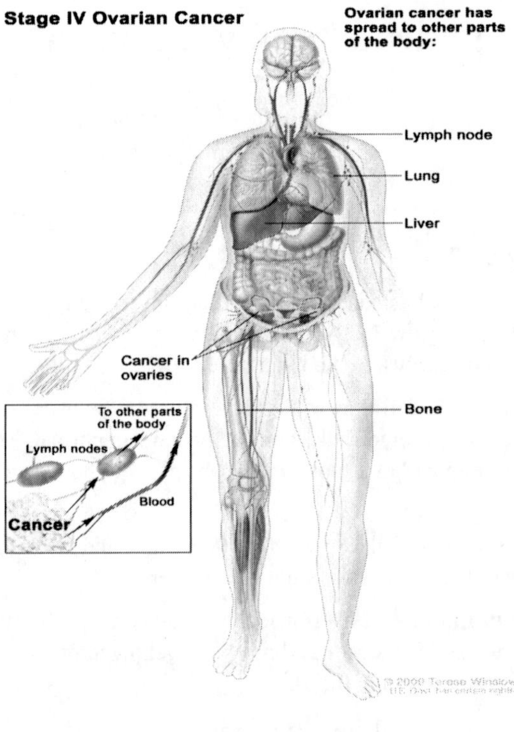

The Ovaries

In women there are many types of reproductive system cancer e.g. cervix, breast, uterus, ovary. The ovaries are part of the female reproductive system, which also includes the fallopian tubes, uterus (womb), cervix (the neck of the uterus), vagina (birth canal) and vulva (external genitals).

The ovaries are two small, grape-shaped organs. They are found in the lower part of the abdomen (the pelvic cavity). There is one ovary on each side of the uterus, close to the end of the fallopian tubes. Each ovary is made up of:

epithelial cells – found on the outside of the ovary in a layer known as the epithelium

germinal (germ) cells – found inside the ovaries, these cells eventually mature into eggs (ova)

stromal cells – form connective (supporting) tissue within the ovaries, and produce the female hormones oestrogen and progesterone.

Each month, the ovaries release an egg (ovum) in a process called ovulation. The egg travels down the fallopian tube into the uterus. If the egg is fertilised by a sperm, it will implant itself into the lining of the uterus and grow into a baby. If the egg is not fertilised by a sperm, the lining is shed and flows out of the body through the vagina. This flow is known as a woman's periods or menses (menstruation).

Two hormones (oestrogen and progesterone) are involved in the process of ovulation (egg release) and menstruation. As a woman gets older, the ovaries gradually produce less of these hormones. When the levels of oestrogen and progesterone fall low enough, a woman's periods become irregular and finally stop. This is known as menopause. After menopause, it is no longer possible to conceive a child. The ovaries also become smaller.

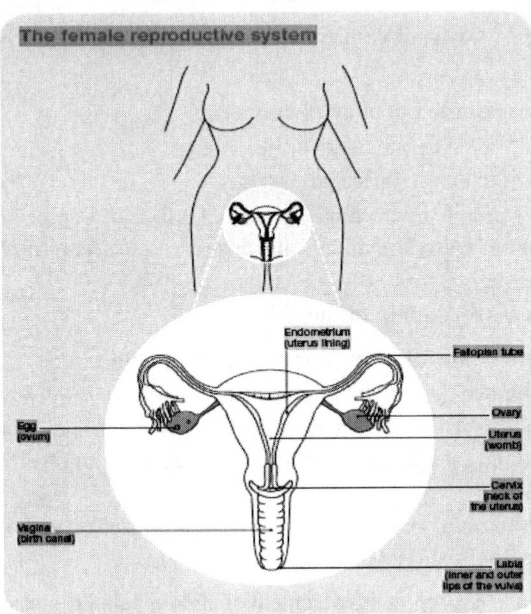

Ovarian cancer

It is a malignant tumour affecting one or both ovaries. It can start in any of the three cell types found in the ovary. Epithelial ovarian, fallopian tube and peritoneal cancers all develop in the same type of cell and are very similar. Many epithelial ovarian cancers start in the fallopian tubes.

Ovarian cancer often spreads from the ovaries to the diaphragm, the lining of the abdomen (peritoneum), and the sheet of fatty tissue that hangs inside the abdomen (omentum).

There are many types of ovarian cancer. The three most common types are epithelial, germ cell and stromal cell tumour. Epithelial cancer is the most common type of ovarian cancer. It originates in fallopian tubes, on the surface of ovary. It usually occurs in women more than 50 years of age.

Germ cell type occurs in women under 40 years of age. It is rare type of ovarian cancer. Stromal cell tumour occurs in cells that produce female hormones. It is also rare and occurs in women between 40 & 60 years.

Some women (usually younger women) are diagnosed with a borderline ovarian tumour. This is not considered to be cancer because, although it can spread, it does not usually invade other organs. For this reason, borderline tumours are also known as low malignant potential tumours.

In medical science, doctors have developed a system of grading cancer of ovary. This helps them to assess treatability and severity of the cancer.

Staging of Ovarian cancer: (International Federation of Gynecology and Obstetrics)

I - Disease limited to ovaries only

I a Limited to one ovary only

I b Both ovaries affected

I c I a or I b with tumour on the surface of one or both ovaries, ruptured capsule, cytologically positive ascites, or positive peritoneal washings

II - Disease extending to the pelvis

II a Disease affecting tubes or uterus or both

II b Extension to other pelvic tissues

II c II a or II b with tumour on the surface of one or both ovaries, ruptured capsule, cytologically positive ascites, or positive peritoneal washings

III - Abdominal disease or affected lymph nodes or both (surface liver disease is still stage III)

III a Microscopic involvement of abdominal peritoneal surfaces.

III b Disease up to 2 cm diameter

III c Disease greater than 2 cm +/" regional lymph nodes

IV - Distant metastases: pleural effusions need to be cytologically positive and liver metastases should be parenchymal

Extent of the problem

Ovarian cancer is fast emerging as the leading cancer of the genital tract in women.

Ovarian cancer is the sixth most common cancer and seventh leading cause of cancer death among women worldwide. In India, it is the third most common gynecological malignancy. But it has poor outcomes making it the leading cause of gynecologic cancer related deaths. The incidence of ovarian cancer is the highest in western nations and lowest in developing countries.

In India there has been a steady increase in prevalence of ovarian cancer. The environmental and /or life-style factors affecting the change had influence on all the age groups. It is due to life style factors, particularly an increase in age at marriage, delay in age at first birth, reduction in parity and improved socio-economic conditions etc.

The burden of various gynaecological cancers in India (2018) according to Globocan (an international cancer agency).(Fig.1)

Ovarian cancer increases from 35 years of age and reaches a peak between the ages 55 and 64. The type of ovarian cancer that is generally found is epithelial in origin. The germ cell variety of ovarian cancer occurs more in young patients. During 2011-2015, in PGIMER Chandigarh, 1052 cases of ovarian cancer were reported. Out of these 93(8.84%) were of germ cell type. Most of the patients reported with involvement of surrounding structures of the ovary.

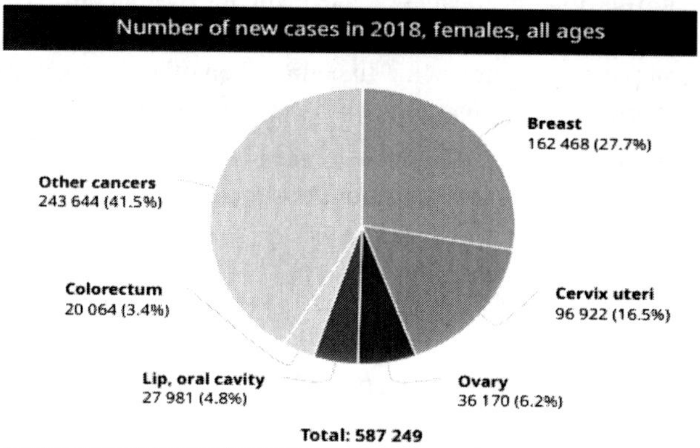

Fig. 1 Globocan 2018 India Fact Sheet.

Prognosis & survival: Five-year relative survival rate of epithelial ovarian cancer ranges from approximately 30% to 50% .Early stage (Stage I &II) diagnosis has better survival chance. However, doctors are able to diagnose only 15% of all ovarian cancers at this early stage. By the time the cancer reaches stage III / IV, it is quite advanced and chances of recovery/ survival are less. Hence, the survival of patients with ovarian cancer can improve by earlier diagnosis. There are higher chances of survival if the patient reports early to the doctor without ignoring symptoms of the disease.

Natural history of disease (Onset, Progress, Stages, Spread)

Ovarian cancer is a deadly disease which continues to be a challenge for doctors (oncologists). It is multifactorial in origin. Therefore, it is important to know its natural history i.e. its origin, evolution, risk factors, pre-clinical perspective, and its clinical manifestations.

Development

The process of origin & development of ovarian cancer is not well characterised, although various mechanisms have been suggested. Ovarian cancer is a disease that belongs to the group of chronic and degenerative diseases with extensive natural history. Unlike breast cancer, it appears in two periods of life, the first one being in youth, and the second one postmenopausal. Over many cycles of ovulation, the ovarian surface epithelium undergoes repeated disruption and repair. The epithelial cells are stimulated to multiply. This increase the chances of spontaneous mutations or after ovulation, these cells may become trapped within the connective tissue surrounding the ovary. This can lead to the formation of inclusion cysts which may increase the rate of DNA damage. This affects the cancer risk.

Most ovarian cancers occur spontaneously, although 5–10 per cent of cases develop due to a genetic reason, like involving dysfunctional BRCA1 or BRCA2 genes. This produces high-grade carcinomas, with a poorer prognosis. Despite complete reduction with first-line chemotherapy (CT), ovarian epithelial cancer occurs again in over 50% of women.

The risk factors of epithelial ovarian cancer are typical of perimenopausal and postmenopausal women. Its frequency increases with the number of decades.

Heredity risks of ovarian cancer

1. Family history of ovarian cancer.
2. BRCA 1 and BRCA 2 mutations: Risk for ovarian cancer in positive cases is from 27–44% as compared to 1% of the general population

Non heredity factors:

- *Age*: It generally occurs in women > 45 years of age. But its more malignant variety occurs in young women.
- Medium-high socioeconomic status
- *Early menarche & late menopause*: In women having their periods at early age, the risk of ovarian cancer increases as the period of ovulation increases. This is same for the women in whom periods continue at later age groups and they get menopause after 55 years.
- *Nulliparity*: Pregnancy reduces the risk of ovarian cancer. Thus women who don't conceive are at greater risk of ovarian cancer.
- Polycystic ovaries
- History of breast, colon, or endometrial cancer (hormone-dependent tumours).
- Infertility treatment with no full-term pregnancy: The use of clomiphene citrate is associated with risk compared with infertile women who do not use it.
- Obesity: In women with a high BMI >30, aged over 18 years.
- Use of hormone replacement therapy for more than five years
- Smoking
- Use of talc and exposure to asbestos / radiation.

The biochemistry of ovarian cancer

There has been a link between polycystic ovary syndrome (PCOS) and ovarian cancer as there is anovulation in PCOS and thus ovulation induction treatments and inducing multifollicular ovulations theoretically increase the risk for ovarian cancer. PCOS is a heterogeneous genetic disorder, characterised by an increased concentration of androgens circulating in the blood. PCOS can evolve into metabolic syndrome, affecting thebody's energy utilisation. PCOS can evolve into metabolic syndrome, affecting the body's energy utilisation. This takes the form of a markedly high rate of insulin synthesis in the blood, abdominal obesity, increased blood pressure, dyslipidemia, insulin resistance, type 2 diabetes mellitus, cardiovascular disease, and endometrial hyperplasia Changes can also take place in the regulation of gonadotropin release, and this interferes with the ovarian steroid inhibition-feedback loop. This results in increased secretion of luteinising hormone in the woman's body. The secretion of follicle-stimulating hormone (FSH) also increases; the stromal cells and ovarian theca cells are hyperactive, and because of this hyperactivity, the secretion of androgens increases; all this allows abnormalities to appear in the biochemistry of the body's metabolism after menopause.

Wake up Call: Diagnosis- Signs & Symptoms (Time to consult doctor) & Investigations (Lab reports) *"Ovarian cancer is not a silent killer, It's just not being heard".*

Diagnosis

In general, ovarian cancer is revealed by increased abdominal volume. But the symptoms are vague and overlooked because the discomfort is not intense and is often confused with gastrointestinal conditions. When the malignant ovarian tumour does become apparent, symptoms will depend on the organ affected. At this time the woman experiences intense gastrointestinal symptoms, with lower abdominal or pelvic pain, and periodic constipation and diarrhoea; vaginal bleeding also occurs. The volume and diameter of the abdomen increases suddenly, through ascites, and this leads to the gradual onset of breathing problem, in line with the amount in litres that is pressing upwards on the diaphragm and affects breathing movement. The patients' body weight increases due to fluid accumulation.

Once the ovarian tumour has been diagnosed as malignant, the prognosis for survival will be related to the following factors:

- *Tumour size.* The smaller the size of tumor the better the prognosis of ovarian cancer.
- *Tumour stage.* Prognosis is better if diagnosed at stage I as the tumor is confined l locally and has not spread.
- *Characteristics of the tumour* by imaging (ultrasound, CT, MRI). The epithelial variety of ovarian cancer is less dangerous than the germ cell type because the latter is malignant.
- Presence or absence of symptoms.
- *Tumour marker values* (cancer-125, cancer 19.9). The higher the values the worse is the prognosis.

Ovarian cancer does lead to symptoms which are often ignored because of their vague nature and it remains undiagnosed for a long time. So treatment is often delayed. Good tools for early diagnosis of high-risk tumours are the ultrasound and immune histochemistry tests. The natural history of ovarian cancer indicates that it will remain as the tumour that takes the life of women in reproductive age for several decades to come.

Ovarian cancer has often been termed 'the silent killer'. But it is being increasingly recognised that the majority of women with ovarian cancer have symptoms[7] which are non-specific since these are also widely experienced among the general population.[7] However, such symptoms assume greater significance in older women (over 50 years of age) and in those with a significant family history (two or more cases of ovarian or breast cancer diagnosed at an early age in first degree relatives). Some factors reduce the risk of developing ovarian cancer. These include having children, breastfeeding, using the combined oral contraceptive pill for several years, tubal ligation or tubectomy.

Even the women actually having ovarian cancer are often suspected of having gastrointestinal disease because of non specific nature of these symptoms, viz., irritable bowel syndrome. As a result, they are not adequately investigated. This results diagnosis delays.[7] Only difference is that these symptoms more frequent, more severe in cancer patients and more persistent than in women who do not have the disease.

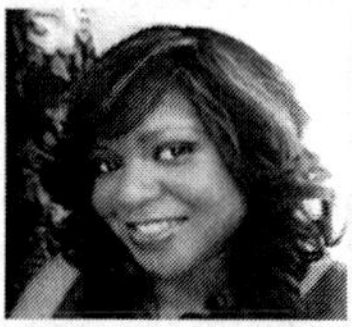

"Ladies, there is no test for ovarian cancer. And until these awesome doctors and researchers come up with one, we have to know our bodies!"

—Tiffany P., Ovarian Cancer Survivor
Age at diagnosis: 32

In such a scenario, doctors advise women to keep a record of how often these symptoms occur. They advise women to discuss with gynaecologist if the symptoms are severe or continue for more than a few weeks. These symptoms can also occur in many other conditions. Having such symptoms do not necessarily mean that woman has ovarian cancer. But it is best to have a check-up.

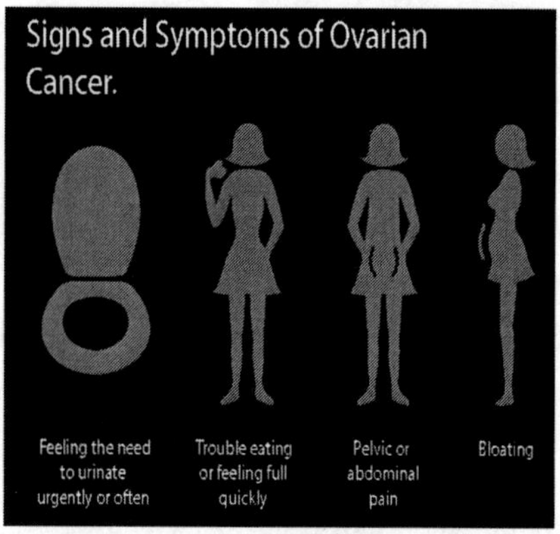

Symptom Index for detection of ovarian malignancy in Indian women-

- *abdominal pain*
- *bloating*
- *increasing abdominal size*
- *difficulty eating or feeling full quickly*
- *pelvic pain*

If any of these symptoms are experienced more than 12 times per month, within last one year were considered to have a positive 'symptom index'

Screening test for ovarian cancer: There is no specific test for this. If there is a suspicion of ovarian cancer, tests and scans may be done. These can show if there are any abnormalities that need to be followed up with a biopsy.

The only way to confirm a diagnosis of ovarian cancer is by taking a tissue sample (biopsy) and looking at the cells under a microscope. This is usually done during surgery. This way, diagnosis and treatment of the cancer is done at the same time.

Pelvic examination

Doctors check for any masses or lumps by feeling your abdomen. They also do vaginal examination using a speculum. An internal examination is not painful but may be uncomfortable. The doctor may also perform a digital rectal examination.

Investigation

To date, there is no suitable regime for detection of ovarian cancer; diagnostic methods are expensive and do not detect malignant tumours in the early stages of disease. However, in women with hereditary risk factors or those identified during a directed history, it is acceptable to do tests with tumour markers. The essential investigation for a suspected adnexal tumour: pelvic ultrasound, preferably using colour Doppler, and better still, by the vaginal route in the early stages.

CA125 blood test

There are some blood tests to check for proteins produced by cancer cells. These proteins are called tumour markers e.g. CA125.

The level of CA125 may be higher in some women with ovarian cancer. However, it can also rise for reasons other than cancer, including ovulation, menstruation, irritable bowel syndrome, liver or kidney disease, endometriosis or fibroids.

The CA125 blood test is not used for screening for ovarian cancer in women who do not have any symptoms. It can be used:

At diagnosis – A CA125 test is more accurate in diagnosing ovarian cancer in women who have been through menopause (postmenopausal) than those who haven't (premenopausal). Women with early-stage ovarian cancer often have normal CA125 levels. This is why doctors will often combine CA125 tests with an ultrasound.

During treatment – If the patient has ovarian cancer that produces CA125, the blood test may be used to check how well the treatment is working. Falling CA125 levels may mean it's working, and rising CA125 may mean the treatment is not working effectively. But the CA125 level is only one item used by the treating team to assess a woman's response to treatment.

After treatment – CA125 blood tests are sometimes included in follow-up tests.

Imaging & Investigations

Doctor may recommend a number of imaging scans and investigations to determine the extent and stage of the disease. Chest x-rays may be done to check the lungs cancer.

Pelvic ultrasound

A pelvic ultrasound uses echoes from sound waves to create a picture of uterus and ovaries on a computer. A sonographer performs the scan. It can be done in two ways:

Abdominal ultrasound –For this patient lies on an examination table while the sonographer moves a small handheld device over abdominal area.

Transvaginal ultrasound – The sonographer inserts a small transducer wand into vagina. It will be covered with a disposable plastic sheath and gel to make it easier to insert. Some women find this procedure uncomfortable, but it should not be painful. The transvaginal ultrasound is often the preferred type of ultrasound, as it provides a clearer picture of the ovaries and uterus.

CT Scan

A CT (computerised tomography) scan uses x-ray beams to take pictures of the inside of the body. It is used to look for signs that the cancer has spread. A CT scan may not be able to detect all ovarian tumours. CT scans are usually done at a hospital or radiology clinic.

Patients are asked not to eat or drink for several hours (fast) before the scan. A liquid dye (called the contrast) is injected into one of the veins to help make the pictures clearer. The contrast makes organs appear white on the scan, so anything unusual can be seen more clearly.

The dye may make the patient feel hot all over and leave a bitter taste in mouth. She may also feel the need to pass urine. These side effects usually ease quickly.

The CT scanner is a large, doughnut-shaped machine. Patient lies on a table that moves in and out of the scanner. The scan takes 10–20 minutes. But it may take extra time to prepare and then wait for the scan. While a CT scan can be noisy, it is painless. Most women can go home as soon as the CT scan is over. The dye used in a CT scan usually contains iodine. If the patient has an allergic reaction to iodine or dyes during a previous scan, she should tell the medical team beforehand and should also let them know if she is diabetic, have kidney disease or is pregnant.

PET Scan

A PET (positron emission tomography) scan highlights abnormal tissues in the body, and it can be more accurate than a CT scan. The results are often used to help with planning before surgery, and to check on how the treatment is working. Before the scan, patient will be injected with a small amount of radioactive glucose solution. This makes cancer cells show up brighter on the scan because they take up more of the glucose solution than normal cells do. Patient will be asked to sit quietly for 30–90 minutes while the glucose solution moves around patient's body, then she will be scanned for high levels of radioactive glucose.

Any radiation will leave patient's body within a few hours. Patient should tell doctor beforehand if she is diabetic, pregnant, think she might be pregnant, or is breastfeeding.

Colonoscopy

A bowel examination (colonoscopy) may also be done to make sure that the symptoms are not caused by a bowel problem. The doctor inserts a thin, flexible tube with a small camera and a light (colonoscope) through the anus into the bowel.

Before the test, patient has to change the diet and take prescribed laxatives to clean out the bowel completely (bowel preparation). The process varies for different people and between hospitals. The doctor gives you specific instructions and talks about what to expect. On the day, patient will probably be given an anaesthetic so that she doesn't feel any discomfort.

A colonoscopy usually takes about 20–30 minutes. Patient will need to have someone take her home afterwards, as she may feel drowsy or weak.

Treatment modalities for ovarian cancer

"Often the biggest hurdle in treatment of cancer is the perception more than the disease."

The treatment for ovarian cancer depends on the type of ovarian cancer you have, the stage of the cancer, general health and fitness of patient, doctors' recommendations, and whether the patient wish to have children.

Treatment options by type of ovarian cancer	
Epithelial	Surgery is the main treatment for all stages of epithelial ovarian cancer. The aim is to remove as much of the cancer as possible. Sometimes, additional treatment is needed. • **Stage I** ovarian cancer is usually treated with surgery alone. Some women will be offered chemotherapy after surgery if there is a high risk of the cancer coming back. • **Stages II, III and IV** are usually treated with a combination of surgery and chemotherapy. New targeted therapy drugs are being offered to women with a BRCA mutation. In some cases, radiation therapy is offered.
Germ cell	This is usually treated with surgery and/or chemotherapy.
Stromal cell	This is usually treated with surgery, sometimes followed by chemotherapy or targeted therapy.
Borderline tumour	This is usually treated with surgery only.

Surgery

Doctors talk about the most suitable type of surgery, as well as the risks and any possible complications. These may include infertility. If having children is important patient need to talk to the doctor before surgery and ask for a referral to a fertility specialist.

Ovarian cancer has many stages. This means that the surgery will help the doctor work out how far the tumour has spread within the pelvic cavity.

Patient is given a general anaesthetic and will have either a laparoscopy (with 3–4 small cuts in your abdomen) or a laparotomy (with a long, vertical cut from your bellybutton to your bikini line). A laparoscopy may be used to see if a suspicious mass is cancerous. However, most women with advanced cancer will have a laparotomy.

The doctor look inside pelvis and abdomen for signs of cancer, and take tissue and fluid samples (biopsy). During the operation, the samples are usually sent to a pathologist, who examines them for signs of cancer. This is called a frozen section analysis or biopsy.

If cancer is present, the doctor will continue the operation and remove as much of the cancer as possible. This is called surgical debulking.

All tissue and fluids removed during surgery are examined for cancer cells by a pathologist. The results will help confirm the type of ovarian cancer, if it has spread (metastasised), and its stage. It may not be possible to remove all the cancerous tissue. Surgery is often followed by chemotherapy, which will shrink or destroy any remaining cancer cells

Types of surgery

Depending on how far the cancer has spread, you may have one or more of the procedures listed below.

Total hysterectomy and bilateral salpingo-oophorectomy	Unilateral salpingo-oophorectomy
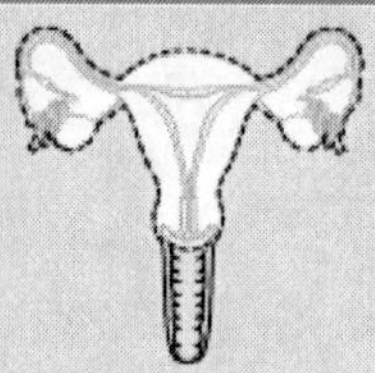 Most women with ovarian cancer will have an operation to remove the uterus and cervix, along with both fallopian tubes and ovaries.	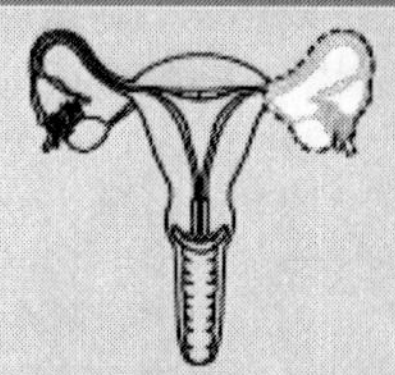 If the cancer is found early and it is only in one ovary, some young women who still wish to have children may have only one ovary and fallopian tube removed.
Omentectomy	**Lymphadenectomy**
The omentum is a sheet of fatty tissue attached to the stomach and bowel. It hangs down in front of the intestines. Ovarian cancer often spreads to the omentum and it may need to be removed.	The pelvis contains large groups of lymph nodes. Cancer cells can spread from your ovaries to nearby lymph nodes. Your doctor may suggest removing some in a lymphadenectomy (also called lymph node dissection).
Colectomy	**Removal of other organs**
If cancer spreads to the bowel, some of the bowel may be removed. A new opening called a stoma may be created (colostomy or ileostomy). This is usually temporary. See page 49 for more details.	Ovarian cancer can spread to many organs in the abdomen. In some cases, parts of the liver, diaphragm, bladder and spleen may be removed if it is safe to do.

What to expect after surgery

After surgery patient will be in a recovery room near the operating theatre. Once she is fully conscious, she will be taken back to the bed on the hospital ward.

Tubes and drips – Patient will have several tubes in place, which will be removed as she recovers. A drip is inserted into a vein in arm (intravenous drip) to give fluids, medicines and pain relief. A small plastic tube (catheter) may be inserted into bladder to collect urine in a bag. A tube may be inserted down nose into the stomach (nasogastric tube) to drain stomach fluid and prevent vomiting

Tubes may be inserted in abdomen to drain fluid from the site of the operation.

Pain – After an operation, it is common to feel some pain, but this can be controlled. For the first day or two, patient may be given pain medicine through a drip or via a local anaesthetic injection into the abdomen (a transverse abdominis plane or TAP block) or spine (an epidural). Let the doctor or nurse know if patient is in pain so they can adjust the medicine. Managing pain will help patient to recover and move around more quickly.

Injections – It is common to have daily injections of a blood thinner to reduce the risk of blood clots. These injections may continue for some time after the operation and while you're having chemotherapy.

Compression devices and stockings – Some women have to use compression devices or wear elastic stockings to keep the blood in their legs circulating. Once patient starts moving around, compression devices will be removed so that she can get out of bed, but she may still wear the stockings for a couple of weeks.

Wound care – Patient can expect some light vaginal bleeding after the surgery, which should stop within two weeks. Doctor will talk about how to keep the wound clean once the patient goes home to prevent it becoming infected.

Length of stay – Patient will probably stay in hospital for 4–7 days for a big operation, less for a laparoscopy or smaller operation.

Further treatment : Doctor should have all the test results within two weeks of surgery. Further treatment will depend on the type of ovarian cancer, the stage of the disease and the amount of any remaining cancer. If the cancer is advanced, it's more likely to come back, so surgery will usually be followed by chemotherapy, and occasionally by targeted therapy. Radiation therapy is not often recommended.

Taking care of yourself at home after surgery

Your recovery time will depend on the type of surgery you had, your general health and your support at home. Most women are able to fully return to their usual activities after 4-8 weeks.

Rest

Take things easy and do what is comfortable. You may try to do meditation and some relaxation technique to relieve stress.

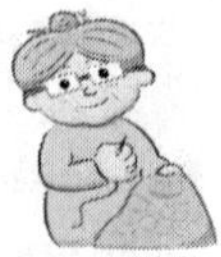

Work

Depending on the nature of work you will probably need leave for 4-6 weeks.

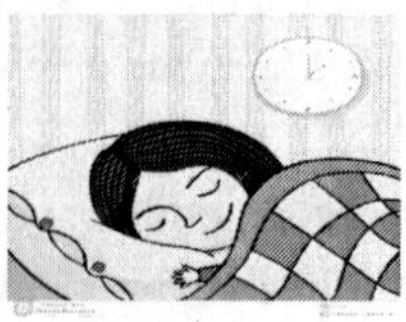

Lifting

Avoid lifting heavy objects (more than 3-4 kg). If you have a partner or children ask them to help around.

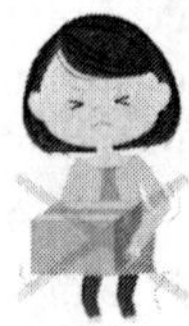

Driving

You will most likely need to avoid driving for few weeks after surgery.

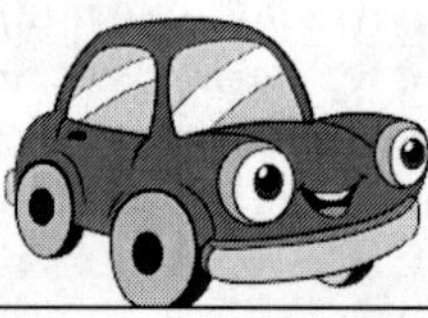

Chemotherapy

It is the treatment of cancer with anti-cancer (cytotoxic) drugs. The aim is to destroy cancer cells while causing the least possible damage to normal, healthy cells. Chemotherapy may be used at different times:

After surgery – Most women will have chemotherapy after surgery (adjuvant chemotherapy) as there may be some cancer cells still in the body. Chemotherapy usually starts 2–4 weeks after surgery. The drugs patient receives will depend on the stage of the cancer and her general health. For ovarian cancer, a combination of several drugs is usually given in repeating cycles spread over 4–5 months. The treatment team will provide details about the specific schedule.

Before surgery – Some women with stage III or stage IV ovarian cancer have chemotherapy before surgery (neoadjuvant chemotherapy). The aim is to shrink the tumours to make them easier to remove. This usually involves three cycles of chemotherapy, followed by surgery, and then another three cycles.

Primary treatment – Chemotherapy may be recommended as the main treatment if the is not well enough for a major operation or when the cancer cannot be surgically removed.

Having chemotherapy -

Chemotherapy is usually given as a combination of two drugs, or sometimes as a single drug. It's delivered as a liquid drip into a vein (intravenous drip). To reduce the need for repeated needles, some women have a small medical appliance or tube placed beneath their skin through which they receive chemotherapy. This may be a port-a-cath, a peripherally inserted central catheter (PICC), or another type of catheter.

The patient will usually have chemotherapy as an outpatient (also called a day patient), but some women need to stay in hospital overnight.

Let the doctor know if the patient is taking nutritional or herbal supplements as these can interact with chemotherapy and may lessen the effect.

Each chemotherapy treatment is called a cycle and is followed by a rest period to give the body time to recover. Ask the doctor about the treatment plan recommended.

Intraperitoneal chemotherapy

This is a way of giving chemotherapy directly into the abdominal cavity – the space between the abdominal organs and the abdominal wall. The drugs are given through a tube (catheter) that is put in place during surgery and removed once the course of chemotherapy ends. It may be offered to women with stage III disease with less than 1 cm of tumour remaining after surgery. Some studies have shown it may be more effective than giving chemotherapy through an intravenous drip. Ask the doctor for more information about this type of treatment and the advantages and side effects.

Blood tests during chemotherapy

Before each chemotherapy session, the patient will have blood tests to ensure her body's healthy cells have had time to recover. If the blood count has not recovered, the doctor may delay treatment. Some women also have blood tests during treatment to check their tumour markers, such as CA125. If the CA125 level was high before chemotherapy, it can be monitored to see if the treatment is working.

Side effects of chemotherapy

Chemotherapy can affect healthy cells in the body, which may cause side effects. Not all women will have side effects, and they will vary according to the drugs given. The health care team will talk about what to expect and how to manage any side effects.

Fatigue –The red blood cell level (haemoglobin) may drop, which can cause the patient to feel tired and short of breath. Travelling to and from treatment can also be exhausting.

Nausea – Some chemotherapy drugs may make the patient feel sick or vomit. She will generally be given anti-nausea medicines with each chemotherapy session to help prevent or reduce nausea and vomiting. Whether or not she feels sick is not a sign of how well the treatment is working.

Changed bowel habits – Many women become constipated while on chemotherapy. This may be caused by anti-nausea drugs or because what the diet changes. The doctor will talk about taking laxatives. Diarrhoea (loose, watery bowel movements) is another possible side effect.

Hair loss – It is likely the patient will lose head and body hair, depending on the chemotherapy drug. The hair will grow back after treatment is completed. But the hair colour and texture may change.

Risk of infections – Chemotherapy reduces white blood cell level, making it harder for the body to fight infection. Colds and flu may be easier to catch and harder to shake off, and scratches or cuts may get infected more easily. The patient may also be more likely to catch a more serious infection and need to be admitted to hospital. Contact the doctor or go the nearest hospital if the temperature of 38°C or over or other signs of infection.

Joint and muscle pain – This may occur after the treatment session. It may feel like the flu, but the symptoms should disappear within a few days. Taking paracetamol may help.

Numbness or tingling in your hands and feet – This is called peripheral neuropathy, and it can be a side effect of certain chemotherapy drugs. Let the doctor know if this happens, as your dose of chemotherapy may need to be adjusted.

Targeted therapy

Targeted therapy drugs can get inside cancer cells and block particular proteins (enzymes) that tell the cancer cells to grow. These drugs are used to treat some types of ovarian cancer. They may also be used in certain situations (e.g. if chemotherapy has not been successful). Genetic testing (see page 11) will help determine if the patient has a particular faulty gene that may respond to targeted therapy drugs.

Bevacizumab is a targeted therapy drug used to treat advanced epithelial tumours. It works by stopping the cancer developing new blood vessels and growing. Bevacizumab is given with chemotherapy every three weeks as a drip into a vein (infusion). It is commonly given in repeating cycles.

Olaparib is a new treatment for women with high-grade epithelial ovarian cancer who have the BRCA1 or BRCA2 gene mutation. This drug is usually given after chemotherapy to help stop the cancer growing. It is taken as a tablet twice a day.

Side effects of targeted therapy

Although targeted therapy minimises harm to healthy cells, it can still have side effects. It is important to discuss any side effects with the doctor immediately. If left untreated, some can become life-threatening. The doctor will monitor the patient throughout treatment.

The most common side effects experienced by women taking bevacizumab include wound-healing problems, bleeding, high blood pressure and kidney problems. In very rare cases, small tears (perforations) may develop in the bowel wall.

The most common side effects experienced by women taking olaparib include nausea, fatigue, vomiting, and low blood cell counts. More serious side effects include bone marrow or lung problems.

Radiation therapy

Radiation therapy (also known as radiotherapy) uses x-rays to damage cancer cells. The radiation is targeted at cancer sites in the body, with the aim of reducing the cancer's growth and improving symptoms.

Radiation therapy for ovarian cancer may be used to treat the pelvis or other sites of cancer that have spread further away. It may be used after chemotherapy or on its own as a palliative treatment.

Before treatment starts, the radiation oncology team will explain the treatment schedule and the possible side effects. The patient will lie on a table under a machine that delivers radiation to the affected parts of the body. She will not feel anything during the treatment, which will take only a few minutes each time. She may be in the room for a total of 10–20 minutes for each appointment.

The number of radiation therapy sessions you have will depend on the type and size of the cancer. She may have a few treatments or daily treatment for several weeks.

Side effects of radiation therapy

The side effects of radiation therapy vary. Most are temporary and disappear a few weeks or months after treatment. Radiation therapy for ovarian cancer is usually given over the abdominal area, which can irritate the bowel and bladder.

Common side effects include feeling tired, diarrhoea, needing to pass urine more often and burning when the patient passes urine (cystitis), and a slight burn to the skin around the treatment site. More rarely, she may have some nausea or vomiting. If this occurs, she will be prescribed medicine to control it.

Palliative treatment

It helps to improve people's quality of life by managing the symptoms of cancer without trying to cure the disease. It is best thought of as supportive care.

Many people think that palliative treatment is for people at the end of their life, but it may be beneficial for people at any stage of advanced ovarian cancer. It is about living for as long as possible in the most satisfying way.

Key points

- Your treatment will depend on many factors, including the type of ovarian cancer, its stage, whether you wish to have children, whether you have a faulty gene, and your overall health and fitness.
- Ovarian cancer is usually treated with surgery. In most women with ovarian cancer, surgery involves a total hysterectomy, as well as the removal of both fallopian tubes and ovaries, and the omentum (fatty tissue).
- During the operation, the doctor may take tissue samples to check for signs of cancer. This is called a biopsy.
- It will take time to recover from an operation. Recovery times vary depending on the type of surgery you have. You will need to take things easy when you first get home from hospital.
- After surgery, you may have further treatment. Most women have chemotherapy, but they may also have radiation therapy or targeted therapy.
- Chemotherapy is usually given soon after an operation for 4–5 months. Side effects may include tiredness, nausea and vomiting, and hair loss.
- Newer treatments for ovarian cancer include targeted therapy drugs, which can help stop the cancer growing. You may need a genetic test to see if you are likely to respond to these drugs.
- Radiation therapy uses x-rays to damage cancer cells. You may have treatment to your pelvis, but it can also be given to other parts of the body if the cancer has spread.
- Palliative treatment aims to improve your quality of life by relieving the symptoms of cancer.

As well as slowing the spread of cancer, palliative treatment can relieve pain and help manage other symptoms. The treatment may include chemotherapy and radiation therapy. If the patient is experiencing swelling and are uncomfortable, she may have a procedure called paracentesis or ascitic tap to drain the extra fluid from the abdomen. Palliative treatment is one aspect of palliative care, in which a team of health professionals aim to meet the physical, practical, emotional, spiritual and social needs.

Managing side effects of chemotherapy and radiotherapy

Chemotherapy is one of the main treatment options but associated with side effects. However the degree of side effects is different for different patients i.e. some women experience many side effects while others have few. Most side effects are temporary but some may be permanent. Radiotherapy is not so frequently used to treat ovarian cancer though it has also its own side effects. **(Please see chapter on cancer cervix for the tips to manage the discomfort that the side effects may cause)**

Role of a good diet in ovarian cancer: Eat healthy Stay Healthy

Treatments for ovarian cancer can affect patient's body needs for nutrients. They can affect eating habits and how the body digests, absorbs, and uses food. Common symptoms are faced by ovarian cancer patients that may affect nutrition during chemotherapy & radiotherapy. **(Please see chapter on cancer cervix for the tips for a good diet in ovarian cancer cases)**

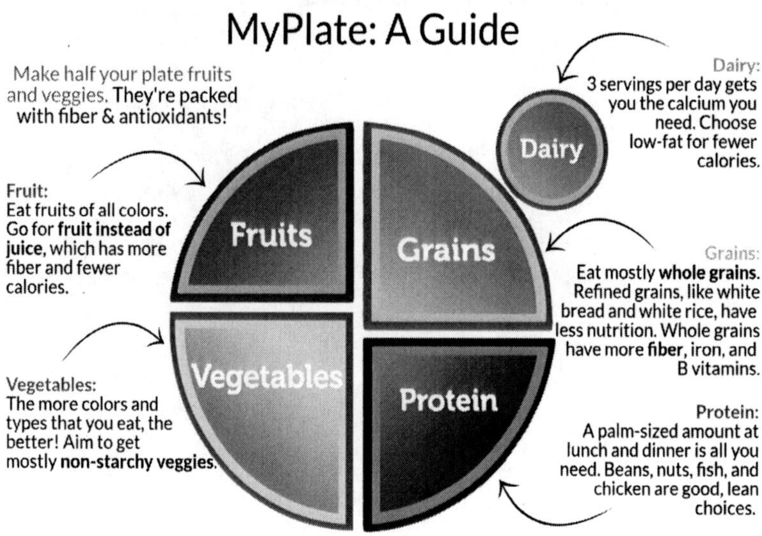

General Cancer Prevention recommendations:

- Maintain your weight within the healthy range and avoid weight gain
- Be physically active as part of everyday life – "walk more sit less"
- Make whole grains, vegetables, fruit and pulses (legumes) such as beans and lentils as a major part of your usual daily diet
- Limit consumption of 'Fast foods' and other processed food high in fat, starches and sugars; It helps control calorie intake and maintain healthy weight
- Limit consumption of red and processed meat
- Limit consumption of sugar sweetened drinks; Drink mostly water and unsweetened drinks
- Limit alcohol consumption
- Do not use supplements
- Aim to meet nutritional needs through diet alone
- For mothers breastfeed your baby
- Reduce intakes of salt, saturated and trans fats, which together will help prevent other non-communicable diseases also.

Clearly established **protective factors** for **ovarian cancer** include:

1. More than one pregnancy carried to term.
2. Use of oral contraceptives and breast-feeding.
3. Tubal ligation not clearly demonstrated.